Guide to Culturally Competent Health Care

Guide to Culturally Competent Health Care

Larry D. Purnell, PhD, RN, FAAN
Professor
College of Health and Nursing Sciences
University of Delaware
Newark, Delaware

Betty J. Paulanka, EdD, RN
Dean and Professor
College of Health and Nursing Sciences
University of Delaware
Newark, Delaware

 F.A. Davis Company • Philadelphia

F. A. Davis Company
1915 Arch Street
Philadelphia, PA 19103
www.fadavis.com

Copyright © 2005 by F. A. Davis Company

Printed in Canada

Last digit indicates print number: 10 9 8 7 6 5 4 3 2 1

Acquisitions Editor: Robert Martone
Developmental Editor: David Carroll
Design Manager: Joan Wendt

As new scientific information becomes available through basic and clinical research, recommended treatments and drug therapies undergo changes. The author(s) and publisher have done everything possible to make this book accurate, up to date, and in accord with accepted standards at the time of publication. The author(s), editors, and publisher are not responsible for errors or omissions or for consequences from application of the book, and make no warranty, expressed or implied, in regard to the contents of the book. Any practice described in this book should be applied by the reader in accordance with professional standards of care used in regard to the unique circumstances that may apply in each situation. The reader is advised always to check product information (package inserts) for changes and new information regarding dose and contraindications before administering any drug. Caution is especially urged when using new or infrequently ordered drugs.

Library of Congress Cataloging-in-Publication Data
Purnell, Larry D.
  Guide to culturally competent health care / Larry D. Purnell, Betty J. Paulanka.
    p. ; cm.
Includes bibliographical references and index.
ISBN 0-8036-1163-3 (softcover : alk. paper)
1. Transcultural medical care—United States. 2. Minorities—Medical care—United States.
[DNLM: 1. Delivery of Health Care—United States. 2. Clinical Competence—United States. 3. Cross-Cultural Comparison—United States. 4. Ethnic Groups—United States. W 84 AA1 P985g 2005] I. Paulanka, Betty J. II. Title.
RA418.5.T73P87 2005
362.1—dc22

2004008057

To the culturally diverse populations in America
who seek health care
                    and
To health-care providers who seek to provide
culturally sensitive health care
to all populations

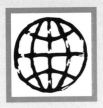

Preface

The Purnell Model for Cultural Competence and its organizing framework are used as a template for each chapter in this guide. The Model's usefulness has been established globally because it recognizes and includes each client's culture in assessment, health-care planning, interventions, and evaluation.

Chapter 1 addresses the need for cultural diversity in the United States and provides population trends and data from the U.S. Bureau of the Census, 2000. Chapter 2 includes (a) the assumptions upon which the Purnell Model for Cultural Competence is based; (b) a description of the primary and secondary characteristics of culture that determine the degree to which one identifies with his/her dominant cultural values, practices, and beliefs; (c) the Purnell Model for Cultural Competence; and (d) a description of the 12 domains of culture. Additionally, Chapter 2 includes 11 boxes, one for each domain of culture, with specific sample questions and observations for assessing an individual's cultural beliefs and practices.

This Guide serves as a useful tool for assessing the most important aspects of an individual's beliefs as they relate to health promotion and wellness, illness and disease prevention, and health maintenance and restoration. Each chapter is organized by the Model's domains of culturally sensitive care and provides key approaches and interventions highlighted in **bold type**. The intent is to provide a quick reference for working with selected culturally diverse groups. These approaches and interventions may need to be adapted based on the individual's and family's personal perspectives and circumstances.

Given the world's diversity and the diversity within cultural groups, it is impossible to include the beliefs and practices of all cultures and subcultures. Because space does not permit a more comprehensive presentation of diverse ethnocultural groups, additional information can be obtained from the textbook, *Transcultural Health Care: A Culturally Competent Approach*, 2nd edition, F. A. Davis Company, Philadelphia, from which much of this information is synthesized. Specific criteria were used for identifying the groups represented in the book and were selected based on a variety of the six criteria that follow:

- The group has a large population in North America, such as people of African American, Appalachian, German, Jewish, Irish, and Mexican heritage.
- The group is relatively new in its migration status, such as people of Arab, Bosnian, and Vietnamese heritage.
- The group is widely dispersed throughout North America, such as people of Chinese, Cuban, Greek, Filipino, Hindu, Iranian, Italian, and Puerto Rican heritage.
- The group has little written about it in the health-care literature, such as people of Brazilian, Egyptian, Haitian, Japanese, Korean, Russian, and Turkish heritage.
- The group holds significant disenfranchised status, such as people of Navajo ancestry, a large American Indian group.
- The group was of particular interest to readers, such as people from Amish heritage.

Larry D. Purnell
Betty J. Paulanka

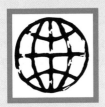

Acknowledgments

We would like to thank and acknowledge a host of people who contributed to either the first or second edition of the textbook: *Transcultural Health Care: A Culturally Competent Approach*, published by F. A. Davis Company. Without these culturally competent people, this handbook would not be possible:

Timor Arslanoglu
Josepha Campinha-Bacote
Marga Simon Coler
Jesse Colin
Mona Counts
Martha From
Cathryn Glanville
Divina Grossman
Homeyra Hafizi
Sandra Hillman
David Hodgins
Jayalakshmi Jambanathan
Teresa Juarbe
Susie Kim
Anahid Dervartanian
   Kulwicki
Juliene Lipson
Linda Matocha
Magelende (Melen) McBride
Afaf Meleis
Mahmoud Meleis

Beatrice Miranda
Ron Nowak
Thu Nowak
Dula Pacquiao
Irena Papadopoulos
Ghislaine Paperwalla
Lauren Regan-Sabet
Janice Selekman
Nancy Sharts-Hopko
Bernard Sorofman
Zen Spangler
Jessica Steckler
Olivia Still
Cara Towle
Toni Tripp-Reimer
Yan Wang
Anna Frances (Fran)
   Wenger
Marion Wenger
Sarah Wilson
Richard Zoucha

We would also like to acknowledge the following people who were consultants for culturally appropriate content:

Caroline Camunas
Lydia DeSantis
William Douglas Galloway
Carol Holtz
Suzan Karong-Edgren
Connie Vance
Diane Weiland

We would also like to thank David Carroll for his assistance in editing and helping bring this book to completion; Robert Martone from F.A. Davis for his unending persistence and patience; and Randee Tobin, who assisted with manuscript preparations.

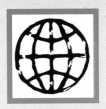

Contents

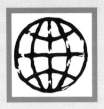

Introduction

Cultural diversity permeates most societies throughout the world. In addition to physical problems, health beliefs and practices of diverse cultures can create serious health problems for health-care providers and their clients. Multicultural holistic health care encompasses diverse populations of clients who need culturally sensitive and culturally competent care from health-care providers. However, it is impossible for health-care providers to be aware of, much less culturally sensitive to, the differences between and among these diverse individuals. A lack of essential knowledge of cultural differences can result in serious threats to the life and quality of health for culturally diverse individuals. Recent efforts to promote global recognition of multiculturalism have encouraged health-care providers to become more aware of cultural differences and to implement this understanding in providing effective health-care interventions. Thus, many individual providers and organizations have made a strong commitment to providing culturally sensitive and competent care to each individual, regardless of the setting in which the care is provided and the backgrounds of the participants in care. As a result of this commitment, health-care organizations and health education programs have begun to recognize the need to prepare health-care professionals with the knowledge, skills, and resources essential to the provision of culturally sensitive and competent care.

Culturally competent individuals value diversity and respect individual differences regardless of one's race, religious beliefs, or ethnocultural background. Thus, the goal of this Guide is to promote cultural sensitivity and culturally competent care that respects each person's right to be understood and treated as a unique individual. However, educational programs and access to resources necessary for cultural competence are not always readily available in a format that is concise and easy to understand. This Guide has been developed to be used in a manner that can be easily accessed and understood. This approach to gaining essential knowledge is designed to help health-care professionals provide the highest quality care for clients and families of diverse backgrounds. This respect is essential to the development of dynamic interpersonal relationships that promote a positive influence on each person's interpretation of and responses to health care in a multicultural environment.

The real challenge for health-care providers is gaining timely access to concise information that facilitates an accurate understanding of cultural beliefs from both the perspective of the client and the provider. This concise Guide uses the Purnell Model as a framework to simplify health assessments and interventions quickly and accurately while enabling culturally relevant care. Although the primary focus of the handbook is on the needs of health-care providers in the United States, the organizing framework and major concepts presented in each chapter are relevant to multicultural health care throughout the world. The small size of this Guide and the outline format of its presentation, with highlighted culturally relevant interventions, make it an essential resource for all health-care providers committed to providing culturally sensitive care, regardless of their practice setting.

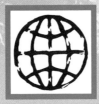

Transcultural Diversity
and Health Care

The Need for Culturally Competent Health Care

For the purposes of this handbook, culture is defined as the totality of socially transmitted behavioral patterns, arts, beliefs, values, customs, and lifeways and all other products of human work and thought characteristics of a population of people that guide their worldview and decision-making. These patterns may be explicit or implicit, are primarily learned and transmitted within the family, are shared by most members of the culture, and are emergent phenomena that change in response to global phenomena. Culture is largely unconscious and has powerful influences on health and illness. Health-care providers must recognize, respect, and integrate clients' cultural beliefs and practices into health prescriptions.

The chapters in this handbook book describe the dominant cultural characteristics of selected ethnocultural groups and provide a guide for assessing cultural beliefs and practices of clients. Practitioners who understand their clients' cultural values, beliefs, and practices are in a better position to participate with their clients and provide culturally acceptable care. Accordingly, there will be improved opportunities for health promotion, illness and disease prevention, and health restoration. To this end, health-care providers need both general and specific cultural knowledge. If practitioners do not have specific knowledge of cultural groups for whom they provide care, they will not know what questions to ask. This information provides a basis for practitioners to assess clients' beliefs and practices. Any generalization made about the behaviors of any individual or group of people is almost certain to be an oversimplification. Within all cultures there are subcultures and ethnic groups that may not hold all the values of their dominant culture. Subcultures, ethnic groups, and ethnocultural populations are groups of people who have experiences different from those of the dominant culture. Subcultures differ from the dominant group and share beliefs according to the primary and secondary characteristics of culture.

The controversial term *race* must be addressed when learning about culture. Race is genetic and includes physical characteristics that are similar among members of the group, such as skin color, blood type, and hair and eye color. Although there is less than 1 percent difference among the races, this difference is significant when conducting physical assessments and prescribing medication, as outlined in culturally specific chapters that follow. People from a given racial group may, but do not necessarily, share a common culture. Culture is learned first in the family, then in school, then in the community and other social organizations.

Primary and Secondary Characteristics of Culture

Major influences that shape peoples' worldview and the extent to which people identify with their cultural group of origin are called the primary and secondary characteristics of culture. The primary characteristics are nationality, race, color, gender, age, and religious affiliation. For example, two people have the same gender, age, nationality, and race, but if one is a devout Roman Catholic and the other is an Orthodox Jew, they may vary significantly in their health-care beliefs and practices

The secondary characteristics include educational status, socioeconomic status, occupation, military experience, political beliefs, urban versus rural residence, enclave identity, marital status, parental status, physical characteristics, sexual orientation, gender issues, reason for migration (sojourner, immigrant, or undocumented status), and amount of time away from the country of origin. Immigration status also influences a person's worldview. For example, people who voluntarily immigrate generally acculturate and more easily assimilate. Sojourners who immigrate with the intention of remaining in their new homeland for only a short time or refugees who think they may return to their home country may not have the need to acculturate or assimilate. Additionally, undocumented individuals (illegal immigrants) may have a different worldview from those who have arrived legally with work visas or as "legal immigrants."

Culture has a powerful unconscious impact on health professionals. Each health-care provider adds a unique dimension to the complexity of providing culturally competent care. The way health-care providers perceive themselves as competent providers is often reflected in the way they communicate with clients. Thus, it is essential for health professionals to take time to think about themselves, their behaviors, and their communication styles in relation to their perceptions of different cultures. Before addressing the multicultural backgrounds and unique individual perspectives of each client, health-care professionals must first address their own personal and professional knowledge, values, beliefs, ethics, and life experiences in a manner that optimizes assessment of and interactions with culturally diverse clients. Self-awareness in cultural competence is a deliberate and conscious cognitive and emotional process of getting to know oneself: one's own personality, values, beliefs, professional knowledge, standards, ethics, and the impact of these factors on the various roles one plays when interacting with individuals who are different from oneself. The ability to understand oneself sets the stage for integrating new knowledge related to cultural differences into the professional's knowledge base and perceptions of health interventions.

The literature reports many definitions for the terms *cultural awareness, cultural sensitivity,* and *cultural competence.* Sometimes these definitions are used interchangeably. However, cultural awareness has more to do with an appreciation of the external signs of diversity, such as arts, music, dress, and physical characteristics. Cultural sensitivity has more to do with personal attitudes and not saying things that might be offensive to someone from a cultural or ethnic background different from that of the health-care provider. Increasing one's consciousness of cultural diversity improves the possibilities for health-care practitioners to provide culturally competent care. Cultural competence, as used in this book, means:

1. Developing an awareness of one's own existence, sensations, thoughts, and environment without letting them have an undue influence on those from other backgrounds.
2. Demonstrating knowledge and understanding of the client's culture, health-related needs, and culturally specific meanings of health and illness.
3. Accepting and respecting cultural differences.
4. Not assuming that the health-care provider's beliefs and values are the same as the client's.
5. Resisting judgmental attitudes such as "different is not as good."
6. Being open to cultural encounters.
7. Being comfortable with cultural encounters.
8. Adapting care to be congruent with the client's culture.
9. Cultural competence is a conscious process and not necessarily linear.

Of the people reporting in the 2000 U.S. census, 75.1 percent were white, 12.5 percent were Spanish/Hispanic/Latino (of any race), 12.3 percent were Black/African American, 0.9 percent were American Indian or Alaskan Native, 3.6 percent were Asian, 0.1 percent were Native Hawaiian or other

Pacific Islander, 5.5 percent were some other race, and 2.4 percent were of two or more races. These numbers total more than 100 percent because the federal government considers race and Hispanic origin to be two separate and distinct categories. Race categories as used in Census 2000 include the following:

1. *White* refers to people having origins in any of the original peoples of Europe, the Near East, the Middle East, and North Africa. This category includes Irish, German, Italian, Lebanese, Turkish, Arab, and Polish.
2. *Black* and *African American* refer to people having origins in any of the black racial groups of Africa and include Nigerians and Haitians and any person who self-designated this category regardless of origin.
3. *American Indian* and *Alaskan Native* refer to people having origins in any of the original peoples of North, South, and Central America and who maintain tribal affiliation or community attachment.
4. *Asian* refers to people having origins in any of the original peoples of the Far East, Southeast Asia, and the Indian subcontinent. This category includes the terms *Asian Indian, Chinese, Filipino, Korean, Japanese, Vietnamese, Burmese, Hmong, Pakistani,* and *Thai.*
5. *Native Hawaiian* and other *Pacific Islander* refer to people having origins in any of the original peoples of Hawaii, Guam, Samoa, Tahiti, the Mariana Islands, and Chuuk.
6. *Some other race* was included for people who are unable to identify with the other categories. Additionally, the respondent could identify, as a write-in, with two races (www.census.gov).

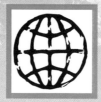

The Purnell Model for Cultural Competence

This chapter describes the Purnell Model for Cultural Competence and its accompanying organizing framework. The model and framework can be used as a guide to assessing the culture of clients. The assumptions on which the Purnell Model is based include the following:

1. All cultures share core similarities.
2. One culture is not better than another culture; they are just different.
3. Cultures change slowly over time.
4. Differences exist within, between, and among cultures.
5. Culture has a powerful influence on one's interpretation of and responses to health care.
6. To be effective, health care must reflect the unique understanding of the values, beliefs, attitudes, lifeways, and worldview of diverse populations and individual acculturation patterns.
7. Learning culture is an ongoing process that develops in a variety of ways, primarily through cultural encounters.

8. Prejudices and biases can be minimized with cultural understanding.
9. Cultural awareness improves the caregiver's self-awareness.
10. Each individual has the right to be respected for his or her uniqueness and cultural heritage.
11. Individuals and families belong to several cultural groups.
12. If clients are coparticipants in their care and have a choice in health-related goals, plans, and interventions, their compliance and health outcomes will be improved.
13. Differences in race and culture often require adaptations to standard interventions.
14. The primary and secondary characteristics of culture determine the extent to which one varies from his/her dominant culture.
15. Caregivers need both culture-general and culture-specific information in order to provide culturally sensitive and competent care.
16. Caregivers who can assess, plan, intervene, and evaluate in a culturally competent manner will improve their care of clients.
17. All health-care professions share the metaparadigm concepts of global society, family, person, and health.
18. All health-care professions need similar information about cultural diversity.
19. Professions, organizations, and associations have their own culture, which can be analyzed using a grand theory of culture.

The Purnell Model

The Purnell Model for Cultural Competence and its organizing framework can be used in all practice settings and by all health-care providers The model is a circle, with an outlying rim representing global society, a second rim representing community, a third rim representing family, and an inner rim representing the person (Fig. 2–1). The interior of the circle is divided into 12 pie-shaped wedges depicting cultural domains (constructs) and their associated concepts. The dark center of the circle represents unknown phenomena. Along the bottom of the model is a jagged line representing the nonlinear concept of cultural consciousness. The 12 cultural domains and their concepts provide the organizing framework. Each domain includes concepts that need to be addressed when assessing patients in various settings. Moreover, health-care providers can use these same concepts to better understand their own cultural beliefs, attitudes, values, practices, and behaviors. An important concept to understand is that no single domain stands alone; they are all interconnected. The 12 domains are overview/heritage, communications, family roles and organization, workforce issues, biocultural ecology, high-risk health behaviors, nutrition, pregnancy and the childbearing family, death rituals, spirituality, health-care practices, and health-care practitioners. For a more complete description of the domains, the reader is referred to the textbook by Purnell and Paulanka, *Transcultural Health Care: A Culturally Competent Approach* (2003, F. A. Davis Company).

ASSESSMENT GUIDE

Following each of the domains and concepts presented below is a box that includes suggested questions to ask and observations to make when assessing clients from a cultural perspective. It is recognized that clinicians are not able to complete a thorough cultural assessment for every client. The list of questions is extensive; thus, the clinician must determine which questions to ask according to the client's presenting symptoms and teaching needs and the potential impact of culture.

DOMAINS AND CONCEPTS

Overview and Heritage. Includes concepts related to the country of origin and current residence; the effects of the topography of the country of origin and the current residence on health, economics, politics, reasons for migration, educational status, and occupations.

Communications. Includes concepts related to the dominant language, dialects, and the contextual use of the lan-

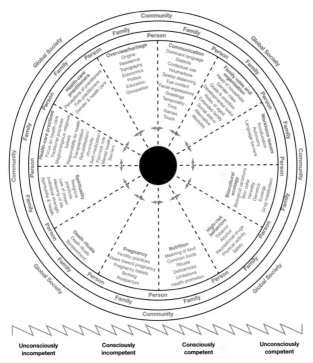

FIGURE 2–1. The Purnell Model for Cultural Competence.

BOX 2–1 • Overview, Inhabited Localities, and Topography

1. Where do you currently live?
2. What is your ancestry?
3. Where were you born?
4. How many years have you lived in the United States (or other country, as appropriate)?

(Continued)

BOX 2–1 • Overview, Inhabited Localities, and Topography *(Continued)*

5. Were your parents born in the United States (or other country, as appropriate)?
6. What brought you (your parents/ancestors) to the United States (or other country, as appropriate)?
7. Describe the land or countryside where you live. Is it mountainous, swampy, etc.?
8. Have you lived other places in the United States/world?
9. What was the land or countryside like when you lived there?
10. What is your income level?
11. Does your income allow you to afford the essentials of life?
12. Do you have health insurance?
13. Are you able to afford health insurance on your salary?
14. What is your educational level (formal/informal/self-taught)?
15. What is your current occupation? If retired, ask about previous occupations.
16. Have you worked in other occupations? What were they?
17. Are there (were there) any particular health hazards associated with your job(s)?

Questions and observations related to the primary and secondary characteristics of culture not previously covered include the following:

1. Have you been in the military? If so, in what foreign countries were you stationed?
2. Are you married?
3. How many children do you have?

guage; paralanguage variations such as voice volume, tone, intonations, inflections, and willingness to share thoughts and feelings; nonverbal communications such as eye contact, gesturing and facial expressions, use of touch, body language, spatial distancing practices, and acceptable greetings; temporality in terms of past, present, and future orientation of worldview; clock versus social time; and the amount of formality in use of names.

BOX 2–2 • Communications

1. What is your full name?
2. What is your legal name?
3. By what name do you wish to be called?
4. What is your primary language?
5. Do you speak a specific dialect?
6. What other languages do you speak?
7. Do you find it difficult to share your thoughts, feelings, and ideas with family? Friends? Health-care providers?
8. Do you mind being touched by friends? Strangers? Health-care workers?
9. How do wish to be greeted? Handshake? Nod of the head, etc.?
10. Are you usually on time for appointments?
11. Are you usually on time for social engagements?
12. Observe the client's speech pattern. Is the speech pattern high- or low-context? Remember, clients from highly contexted cultures place greater value on silence.
13. Observe the client when physical contact is made. Does he/she withdraw from the touch or become tense?
14. How close does the client stand when talking with family members? With health-care providers?
15. Does the client maintain eye contact when talking with the nurse/physician/etc.?

Family Roles and Organization. Includes concepts related to the head of the household, gender roles (a product of biology and culture), family goals and priorities, developmental tasks of children and adolescents, roles of the aged and extended family, individual and family social status in the community, and acceptance of alternative lifestyles such as single parenting, nontraditional sexual orientations, childless marriages, and divorce.

BOX 2–3 • Family Roles and Organization

1. Who makes most of the decisions in your family?
2. What types of decisions do(es) the female(s) in your family make?
3. What types of decisions do(es) the male(s) in your family make?
4. What are the duties of the women in the family?
5. What are the duties of the men in the family?
6. What should children do to make a good impression for themselves and for the family?
7. What should children not do to make a good impression for themselves and for the family?
8. What are children forbidden to do?
9. What should adolescents do to make a good impression for themselves and for the family?
10. What should adolescents not do to make a good impression for themselves and for the family?
11. What are adolescents forbidden to do?
12. What are the priorities for your family?
13. What are the roles of the elderly in your family? Are they sought for their advice?
14. Are there extended family members in your household? Who else lives in your household?
15. What are the roles of extended family members in this household? What gives you and your family status?
16. Is it acceptable to you for people to have children out of wedlock?

17. Is it acceptable to you for people to live together and not be married?
18. Is it acceptable to you for people to admit being gay or lesbian?
19. What is your sexual preference/orientation? (if appropriate, and then later in the assessment after a modicum of trust has been established)

 BOX 2–4 • Biocultural Ecology

1. Are you allergic to any medications?
2. What problems did you have when you took over-the-counter medications?
3. What problems did you have when you took prescription medications?
4. What are the major illnesses and diseases in your family?
5. Are you aware of any genetic diseases in your family?
6. What are the major health problems in the country from which you come (if appropriate)?
7. With what race do you identify?
8. Observe skin coloration and physical characteristics.
9. Observe for physical handicaps and disabilities.

Workforce Issues. Includes concepts related to autonomy, acculturation, assimilation, gender roles, ethnic communication styles, and health-care practices of the country of origin. Because this handbook is intended for use in the clinical setting with patients, this domain is not discussed.

Biocultural Ecology. Includes physical, biological, and physiological variations among ethnic and racial groups such as skin color (the most evident) and physical differences in body habitus; genetic, hereditary, endemic, and topographical diseases; psychological makeup of individuals; and the physiological differences that affect the way drugs are metabolized by the body.

High-Risk Health Behaviors. Includes substance use and misuse of tobacco, alcohol, and recreational drugs; lack of physical activity; increased calorie consumption; nonuse of safety measures such as seat belts, helmets, and safe driving practices; and not taking safety measures to prevent contracting HIV and sexually transmitted diseases.

Nutrition. Includes the meaning of food, common foods and rituals; nutritional deficiencies and food limitations; and the use of food for health promotion and restoration and illness and disease prevention.

Pregnancy and Childbearing Practices. Includes culturally sanctioned and unsanctioned fertility practices; views on pregnancy; and prescriptive, restrictive, and taboo practices related to pregnancy, birthing, and the postpartum period.

Death Rituals. Includes how the individual and the society view death and euthanasia, rituals to prepare for death, burial practices, and bereavement behaviors. Death rituals are slow to change.

Spirituality. Includes formal religious beliefs related to faith and affiliation and the use of prayer; behavior practices that give meaning to life; and individual sources of strength.

 BOX 2–5 • High-Risk Health Behaviors

1. How many cigarettes a day do you smoke?
2. Do you smoke a pipe (or cigars)?
3. Do you chew tobacco?
4. For how many years have you smoked/chewed tobacco?
5. How much do you drink each day? Ask about wine, beer, and spirits.
6. What recreational drugs do you use?
7. How often do you use recreational drugs?
8. What type of exercise do you do each day?
9. Do you use seat belts?
10. What precautions do you take to prevent getting a sexually transmitted disease or HIV/AIDS?

BOX 2–6 • Nutrition

1. Are you satisfied with your weight?
2. Which foods do you eat to maintain your health?
3. Do you avoid certain foods to maintain your health?
4. Why do you avoid these foods?
5. Which foods do you eat when you are ill?
6. Which foods do you avoid when you are ill?
7. Why do you avoid these foods (if appropriate)?
8. For what illnesses do you eat certain foods?
9. Which foods do you eat to balance your diet?
10. Which foods do you eat every day?
11. Which foods do you eat every week?
12. Which foods do you eat that are part of your cultural heritage?
13. Which foods are high-status foods in your family/culture?
14. Which foods are eaten only by men? Women? Children? Teenagers? Older people?
15. How many meals do you eat each day?
16. What time do you eat each meal?
17. Do you snack between meals?
18. What foods do you eat when you snack?
19. What holidays do you celebrate?
20. Which foods do you eat on particular holidays?
21. Who is present at each meal? Is the entire family present?
22. Do you primarily eat the same foods as the rest of your family?
23. Where do you usually buy your food?
24. Who usually buys the food in your household?
25. Who does the cooking in your household?
26. How frequently do you eat at a restaurant?
27. When you eat at a restaurant, in what type of restaurant do you eat?
28. Do you eat foods left from previous meals?
29. Where do you keep your food?

(Continued)

BOX 2–6 • Nutrition *(Continued)*

30. Do you have a refrigerator?
31. How do you cook your food?
32. How do you prepare meat?
33. How do you prepare vegetables?
34. What type of spices do you use?
35. What do you drink with your meals?
36. Do you drink special teas?
37. Do you have any food allergies?
38. Are there certain foods that cause you problems when you eat them?
39. How does your diet change with each season?
40. Are your food habits different on days you work versus when you are not working?

BOX 2–7 • Pregnancy and Childbearing Practices

1. How many children do you have?
2. What do you use for birth control?
3. What does it mean to you and your family when you are pregnant?
4. What special foods do you eat when you are pregnant?
5. What foods do you avoid when you are pregnant?
6. What activities do you avoid when you are pregnant?
7. Do you do anything special when you are pregnant?
8. Do you eat nonfood substances when you are pregnant?
9. Who do you want with you when you deliver your baby?
10. In what position do you want to be when you deliver your baby?
11. What special foods do you eat after delivery?
12. What foods do you avoid after delivery?

13. What activities do you avoid after you deliver?
14. Do you do anything special after delivery?
15. Who will help you with the baby after delivery?
16. What bathing restrictions do you have after you deliver?
17. Do you want to keep the placenta?
18. What do you do to care for the baby's umbilical cord?

BOX 2–8 • Death Rituals

1. What special activities need to be performed to prepare for death?
2. Would you want to know about your impending death?
3. What is your preferred burial practice? Interment, cremation?
4. How soon after death does burial occur?
5. How do men grieve?
6. How do women grieve?
7. What does death mean to you?
8. Do you believe in an afterlife?
9. Are children included in death rituals?

BOX 2–9 • Spirituality

1. What is your religion?
2. Do you consider yourself deeply religious?
3. How many times a day do you pray?
4. What do you need in order to say your prayers?
5. Do you meditate?
6. What gives strength and meaning to your life?
7. In what spiritual practices do you engage for your physical and emotional health?

Health-Care Practices. Includes the focus of health care (acute versus preventive); traditional, magicoreligious, and biomedical beliefs and practices; individual responsibility for health; self-medicating practices; and views on mental illness, chronicity, rehabilitation, acceptance of blood and blood products, and organ donation and transplantation.

Health-Care Practitioners. Includes the status, use, and perceptions of traditional, magicoreligious, and biomedical health-care providers and the gender of the health-care provider.

BOX 2–10 • Health-Care Practices

1. In what prevention activities do you engage to maintain your health?
2. Who in your family takes responsibility for your health?
3. What over-the-counter medicines do you use?
4. What herbal teas and folk medicines do you use?
5. For what conditions do you use herbal medicines?
6. What do you usually do when you are in pain?
7. How do you express your pain?
8. How are people in your culture viewed or treated when they have a mental illness?
9. How are people with physical disabilities treated in your culture?
10. What do you do when you are sick? Stay in bed, continue your normal activities, etc.?
11. What are your beliefs about rehabilitation?
12. How are people with chronic illnesses viewed or treated in your culture?
13. Are you averse to blood transfusions?
14. Is organ donation acceptable to you?
15. Are you an organ donor?
16. Would you consider having an organ transplant if needed?

17. Are health-care services readily available to you?
18. Do you have transportation problems accessing needed health-care services?
19. Can you afford health care?
20. Do you feel welcome when you see a health-care professional?
21. What traditional health-care practices do you use? Acupuncture, acupressure, cai gao, moxibustion, aromatherapy, coining, etc.?
22. What home difficulties do you have that might prevent you from receiving health care?

BOX 2–11 • Health-Care Practitioners

1. What health-care providers do you see when you are ill? Physicians, nurses?
2. Do you prefer a same-sex health-care provider for routine health problems? For intimate care?
3. What healers do you use beside physicians and nurses?
4. For what conditions do you use healers?

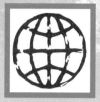

CHAPTER 3

People of African American Heritage

Overview and Heritage

Over 34,500,000 African Americans (12.1 percent of the population) live in the United States (www.census.com, 2002). Most are of African ancestry; however, many have non-African ancestors. African Americans are largely the descendants of Africans who were forcibly brought to this country as slaves between 1619 and 1860. Over half live in the South, 19 percent in the North and Northeast, 9 percent in the West, and 19 percent in the Midwest. The highest concentration can be found in metropolitan areas.

Younger blacks prefer the term *African American,* whereas older African Americans may use the terms *Negro* or *colored.* Middle-aged African Americans usually refer to themselves as black or black American. The primary and secondary characteristics of culture (see Chapter 1) describe variables that contribute to the diversity of the African American population. To avoid stereotyping, health-care providers must assess and plan interventions on an individual basis.

Most families place a high value on education and make

great sacrifices so at least one child can go to college. However, many African Americans continue to be underrepresented in managerial and professional positions, overrepresented in the working class, and are more likely to be employed in hazardous occupations, resulting in occupation-related diseases and illness.

COMMUNICATIONS

- The dominant language of African Americans is English. However, many refer to an informal language known as Black English, or Ebonics. For example, some may pronounce *th* as *d*. Therefore, the word *these* may be pronounced *dese*. Health-care professionals must not stereotype African Americans as speaking only in Black English because most African Americans are articulate and competent in the formal English language.
- Many tend to be high-keyed, animated, confrontational, and interpersonal, expressing their feelings openly to trusted friends or family. What transpires within the family is viewed as private and not appropriate for discussion with strangers. A common phrase that reflects this perspective is, "Don't air your dirty laundry."
- Speech volume is often loud compared with other cultural groups. Speech is dynamic and expressive. Body movements are involved when communicating with others. Facial expressions can be very demonstrative.
- Health-care providers must not misunderstand this loud volume; people may not necessarily be reflecting anger, but merely expressing their thoughts in a dynamic manner.
- Most individuals are comfortable with a close personal space. However, health-care providers should be aware that maintaining direct eye contact may be misinterpreted as aggressive behavior by some.
- In general, most individuals are more present- than past- or future-oriented. Younger and middle-aged people are more present-oriented, with evidence of becoming more

future-oriented as indicated by the value placed on education. Some are more relaxed about time. It is more important to make an appointment than to be on time for the appointment. Therefore, flexibility in timing appointments may be necessary for those who have a circular sense of time rather than the dominant culture's linear sense of time.

- Most prefer to be greeted formally as Mr., Mrs., Ms., or Miss. They prefer their surname because the "family name" is highly respected and connotes pride in their family heritage. Youths commonly address unrelated African Americans who live in the community as uncle, aunt, or cousin. Greet clients by the last name, using the appropriate title until told to do otherwise.

FAMILY ROLES AND ORGANIZATION

- A high percentage of families are matriarchal and live below the poverty level. A single head-of-household is accepted without stigma. When nuclear families are unable to provide emotional and physical support for their children, grandmothers, aunts, and extended or augmented families readily provide assistance or take responsibility for the children.
- Families are usually pluralistic in nature; gender roles and childrearing practices vary widely depending on ethnicity, socioeconomic class, rural versus urban location, and educational achievement. The diverse family structure extends the care of family members beyond the nuclear family to include relatives and nonrelatives. Many family tasks such as cooking, cleaning, child care, and shopping are shared, requiring flexibility and adaptability of roles. The extended family structure is important for teaching health strategies and providing support. Recognize the importance of including women in decision-making and disseminating health information.
- Given their strong work and achievement orientation, most value self-reliance and education for their children. Because parents often do not expect to get full benefit

from their efforts because of discrimination, many families tend to be more protective of their children and act as a buffer between their children and the outside world.

- Respect, obedience, conformity to parent-defined rules, and good behavior are stressed for children. The belief is that a firm parenting style, structure, and discipline are necessary to protect children from danger outside of the home. In violence-ridden communities, mothers try to keep young children off the streets and encourage them to engage in productive activities. Adolescents are assigned household chores as part of their family responsibility, and many seek employment for pay when they are old enough, thus learning "survival skills" very early.

- Older people, especially grandmothers, are respected for their insight. The role of the grandmother is one of the most central roles in the family, providing economic support and playing a critical role in child care. Include grandmothers when providing support and health teaching.

- Social status is important within the community. Occupations such as medicine, dentistry, nursing, and the clergy are highly respected.

- Those who move up the socioeconomic ladder often find themselves caught between two worlds, with roots in the African American community but at times interacting more within the European American community. Some refer to these individuals as *oreos*—a derogatory term that means "black on the outside, white on the inside."

- Although there has been a decline in the incidence of teen pregnancy, it continues to be a problem in many communities. Poor pregnancy outcomes, such as premature and low-birth-weight infants and obstetrical complications are common outcomes of teen pregnancy. Premarital teenage pregnancy is not condoned; rather, it is accepted after the fact. Furthermore, the teenage mother is expected to assume primary responsibility for her child, with the extended family providing a strong support system. In other instances, the infant may be informally adopted, and someone other than the mother may become the primary caregiver.

- Acceptance of same-sex relationships varies between and among families. Personal disclosure to friends and family may jeopardize relationships, thereby forcing some to remain closeted. Do not disclose same-sex relationships to others.

BIOCULTURAL ECOLOGY

- African Americans encompass a gene pool of more than 100 racial strains. Therefore, skin color among African Americans can vary from light to very dark. Pallor in dark-skinned people can be observed by the absence of the underlying red tones that give brown and black skin its "glow" or "living color." Lighter-skinned people appear more yellowish brown, whereas darker-skinned African Americans appear ashen.
- To assess conditions such as inflammation, cyanosis, jaundice, and petechiae, palpate the skin for warmth, edema, tightness, or induration. To assess for cyanosis in dark-skinned blacks, observe the oral mucosa or conjunctiva. Jaundice is assessed more accurately by observing the sclera of the eyes, the palms of the hands, and the soles of the feet, which may have a yellow discoloration.
- Keloid formation, common among dark-skinned people, is one example of the tendency toward overgrowth of connective tissue. Diseases such as lymphoma and systemic lupus erythematosus may occur in African Americans as a result of this overgrowth of connective tissue.
- African Americans have a greater bone density than European Americans, Asians, and Hispanics, resulting in a lower incidence of osteoporosis.
- Pseudofolliculitis ("razor bumps") is more common among males, whereas melasma ("mask of pregnancy") is more common among darker-skinned females during pregnancy. Many experience a disproportionate amount

of pigment discoloration, with vitiligo being the most common. This is an autoimmune disease that causes skin discoloration and is associated with diabetes and thyroid disorders. If left untreated, it can cause skin cancer.

- Birthmarks are more common in this population. Mongolian spots, which are found more often in newborns, disappear over time.

- African Americans suffer from genetic conditions such as sickle cell disease, sickle cell anemia, sickle cell hemoglobin C disease, beta–thalassemia, and glucose-6-phosphate dehydrogenase deficiency.

- The pathophysiology of hypertension in African Americans is related to volume expansion, decreased renin, and increased intracellular concentration of sodium and calcium, making African Americans more genetically prone than whites to retain sodium.

- African Americans have a lower life expectancy, with a 65-year average for males and 74 years for females. Disparities in health care are multifactorial. Although there has been a decline in leading causes of death such as accidents, cancer, infant mortality, and cardiovascular diseases, the adjusted death rates for African Americans are higher than for whites. Other causes of death are homicide, cirrhosis, malnutrition, chemical dependency, and diabetes.

- The leading causes of death among women are cancer, stroke, chronic obstructive pulmonary disease, pneumonia, unintentional injuries, diabetes, suicide, alcohol use, illicit drug use, and HIV/AIDS. Living in urban industrial areas also exposes them to pollution, increasing their risk for developing diseases associated with environmental hazards.

- African Americans are at a higher risk of misdiagnosis for psychiatric disorders and, therefore, may be treated inappropriately with drugs.

- African Americans respond to or metabolize alcohol, antihypertensives, beta-blockers, psychotropic drugs, and caffeine differently than European Americans. Psychiatric clients experience a higher incidence of extrapyramidal effects with haloperidol decanoate than European Americans. They are more susceptible to tricyclic antidepressant delirium, showing higher blood levels and a faster therapeutic response. As a result, they experience more toxic side effects. Observe African American clients closely for side effects related to tricyclics and other psychotropic medications. Light eyes dilate wider in response to mydriatic drugs than do dark eyes. This difference in response to mydriatic drugs must be taken into consideration when treating African Americans.

HIGH-RISK HEALTH BEHAVIORS

- Because significant numbers of African Americans are poor and live in inner cities, they tend to concentrate their efforts on day-to-day survival. Health care often takes second place to basic needs of the family, such as food and shelter. In addition, the role of the family has an impact on their health-seeking behaviors. Because of strong family ties, individuals are frequently taught to seek health care from the family rather than from health-care professionals. This cultural practice may contribute to the failure of some to seek treatment at an early stage. Screening programs may best be initiated in community and church activities where the entire family is present.

NUTRITION

- Food is used to celebrate special events, holidays, and birthdays and is a symbol of health and wealth. Food is usually offered to guests when they enter or leave a household. One is expected to accept the "gift" of food. Be sensitive to the meaning attached to food because individuals who reject the food are also perceived as rejecting the giver of the food.
- Food may be perceived negatively in the context of witchcraft. It is thought that witchcraft promotes intentional poisoning by food. Thus, it is important

to watch carefully what one eats and who gives them food.

- Diets are frequently high in fat, cholesterol, and sodium and low in fiber, fruits, and vegetables. The diet is referred to as soul food. Salt pork (fatback or "fat meat") is a key ingredient in the diet of many individuals. Salt pork is inexpensive and therefore more affordable. However, a person with *high blood* (a term often used for high blood pressure) should avoid or reduce intake of salt, pork, red meats, and fried foods. A diet of liver, greens, eggs, fruits and vegetables, vinegar, lemon, and garlic is recommended to remedy "low blood."

- Being overweight is seen as positive. In the African American community it is common to view individuals who are at an ideal body weight as "not having enough meat on their bones." It is important to have meat on one's bones to be able to afford weight loss during times of sickness. Negotiate with clients to determine an acceptable weight.

- Parents are encouraged by their elders to begin feeding solid foods, such as cereal, at an early age (usually before 2 months). The cereal is mixed with formula and given to the infant in a bottle. Many believe that giving only formula will starve the baby and that the infant needs the added cereal to sleep through the night. Health-care providers, working with family planning and child-care clinics, can provide factual knowledge regarding the deleterious effects of giving infants solid foods at an early age.

- Some believe that too much red meat causes high blood pressure. Foods such as milk, vegetables, and meat are referred to as "strength foods." However, religious affiliations may lead a person to engage in a diet that does not include such foods. For example, in a Muslim *halal* diet, pork or pork products are not allowed. In fact, some Muslims even refuse pork-based insulin because of their beliefs that pork-based medicines are filthy and that "you are what you eat."

- Lactose intolerance occurs in 75 percent of this

African American

population. Low levels of thiamine, riboflavin, vitamins A and C, and iron are commonly associated with a poor diet as a result of low socioeconomic status. Complete an individual diet assessment before making recommendations in order to determine what are acceptable and unacceptable food choices and preparation practices.

PREGNANCY AND CHILDBEARING PRACTICES

- Although oral contraceptives may be the most popular choice of birth control, Catholics tend to choose the rhythm method. Many oppose abortion because of religious, moral, cultural, or Afrocentric beliefs, resulting in a delay in making a decision until it is no longer safe to have an abortion.
- Women usually respond to pregnancy based on their satisfaction with self, economic status, and career goals.
- The family network guides many of the practices and beliefs of pregnant women, including the common practice of geophagia, the eating of earth or clay. This natural craving is believed to alleviate several mineral deficiencies and serve the belief that the unborn child "needs" this supplement. However, geophagy can lead to potassium deficiency, constipation, and anemia.
- Some claim that the baby signals what it wants from the mother via a food craving and that if the mother does not consume the specific food, the child is birth-marked with that particular food. Health-care providers need to provide factual information regarding the consequences of eating nonfood substances that may be harmful to the mother or fetus.
- Taboo practices during pregnancy include pregnant women not taking pictures because it may cause a stillbirth and not having their picture taken because it captures their soul. Some also believe that it is not wise to reach over their heads because the umbilical cord will wrap around the baby's neck. Another taboo is related to the belief that purchasing clothing for the infant prior to his or her birth can cause a stillbirth. Just because

someone seems to not have prepared for the newborn does not mean that the baby is not wanted.

- Home practices related to initiating labor include taking a ride over a bumpy road, ingesting castor oil, eating a heavy meal, or sniffing pepper.
- If a baby is born with the amniotic sac (referred to as a "veil") over its head or face, the neonate is thought to have special powers. In addition, a child born after a set of twins, one born with a physical problem or disability, or a child who is the seventh son in a family is thought to have special powers from God.
- The postpartum period is greatly extended due to the belief that the mother is at greater risk than the baby. She is cautioned to avoid cold air and is encouraged to get adequate rest to restore the body to normal.
- Postpartum practices for child care can involve the use of a bellyband or a coin placed on top of the infant's umbilical area to prevent the umbilical area from protruding outward. Teach methods for keeping equipment and objects clean that are used on the umbilicus.

DEATH RITUALS

- For most individuals, death does not end the connection among people, especially families. Relatives communicating with the deceased's spirit are one example of this endless connection. Some believe in "voodoo death," a belief that illness or death may come to an individual via a supernatural force. Voodoo is more commonly known as "root work," "hex," "fix," "conjuring," "tricking," "mojo," "witchcraft," "spell," "black magic," or "hoodoo" (Campinha-Bacote, 1992).
- Many African Americans do not know about or complete advance directives. This is attributed, in part, to the fact that end-of-life decisions are usually made by the family. A culturally relevant discussion and education in the African American community is needed regarding advance directives and durable power of attorney.

- Most families do not rush to bury the deceased, allowing time for relatives to travel from far away to attend funeral services. Therefore, it is common for the burial service to be held 5 to 7 days after death.
- The body must be kept intact after death. For example, it is common to hear "I came into this world with all my body parts, and I'll leave this world with all my body parts!" Explain the legal requirements of autopsy.
- One response to hearing about a death of a family member is falling out, which is manifested by sudden collapse and paralysis and the inability to see or speak. However, the individual's hearing and understanding remain intact. Health-care providers must understand that this condition is a cultural response to the death of a family member or severe emotional shock and not a medical condition requiring emergency intervention.
- Some individuals are less likely to express grief openly and publicly. However, they do express their feelings openly during the funeral. Funeral services encourage emotional expression and catharsis by incorporating religious songs into the ceremony and by providing a visual display of the body. Accept varied responses to bereavement.

SPIRITUALITY

- Most African American Christians are affiliated with the Baptist and Methodist denominations. However, many other distinct religious groups are represented, including African, Episcopal, Jehovah's Witnesses, Church of God in Christ, Seventh-Day Adventist, Pentecostal, Apostolic, Presbyterian, Lutheran, Roman Catholic, Nation of Islam, and other Islamic sects. Determine specific church affiliation at the time of the intake interview.
- Churches play a major role in the development and survival of African Americans. There is no disjunction between the black Church and the black community; whether one is a church member or not is beside the

point. In any assessment, determine the importance and meaning of the black Church to clients.

- Most individuals take their religion seriously and expect to receive a message in preaching that helps them in their daily lives. Religious involvement is associated with positive mental health. Furthermore, most people take an active part in religious activities. Participation may involve group singing, creating original words to songs, spontaneous testimony of a personal spiritual view, or expression of deep emotion. Singers might be encouraged with cries of "Sing it, sister!" or "That's all right."
- Most individuals strongly believe in the use of prayer for all situations they encounter. They use prayer for the sake of others who are experiencing problems. Prayers reflect the trust and faith one has in God.
- Many also believe in the "laying on of hands" while praying. Certain individuals are believed to have the power to heal the sick by placing hands on them. African Americans may pray in a language that is not understood by anyone but the person reciting the prayer. This expression of prayer is referred to as "speaking in tongues."
- Having faith in God is a major source of inner strength. Whatever happens is "God's will." Because of this belief, many are perceived to have a fatalistic view of life. This does not mean that individuals do not care about their health or are not willing to practice illness prevention measures.
- Most individuals consider themselves spiritual beings; sickness is viewed as a separation between God and man. Furthermore, God is thought to be the supreme healer; thus, health-care practices center on religious and spiritual activities such as going to church, praying daily, laying on of hands, and speaking in tongues.
- Some people associate illness or genetic/hereditary disorders in children with the sins of their parents. In this instance, they believe that healing can occur only through the prayers of a faith healer. Provide factual information about genetic/hereditary disorders.

African American

HEALTH-CARE PRACTICES

- Many individuals are pessimistic about human relationships and believe that it is more natural to do evil than to do well. Belief systems emphasize three major themes: (1) the world is a very hostile and dangerous place in which to live; (2) the individual is open to attack from external forces; (3) the individual is considered to be a helpless person when he or she has no internal resources to combat such an attack and, therefore, needs outside assistance.

- Because some people tend to be suspicious of health-care professionals, many may see a physician or nurse only when absolutely necessary. Some older people use the *Farmers' Almanac* to choose what are thought to be good times for medical and dental procedures.

- Many believe in natural and unnatural illnesses. Natural illness occurs in response to normal forces from which individuals have not protected themselves. Unnatural illnesses come via different people or spirits. Health is viewed as harmony with nature, whereas illness is seen as a disruption in this harmonic state due to demons, "bad spirits," or both. In treating an unnatural illness, health-care providers should seek clergy for assistance and encourage the client to pray to a supreme being.

- Individuals commonly use home remedies, consult folk healers (root doctors), and receive treatment from Western health-care professionals. To render services that are effective and culturally acceptable, health-care providers should do a thorough cultural assessment and become partners with the community. Focus groups can provide health-care professionals with insight into health-care practices acceptable to African Americans.

- When taking prescribed medications, it is common practice to take the medications differently than prescribed. For example, in treating hypertension, some take their antihypertensive medication on an "as needed" basis. Other helpful medical treatment modalities in treating hypertension include relaxation

techniques and transcendental meditation. Explain the
importance of taking medications as prescribed.

- Needed health-care services may not be affordable for
those in lower socioeconomic groups. Some services,
although accessible, may not be culturally relevant. For
example, a health-care professional may prescribe a
strict diabetic diet to a newly diagnosed diabetic African
American client without taking into consideration the
dietary habits of this person. Such therapeutic interventions developed by health-care professionals may be
underutilized or ignored. Always include the client and
family when doing dietary counseling.

- There is a general distrust of health-care professionals,
practitioners, and the health-care system. The unequal
distribution or underrepresentation of ethnic minority
health-care providers is a barrier to care. When possible,
encourage the support of similar ethnic minorities to
promote healthy interactions.

- Some perceive pain as a sign of illness or disease; thus,
regularly prescribed medicine may not be followed if
individuals are not in pain. Some believe that suffering
and pain are inevitable and must be endured, thus
contributing to their high tolerance level for pain.
Prayers and the laying on of hands are thought to free
the person from all suffering and pain, and people who
still experience pain are considered to have little faith.
Dispel myths about the need for pain medications.

- Low educational levels may limit access to information
about the etiology and treatment of mental illness. The
high frequency of misdiagnosis among blacks/African
Americans contributes to their reluctance to trust mental health professionals. Many are more likely to report
hallucinations when suffering from an affective disorder,
which may lead to the misdiagnosis of schizophrenia.

- Close family and spiritual ties allow one to enter the
sick role with ease. Extended and nuclear family
members willingly care for sick individuals and assume
their responsibilities without hesitation. Sickness and
tragedy bring families together, even in the presence of
family conflict. Engage extended family members in the

African American

care of family members when self-care becomes a concern.

- Blood transfusions are generally accepted unless the client belongs to a religious group, such as Jehovah's Witnesses, that does not permit this practice.
- Low levels of organ donation may be related to social practices, religious beliefs, and cultural expectations. Five reasons for the low level of organ donation include lack of information about kidney transplantation, religious fears and superstitions, distrust of health-care providers, fear that donors would be declared dead prematurely, and racism (African Americans prefer to give their organs to other African Americans).

HEALTH-CARE PRACTITIONERS

- Physicians are recognized as heads of the health-care team, with nurses having lesser importance. However, as nurses are becoming more educated, African Americans are holding them in higher regard.
- Folk practitioners can be spiritual leaders, grandparents, elders of the community, voodoo doctors, or priests. Voodoo doctors are consulted for unnatural illnesses or for removing a hex. An individual may place a hex on a person because of resentment of achievement, sexual jealousy, love, or envy. A hex can be placed on the victim by using a piece of the individual's hair, fingernail, blood, or some other personal item of the victim. Victims usually seek help from a voodoo or conjure doctor to have the hex removed with magic or religious powers. Include spiritual leaders and voodoo practitioners in care if the client wishes.
- Folk practitioners are respected and valued in the African American community and are used by all socioeconomic levels. Many perceive health-care professionals as outsiders, and they may be suspicious and cautious of health-care practitioners they have not heard of or do not know. Because interpersonal relationships are highly valued in this group, it is

important initially to develop a sound, trusting relationship.

- Whereas some individuals may prefer a health provider of the same gender for urologic and gynecologic conditions, gender is generally not a major concern in selection of a health-care provider. Men and women can provide personal care to the opposite sex. On occasion, young men prefer that another man or older woman give personal care. Some women prefer female primary care physicians. The health-care provider should respect these wishes and provide same-gender care providers when possible.

African American

References

Campinha-Bacote, J. (1992). Voodoo illness. *Perspectives in Psychiatric Nursing, 28*(1), 11–19.

Glandville, C. (2003). People of African American heritage. In L. Purnell and B. Paulanka (Eds.), *Transcultural health care: A culturally competent approach* (2nd ed., pp. 40–54). Philadelphia: F.A. Davis.

Glazer, W.M., Morganstern, H., & Doucette, J.T. (1993). Predicting the long-term risk of tardive dyskinesia in outpatients maintained on neuroleptic medications. *Journal of Clinical Psychiatry, 54*(4), 133–139.

Levy, R. (1993). Ethnic and racial differences in response to medicines: Preserving individualized therapy in managed pharmaceutical programmes. *Pharmaceutical Medicine*, 7, 139–165.

Plawecki, H., & Plawecki, J. (1992). Improving organ donation rates in the black community. *Journal of Holistic Nursing, 10*(1), 34–46.

Waters, C. (2000). End-of-life directives among African Americans: A need for community-centered discussion and education. *Journal of Community Health Nursing, 17*(1), 25–37.

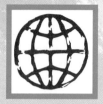

The Amish

Overview and Heritage

Today's Amish live in rural areas in a band of more than 20 states, stretching westward from Pennsylvania, Ohio, and Indiana to as far west as Montana, with some scattered settlements in Florida and the province of Ontario, Canada. More than half live in Pennsylvania, Ohio, and Indiana (Kraybill, 2001). The **Old Order Amish**, so-called for their strict observance of traditional ways that distinguish them from other, more progressive "plain folk," are the largest and most notable group. The Amish emerged after 1693, when they parted ways with the **Anabaptist** movement that originated in Switzerland in 1525. After experiencing severe persecution and martyrdom in Europe, the Amish and related groups immigrated to North America in the 17th and 18th centuries. Some variant groups are named after their factional leaders (for example Egli and Beachy Amish); some are called conservative Amish Mennonites; and other, New Order Amish. No Amish live in Europe today.

The Amish have transplanted and preserved a way of life that has the appearance of preindustrial European peasantry. In the modern, industrial United States, they have persisted in relative social isolation based on religious principles. Over time, the Amish have continued to adapt and change at their own pace, accepting innovations selectively. Although most Amish homes do not have electric and electronic labor-saving devices and appliances, that does not preclude their openness to using state-of-the-art medical technology necessary for health promotion.

COMMUNICATIONS

- English is the language of school, of written and print communications, and of contact with most non-Amish outsiders.
- At home and in the immediate Amish communities, Deitsch, or Pennsylvania German, is used. In this highly contextual culture, less overt verbal communication is required, and more reliance is placed on implicit, often unspoken, understandings. Much of what passes for "general knowledge" in our information-rich popular culture is screened, or filtered, out of Amish awareness.
- Health-care providers can expect all their Amish clients of school age and older to be fluently bilingual. They can readily understand spoken and written directions and answer questions presented in English, although their own terms for some symptoms and illnesses may not have exact equivalents in Deitsch and English.
- The Amish have severely restricted their own access to print media, permitting only a few newspapers and periodicals. Most have also rejected electronic media such as radios, television, and entertainment and information applications of film and computers.
- The Amish are clearly not outwardly demonstrative or exuberant. Fondness and love of family members is held deeply but privately. *Demut*, humility, is a priority value, the effects of which may be observed in public as a modest and unassuming demeanor. *Hochmut,* pride or arrogance, is avoided because of frequent verbal warnings.
- The expression of joy and suffering is not entirely subdued by dour or stoic silence.

- The Amish present in an unpretentious, quiet manner, with modest outward dress in plain colors lacking any ornament, jewelry, or cosmetics.
- They are unassertive and nonaggressive and avoid confrontational speech styles and public displays of emotion.
- Amish self-perception is grounded in the present. In public, Amish avoid eye contact with non-Amish, but in one-on-one clinical contacts, clients can be expected to express openness and candor with unhesitating eye contact.
- They are generally punctual and conscientious about keeping appointments.
- Using first names with Amish people is appropriate because there is only a limited number of surnames. For example, it is preferable to use John or Mary during personal contacts rather than Mr. or Mrs. Miller. Within Amish communities, individuals are identified further by nicknames, residence, or a spouse's given name. Health-care workers should greet Amish clients with a handshake and a smile.
- Telephones (a few Amish businesses have them) and automobiles are generally owned by nearby non-Amish neighbors and used by Amish only when it is deemed essential, such as for reaching health-care facilities.

FAMILY ROLES AND ORGANIZATION

- Amish society is patriarchal, but women are accorded high status and respect. Practically speaking, husband and wife may share equally in decisions regarding the family farming business. In public, the wife may assume a retiring role, deferring to her husband, but in private they are typically partners.
- The Amish family pattern is the three-generational family. This kinship network includes consanguine relatives consisting of the parental unit and households of married children and their offspring.
- The highest priority for parents is childrearing, a charge given them by the church. Babies are welcomed as a gift from God.

- Young people older than 16 years may experiment with non-Amish dress and behavior, but the expectation is that they will be baptized Amish before marriage. Unmarried children live in the parents' home until marriage. Single adults are included in the social fabric of the community.
- Families are the units that make up church districts. The size of church districts is measured by the number of families rather than by the number of church members.
- Grandparents have respected status as elders; they provide valuable advice, material support, and services that include childcare to the younger generation. Family emotional and physical proximity to older adults facilitates elder care.

BIOCULTURAL ECOLOGY

The Amish are essentially a closed population, with exogamy occurring very rarely. Most are of German and Swiss descent; therefore, their physical characteristics differ, with skin variations ranging from light to olive tones. Hair and eye colors vary accordingly. A range of recessive genetic tendencies occurs in the Amish as shown in Box 4–1.

HIGH-RISK HEALTH BEHAVIORS

- Farm and traffic accidents are major health concerns because of horse-drawn vehicles. Transportation-related injuries involving farm animals are the largest group. Falls from ladders and down hay holes result in numerous orthopedic injuries. Encourage close monitoring of children who operate farm equipment and transportation vehicles. Teach them about safety factors.

NUTRITION

- Most Amish families grow their own produce. Typical meals include meat; potatoes or noodles or both; a cooked vegetable; bread; something pickled, such as red beets; cake or pudding; and coffee.

Amish

BOX 4–1 • Recessive Genetic Tendencies

- Dwarfism
- Ellis–van Creveld syndrome is characterized by short stature and an extra digit on each hand, congenital heart defects, and nervous system involvement resulting in some amount of mental deficiency
- *Cartilage hair hypoplasia,* also a dwarfism syndrome, is characterized by short stature; fine, silky hair; and deficient cell-mediated immunity that increases susceptibility to viral infections
- *Pyruvate kinase anemia,* a rare blood-cell disease with jaundice and anemia
- *Hemophilia B*
- *Phenylketonuria* (PKU) results in an inability to metabolize the amino acid phenylalanine, evidenced as high blood levels of the substance and eventually severe brain damage if the disorder is untreated
- *Glutaric aciduria*, a progressive neurologic disease, which can be prevented by screening individuals at risk, restricting dietary protein, and thus limiting protein catabolism, dehydration, and acidosis during illness episodes
- **Health-care providers need to plan for family and community education about genetic counseling and screening of newborns for genetic conditions.**

- At mealtimes, all members of the household are expected to be present unless they are working away from home.
- In general, snacks and meals tend to be high in fat and carbohydrates. Common snacks are large, home-baked cookies about 3 inches in diameter, ice cream, pretzels, and popcorn.
- When asking about weight control, suggest reducing portion size, decreasing the amount of sugar used in

baking, limiting fatty meats, and altering food preparation practices.

PREGNANCY AND CHILDBEARING PRACTICES

- Children are considered gifts from God. The average
  number of live births per family is seven. Birth control is
  viewed as interfering with God's will and thus should be
  avoided. Nevertheless, some Amish women do use
  intrauterine devices, but this practice is uncommon.
  Approaching the subject of birth control obliquely may
  make it possible for an Amish woman or man to sense
  the health professional's respect for Amish values and
  thus encourage discussion. "When you want to learn
  more about birth control, I would be glad to talk to
  you" is a suggested approach.
- Women participate in prenatal classes, often with their
  husbands. Women are interested in learning about all
  aspects of perinatal care, but they may choose not to
  participate in sessions when videos are used. Prenatal
  class instructors should inform them ahead of time
  when videos or films will be used so they can decide
  whether to attend.
- Most Amish women prefer home births and choose to
  use Amish or non-Amish lay midwives who promote
  childbearing as a natural part of the life cycle. The
  Amish have no major taboos or requirements for birthing. Men may be present, and most husbands choose to
  be involved; however, they are likely not to be demonstrative in showing affection verbally or physically.
- The laboring woman cooperates quietly, seldom audibly
  expressing discomfort. Women sometimes use herbal
  remedies to promote labor. Knowledge about and
  respect for Amish health-care practices alert physicians
  and nurses to the possibility of simultaneous treatments
  that may or may not be harmful.
- The postpartum mother resumes her family role
  managing, if not doing, all the housework, cooking,
  and child care within a few days after childbirth.
  Grandmothers often come to stay with the new family

Amish

for several days to help with care of the infant and give support to the new mother. Older siblings are expected to help care for the younger children and to learn how to care for the newborn.

- When hospitalized, the family may want the patient to spend the least allowable time in the hospital.

DEATH RITUALS

- Families are expected to care for the aging and the ill in the home. However, when hospitalization is required, make private arrangements for family members to stay overnight in the hospital. A wake-like "sitting up" through the night is expected for the seriously ill and dying.
- The funeral ceremony is simple and unadorned, with a plain wooden coffin. Although grief and loss are keenly felt, verbal expression may seem muted as if to indicate stoic acceptance of suffering.

SPIRITUALITY

- Amish settlements are subdivided into church districts similar to rural parishes, with 30 to 50 families in each district. Local leaders are chosen from their own religious community and are generally untrained and unpaid. No regional or national church hierarchy exists to govern internal church affairs. To maintain harmony within a group, individuals often forgo their own wishes. In addition to Sunday services, silent prayer is always observed at the beginning of a meal, and in many families, a prayer also ends the meal.
- When choosing among health-care options, families usually seek counsel from religious leaders, friends, and extended family, but the final decision resides with the immediate family.

HEALTH-CARE PRACTICES

- The body is considered to be the temple of God, and human beings are stewards of their bodies. Medicine and health care should always be used with the understanding that it is God who heals. Nothing in the Amish understanding of the Bible forbids them from using preventive or curative medical services. They are highly involved in the practices of health promotion and illness prevention. Men are involved in major health-care decisions and often accompany the family to the chiropractor, physician, or hospital. Health-care decision-making is influenced by three factors: (1) type of health problem, (2) accessibility of health-care services, and (3) perceived cost of the service. Grandparents are frequently consulted about treatment options.

- Many Amish do not carry health insurance. Some have formalized mutual aid, such as the Amish Aid Society.
- Providers must be aware that some individuals may withhold important medical information from medical professionals by neglecting to mention folk and alternative care being pursued at the same time.
- When the Amish use professional health-care services, they want to be partners in their health care and want to retain their right to choose from all culturally sanctioned health-care options.
- Care is expressed in culturally encoded expectations, which the Amish best describe in their dialect as abwaarde, meaning "to minister to someone by being present and serving when someone is sick in bed."
- Some accept medical advice regarding the need for high-technology treatments such as transplants or other high-cost interventions.
- The client's family seeks prayers and advice from the bishop and deacons of the church, the extended family, and friends, but the decision is generally a personal family choice. Family members may also seek care from Amish healers and other alternative care practitioners, who may suggest nutritional supplements.
- Herbal remedies include those handed down by successive generations of mothers and daughters.
- Common folk illnesses are described in Box 4–2.

Amish

BOX 4–2 • Common Folk Illnesses

- **Brauche,** sometimes referred to as sympathy curing or powwowing, is referred to as "warm hands" and includes the ability to feel when a person has a headache or a baby has colic.
- **Abnemme** is a condition in which the child fails to thrive and appears puny. Specific treatments for the child may include incantations.
- **Aagwachse,** or livergrown, meaning "hide-bound" or "grown together," includes crying and abdominal discomfort that is believed to be caused by jostling in rough buggy rides.

- Health-care knowledge is passed from one generation to the next through women.
- Health-care providers must inquire about the full range of remedies being used. For the Amish client to be candid, the provider must develop a context of mutual trust and respect.
- When catastrophic illness occurs, the Amish community responds by being present, helping with chores and relieving family members so they can be with the afflicted person in the acute care hospital.
- The Amish are unlikely to display pain and physical discomfort. The health-care provider may need to remind Amish clients that medication is available for pain relief if they choose to accept it.
- There are no cultural or religious rules or taboos prohibiting blood transfusions or organ transplantation and donation. Some may opt for organ transplantation after the family seeks advice from church officials, extended family, and friends, but the patient or immediate family generally makes the final decision.
- Children with mental or physical differences are sometimes referred to as "hard learners" and are expected to go to school and be incorporated into the classes with assistance from other student "scholars" and parents.

The mentally ill are generally cared for at home whenever possible.

HEALTH-CARE PRACTITIONERS

- Amish hold all health-care providers in high regard. Health is integral to their religious beliefs, and care is central to their worldview. They tend to place trust in people of authority when they fit Amish values and beliefs.
- Amish usually refer to their own healers by name rather than by title, although some say brauch-doktor or braucher. In some communities, both men and women provide these services. Amish folk healers use a combination of treatment modalities, including physical manipulation, massage, brauche, herbs and teas, and reflexology. Most prefer professionals who discuss health-care options, giving consideration to cost, need for transportation, family influences, and scientific information.
- Because Amish are not sophisticated in their knowledge of physiology and scientific health care, health-care professionals should bear in mind that the Amish respect authority and that they may unquestioningly follow orders.
- Make sure that clients understand instructions and reasons why interventions are offered.

References

Hostetler, J. A. (1993). *Amish society,* 4th. ed. Baltimore: Johns Hopkins University Press.

Huntington, G. E. (1993). Health care. In D. B. Kraybill (Ed.), *The Amish and the state.* Baltimore: Johns Hopkins University Press.

Kraybill, D. B. (2001). *The riddle of Amish culture,* rev. ed. Baltimore: Johns Hopkins University Press.

Wenger, A. F. Z., & Wenger, M. R. (2003). The Amish. In L. Purnell and B. Paulanka (Eds.), *Transcultural health care: A culturally competent approach* (2nd ed., pp. 54–73). Philadelphia: F.A. Davis Company.

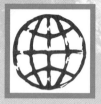

People of Appalachian Heritage

The term *Appalachian* describes people born in the Appalachian mountain range and their descendants, who live in or near Appalachia. With a population of more than 22 million, Appalachia comprises 406 counties in 13 states—Georgia, Alabama, Mississippi, Virginia, West Virginia, North Carolina, South Carolina, Kentucky, Tennessee, Ohio, Maryland, New York, and Pennsylvania. Most of the region is rugged, mountainous terrain that is partially responsible for its residents' values and traditions. Substandard secondary and tertiary roads as well as limited public bus, rail, and airport facilities prevent easy access to the area. Although the region includes several large cities, most Appalachians live in small, isolated settlements that preserve their unique identity. German, Scotch-Irish, Welsh, French, and English are the primary groups who settled the region between the 17th and 19th centuries. Like many disenfranchised groups, the people of Appalachia have been described in stereotypically negative terms (e.g., "poor white trash") that in no way represent the people or the culture as a whole. Appalachians are loyal, caring, family-oriented, religious, hardy, independent, honest, patriotic, and resourceful. The concept of "home" is associated with the land and the family, not a physical structure. Although many are well educated, for some education beyond elementary levels is not considered important because it is not viewed as necessary to earning a living in their traditional occupations.

COMMUNICATIONS

- The dominant language among Appalachians is English, with many words derived from 16th-century Elizabethan English. This can cause communication difficulties with health-care practitioners who are not familiar with the dialect. Many drop the *g* on words ending in *ing*. For example, *writing* becomes *writin'*, *reading* becomes *readin'*, and *spelling* becomes *spellin.'* Consonants may be added, and vowels may be pronounced with a diphthong that can cause difficulty to one unfamiliar with this dialect; hence, *poosh* for *push, boosh* for *bush, warsh* for *wash, hiegen* for *hygiene, deef* for *deaf, welks* for *welts, whar* for *where, hit* for *it, hurd* for *heard,* and *your'n* for *your.* If unfamiliar with the exact meaning of a word, it is best to ask the client to elaborate.
- Appalachians practice the *ethic of neutrality*, which helps shape communication styles, their worldview, and other aspects of the culture.
- The themes of ethic neutrality are described in Box 5–1.
- Many Appalachians are less precise in describing emotions and are more concrete in conversations; many answer questions in a direct manner. Health-care practitioners should use more open-ended questions when obtaining health information and eliciting opinions and beliefs about health-care practices.
- Many Appalachians do not easily trust or share their thoughts and feelings with outsiders and are sensitive to

> **BOX 5–1 • Four Dominant Themes of the Ethic of Neutrality**
>
> - Avoid aggression and assertiveness.
> - Do not interfere with others' lives unless asked to do so.
> - Avoid dominance over others.
> - Avoid arguments, and seek agreement.

direct questions about personal issues. Sensitive topics are best approached with indirect questions and suggestions.
- Because of past experiences with large mining and timber companies, many dislike authority figures and institutions that attempt to control behavior. It may be helpful to "sit a spell" and "chat" before getting down to the business of collecting health information. To establish trust, it is necessary to demonstrate an interest in the client's family and other personal matters, drop hints instead of giving orders, and solicit clients' opinions and advice.
- More traditional individuals may stand at a distance when talking with people in health-care situations.
- Direct eye contact from strangers may be considered as aggression or hostility.
- Most Appalachians are comfortable with silence and when talking are likely to speak without emotion, facial expression, or gestures.
- Calling a person by his or her first name with the title Miss (pronounced "miz," similar to "Ms.," when referring to women, whether single or married) or Mr. (for example, Miss Lillian or Mr. Bill) denotes familiarity with respect. Miss Lillian may or may not be married.
- Some individuals may respond better to verbal instructions and education, with reinforcement from videos rather than from printed communications.
- Based on their fatalistic view, individuals believe they have little or no control over nature and that the time of

death is "predetermined by God." Thus, one frequently hears expressions such as "I'll be there, God willing, or if the crick (creek) don't rise."

- When individuals are not seen because they are late for an appointment and are asked to reschedule, they may not return because of difficult transportation or feelings of rejection. Health-care practitioners should be flexible with appointments.

FAMILY ROLES AND ORGANIZATION

- The traditional household continues to be patriarchal, with many families becoming more egalitarian in beliefs and practices, especially if the woman earns more money than the man.
- Large families are common, and children are usually accepted regardless of their negative behaviors in school or with authority figures. Publicly, parents impose strict conformity for fear of community censure. However, permissive behavior at home is unacceptable, and hands-on physical punishment, to an extent that some perceive as abuse, is common. Health-care providers may need to work with parents to explain current laws of child abuse.
- Older people and pregnant women are treated with increased status in the family, church, and community.
- Grandparents frequently care for grandchildren, especially if both parents work. Elders usually live close to or with their children when they are no longer able to care for themselves. Many adult children do not consider nursing home placement for their parents because it is perceived as the equivalent of a death sentence. The family network can be a rich resource for health-care providers when health teaching and assistance with personalized care are needed. The family rather than the individual must be considered as the basic treatment unit.
- Although alternative lifestyles are usually readily accepted in the Appalachian culture, the health-care provider must still take precautions not to disclose same-sex relationships to others.

Appalachian

BIOCULTURAL ECOLOGY

- The influence of Native Americans can be observed in olive-toned skin.
- Those of Scotch-Irish background and others with light skin tones are at increased risk for skin cancer and need to take precautions to protect themselves from the harmful effects of the sun.
- Predominant occupations such as farming, textile manufacturing, mining, furniture-making, and logging place residents at increased risk for respiratory diseases such as black lung, brown lung, and emphysema.
- The incidence of hypochromic anemia, otitis media, cardiovascular diseases, female obesity, noninsulin-dependent diabetes mellitus, and parasitic infections is greater than the national norm.
- Children are at greater risk for sudden infant death syndrome, congenital malformations, and infections. Only 70 percent of children are immunized, compared with 90 percent for the nation as a whole. The area also has an incidence of childhood injuries due to burns, trauma, poisoning, child neglect, and abuse that is higher than average.

HIGH-RISK HEALTH BEHAVIORS

- High smoking rates continue throughout Appalachia. Use of smokeless tobacco is the highest in the country. Underage use of alcohol is widespread among teens. A low rate of exercise and diets high in fats and refined sugars are also important risk factors.
- A 10-step pattern of health-seeking behaviors has been identified and is shown in Box 5–2.

NUTRITION

- Wealth means having plenty of food for family, friends, and social gatherings. Eating habits include high-cholesterol organ meats such as tongue, liver, heart, lungs (called lights), and brains.

BOX 5–2 • Health-Seeking Behaviors Among Appalachians

1. At the onset of symptoms, self-care practices that are usually learned from mothers are implemented.
2. When the symptoms persist, they call their mother, if she is available.
3. If the mother is unavailable, they call the female in their kin network that is perceived as knowledgeable regarding health. If a nurse is available, they may seek the nurse's advice.
4. If relief is not achieved, they use over-the-counter (OTC) medicine they have seen advertised on television for symptoms that most closely match their own.
5. If that is ineffective, they use some of a neighbor's medicine.
6. Next, they ask the local pharmacist for a recommendation; this usually marks the first encounter with a professional health provider. (Of course, they usually do not tell the pharmacist that they tried the neighbor's medicine.) The pharmacist may strongly suggest that they see a health-care provider; however, on their insistence, the pharmacist may recommend another OTC medication.
7. When no relief is achieved, they seek a local health-care provider. The provider treats them to the best of his or her ability.
8. If the condition does not resolve, the local health-care provider refers them to a specialist in the area.
9. The specialist treats the condition to the best of his or her ability.
10. If unsuccessful, the specialist refers them to the closest tertiary medical center.

Appalachian

(Continued)

BOX 5–2 • Health-Seeking Behaviors Among Appalachians *(Continued)*

These 10 steps may not always follow the sequence presented here; some steps may be skipped, and not all steps are always completed. The time around these 10 steps may be several years. Often by the time they are referred for definitive treatment, compensatory reserves have been depleted, and they die at large medical centers. **It is essential to inquire in a nonjudgmental way about all treatments used for an illness.**

- Common foods are sweet potato pie; molasses candy; apple beer; gooseberry pie; pumpkin cake; and pickled beans, fruit, corn, beets, and cabbage, all of which are high in sodium.
- Bone marrow is used to make sauces, and stomach, intestines (chitlins or chitterlings), pigs' feet, tail, and ribs are also commonly eaten.
- Many recipes contain lard, and meats are preserved with salt. Low-fat game meat is usually breaded and fried with lard or animal fat, negating the overall gains from these low-fat meat sources.
- Most diets include sweet prepackaged drinks, Kool-Aid with added sugar, very sweet iced tea, and soda.
- Explain the benefits of low-fat preparation practices and the potential harmful effects of excess salt and sugar.
- Babies from the first month are fed grease, sugar, and coffee to promote hardiness. Many believe that the sooner a baby can take foods other than milk, the healthier it will be.
- Factual information that describes health risks with early feeding of solid foods may help prevent later nutritional allergies in children.
- Many children replace meals with snacks. The most common snacks are candy, salty foods, desserts, and

carbonated beverages. Many adolescents skip breakfast and lunch entirely, preferring to eat snack foods. This pattern of snacking can result in deficiencies in vitamin A, iron, and calcium.

PREGNANCY AND CHILDBEARING PRACTICES

- Fertility control methods include birth control pills, condoms, and tubal ligation; abortion is an individual choice.
- A popular belief is that taking laxatives facilitates an abortion.
- A disproportionate number of teenage pregnancies occur at a younger age among Appalachians when compared with non-Appalachians. Fertility practices and sexual activity, both sensitive topics for many teenagers, are areas in which outsiders unknown to the family may be more effective than health-care practitioners who are known.
- Beliefs about pregnancy are shown in Box 5–3.

BOX 5–3 • Beliefs About Pregnancy

- Boys are carried higher and the mother's belly appears pointy, whereas girls are carried low.
- Picture-taking can cause a stillbirth.
- Reaching over one's head can cause the cord to strangle the baby.
- Wearing an opal ring during pregnancy may harm the baby.
- Being frightened by a snake or eating strawberries or citrus fruit can cause birthmarks.
- If the mother experiences a tragedy, a congenital anomaly may occur.
- If the mother craves a particular food during her pregnancy, then she should eat that food or the baby will have a birthmark similar to the craved food.

Appalachian

- The birthing mother is expected to accept childbirth as a short, intense, natural process that will bring her closer to the Earth and must be endured. Let the birthing mother know that pain medicine is available if she desires.

DEATH RITUALS

- When death is expected, family and friends may stay through the night.
- Funeral services can last for 3 hours. The amount of time for a service varies according to the age of the deceased. For example, the service for an elderly person is usually longer than for a younger person. The body is displayed for hours, either in the home or at the church, so that all those who wish to view the body may do so.
- At the end of the service, all who wish to view the body again may, with the closest relative being the last to view the body.
- The deceased is usually buried in his or her best clothes. A common practice is to bury the deceased with personal possessions.
- After the funeral services are completed, elaborate meals are served either in the home or at the church. Services are accompanied by singing before, during, and after the service.
- Clergy help families through the grieving process by providing counseling and support to family members.

SPIRITUALITY

- Most churches in the region stress fundamentalism in religious practices and use the King James Bible.
- Prayer for many Appalachians is a primary source of strength. Prayer is personally designed around specific church and religious beliefs and practices, which vary widely throughout the region and between and among churches of similar faith.
- Churches in many parts of Appalachia serve as the social centers of the community and are a good location for health teaching.

- Many small churches have lay preachers instead of trained ministers. Most believe that to be a preacher, a person must have a divine calling.
- Many of the Baptist faiths believe that baptism must be performed in a river, pond, or lake so that the body can be submerged. Feet-washing (men wash men's feet, and women wash women's feet) demonstrates humility.
- Some free-will churches (for example, The Holiness Church) preach against attending movies, ball games, and social functions where dancing occurs. Other sects believe in handling poisonous snakes, although this is rare; it is believed that the snake will not bite those who have faith.
- Some ingest strychnine in small doses during religious services to increase sensory stimuli. This practice can precipitate convulsions if ingested in large enough amounts.
- Fire-handling is still practiced by some groups, with the belief that the hot coals will not burn those who have faith.
- Within the context of *fatalism* comes the belief that what happens to the individual is largely a result of God's will.
- Meaning in life comes from the family and "living right," which is defined by each person and usually means living right with God and in the beliefs of a chosen church.
- Forming partnerships between health-care providers and faith-related organizations for health promotion, wellness, illness, and disease prevention has strong potential for improving the health status of Appalachians. Respect the spiritual beliefs of Appalachians without expressing negative comments.

HEALTH-CARE PRACTICES

- Because self-reliance activities and nature predominate over people, many believe that it is best to let nature heal.

Appalachian

- For some who do not believe in owing money, seeing a health-care provider may be postponed until the condition is severe.
- Many may not see formal biomedical health-care practitioners until self-medicating and folk remedies have been exhausted. When they finally seek formal health care, the conditions have become severe, take longer to treat, and have a less favorable outcome.
- Individuals may feel powerless regarding their own health and abdicate self-responsibility in favor of high expectations and unrealistic dependence on the health-care system, with the physician taking charge of their care completely.
- Offering transportation on a regular schedule and by appointment may improve access.
- A major health concern for many Appalachians is the state of their blood, which is described as being thick or thin, good or bad, and high or low; these conditions can be regulated by diet. Some individuals fear "being cut on" or "going under the knife" and feel that the hospital is a place where one goes to give birth or die. Provide explanations and instructions in an unhurried manner.
- When older people see a health-care provider, many expect immediate help. Physicians who dispense medications in their offices are considered helpful.
- A strong belief in folk medicine is a traditional part of the culture. Using herbal medicines, poultices, and teas is common practice among individuals of all socioeconomic levels. Although many of these home remedies are not harmful, some may have deleterious effects when used to the exclusion of, or in combination with, prescription medications.
- Ascertain if individuals intend to use folk medicines simultaneously with prescription medications and treatment regimens so that these remedies can be incorporated into the plan of care and dialogue can be undertaken to prevent adverse effects.

- Health-care providers who integrate folk medicine into allopathic prescriptions have a greater chance of improving clients' compliance with health prescriptions and interventions.
- Bureaucratic forms foster fear and suspicion of health-care providers. Help clients complete bureaucratic forms if needed.
- Be aware that clients may be especially sensitive to criticism. If the provider uses language that the client does not understand, the provider may be perceived as "stuck up." Decrease language barriers by decoding the jargon of the health-care environment.
- Individuals with mental impairments or physical handicaps are readily accepted and not turned away. The mentally handicapped are perceived not as crazy but rather as having "bad nerves" or being "quite turned" or "odd turned."
- The traditional belief is that disability is a natural and inevitable part of the aging process.
- For many, pain is something that is to be endured and accepted stoically. When a person becomes ill or has pain, personal space collapses inward, and the person expects to be waited on and cared for by others. Explain that self-care activities and taking pain medicine will hasten the healing process.

HEALTH-CARE PRACTITIONERS

- Folk practitioners are primarily older women but may be men. Grannies and herb doctors are trusted and known to individuals and the community for giving more personalized care.
- For clients to become more accepting of biomed-ical care, it is important for health-care providers to approach individuals in an unhurried manner and engage clients in decision-making and care-planning.
- Generally, there is no problem providing care to oppo-site gender clients.

Appalachian

References

Purnell, L. (2003). People of Appalachian heritage. In L. Purnell and B. Paulanka (Eds.), *Transcultural health care: A culturally competent approach* (2nd ed., pp. 73–90). Philadelphia: F.A. Davis Company.

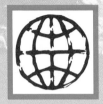

People of Arab Heritage

Overview and Heritage

Arabs trace their ancestry and traditions to the nomadic desert tribes of the Arabian Peninsula. They share a common language, Arabic. Most are united by Islam, a major world religion that originated in 7th-century Arabia. Despite these common bonds, great diversity exists among Arabs related to religious preference and other primary and secondary characteristics of culture discussed in Chapter 1. More than 3 million Arab Americans disappear in national studies annually because they are counted as white in census data. The September 11, 2001, al Qaeda terrorist attack on the United States has increased the number and intensity of negative comments about Arabs. Health-care providers need to understand that few Arab Americans support terrorist attacks and that it is inappropriate to pigeonhole people by their cultural background.

The 22 Arab countries include Algeria, Bahrain, Comoros, Djibouti, Egypt, Iraq, Jordan, Kuwait, Lebanon, Libya, Mauritania, Morocco, Oman, Palestine, Qatar, Saudi Arabia, Somalia, Sudan, Syria, Tunisia, United Arab Emirates, and

Yemen. First-wave immigrants, primarily Christians, came to the United States between 1887 and 1913 seeking economic opportunity. Most were male, illiterate, and unskilled mountain or rural immigrants who valued assimilation. First-wave immigrants and their descendants typically resided in urban centers of the Northeast. Most post-1965 immigrants are Muslims. Arabism and Islam are intrinsically interwoven with some elements of Christianity so that Arabs, whether Christian or Muslim, share some basic traditions and beliefs. Consequently, knowledge of their religion is critical to understanding the Arab American client's cultural frame of reference when providing care that has implications for religious beliefs and practices. Second-wave immigrants entered the United States after World War II. Most are refugees from nations beset by war and political instability. This group includes a large number of professionals and individuals seeking educational degrees who have subsequently remained in the United States. Most are Muslims and favor professional occupations. Many second-wave Arab Americans have settled in Texas and Ohio.

COMMUNICATIONS

- Arabic is the official language of the Arab world. Modern or classical Arabic is a universal form of Arabic used for all writing and formal situations ranging from radio newscasts to lectures.
- Although English is a common second language, language and communication can pose formidable problems in health-care settings. Speak clearly and slowly, giving time for translation. Obtain an interpreter if necessary.
- Communication is highly contextual, where unspoken expectations are more important than the actual spoken words. Conversants stand close together, maintain steady eye contact, and touch (only between members of the same sex) the other's hand or shoulder.
- Speech is loud and expressive and is characterized by repetition and gesturing, particularly when involved in serious discussions. Observers witnessing impassioned

communication may incorrectly assume that Arabs are argumentative, confrontational, or aggressive.

- Privacy is valued, and many resist disclosure of personal information to strangers, especially when it relates to familial disease conditions. Among friends and relatives, Arabs express feelings freely.

- Good manners are important in evaluating a person's character. Inquire first about well-being, and exchange pleasantries. Etiquette requires shaking hands on arrival and departure. Devout Muslim men may not shake hands with women. When a man meets a woman, wait for the woman to extend her hand. Sitting and standing properly is critical; to do otherwise is taken as a lack of respect.

- Box 6–1 describes techniques for communicating with Arab Americans.

- Punctuality is not taken seriously except in cases of business or professional meetings. Explain the importance of punctuality in the American health-care system. Maintain flexibility with appointments when possible.

- Titles are important and are used in combination with the person's first name (e.g., Mr. Khalil or Dr. Ali). Some may prefer to be addressed as mother (*Um*) or father (*Abu*) of the eldest son (e.g., Abu Khalil, "father of Khalil").

FAMILY ROLES AND ORGANIZATION

- Muslim families have a strong patrilineal tradition. Women are subordinate to men, and young people are subordinate to older people. The man is the head of the family, and his influence is overt. In public, a wife's interactions with her husband are formal and respectful. However, behind the scenes she typically wields tremendous influence, particularly in matters pertaining to the home and children.

- Older male figures assume the role of decision-maker. Women attain power and status in advancing years, particularly when they have adult children.

Arab

BOX 6–1 • Guidelines for Communicating with Arab Americans

- Employ an approach that combines expertise with warmth.
- Minimize status differences, and pay special attention to the person's feelings.
- **Take time to get acquainted before delving into business. If sincere interest in the person's home country and adjustment to American life is expressed, he or she is likely to enjoy relating such information, much of which is essential to assessing risk for a traumatic immigration experience and understanding the person's cultural frame of reference.**
- Sharing a cup of tea gives an initial visit a positive beginning.
- **Clarify role responsibilities regarding taking a history, performing physical examinations, and providing health information.**
- **Perform a comprehensive assessment. Explain the relationship of the information needed for physical complaints.**
- A spokesperson may answer questions directed to the client, but family members may edit some information that they feel is inappropriate.
- Family members or an influential intermediary may act as the client's advocate. They may attempt to resolve problems by taking appeals "to the top" or by seeking the help of an influential intermediary.
- Convey hope and optimism. The concept of "false hope" is not meaningful to Arabs because they regard God's power to cure as infinite.

- Gender roles are clearly defined and regarded as a complementary division of labor. Men are breadwinners, protectors, and decision-makers. Women are responsible for the care and education of children and for the maintenance of a successful marriage by tending to their husbands' needs.

- Although women in more urbanized Arab countries often have professional careers, with some women advocating for women's liberation, the family and marriage remain primary commitments for most. The authority structure and division of labor within Arab families are often misinterpreted, fueling common stereotypes of the overtly dominant male and the passive and oppressed woman. Do not be judgmental with family decision-making and roles.

- Family reputation is important; children are expected to behave in an honorable manner and not bring shame to the family.

- Children are dearly loved, indulged, and included in all family activities. A child's character and successes (or failures) in life are attributed to upbringing and parental influence.

- Childrearing patterns also include great respect for parents and elders. Children are raised not to question elders and to be obedient to older brothers and sisters. Discipline includes physical punishment and shaming.

- The father is the disciplinarian, whereas the mother is an ally and mediator, an unfailing source of love and kindness. Children are made to feel ashamed because others have seen them misbehave rather than to experience guilt arising from self-criticism and inward regret. Explain child abuse laws in the United States.

- Adolescents are pressed to succeed academically. Academic failure, sexual activity, illicit drug use, and juvenile delinquency bring shame to the family. For girls in particular, chastity and decency are required.

- Women value modesty, especially devout Muslims, for whom modesty is expressed with their attire. Many Muslim women view the *hijab*, "covering the body except for one's face and hands," as offering them protection in situations in which the sexes mix. It is a recognized symbol of Muslim identity and good moral character. Ironically, many Americans associate the *hijab* with oppression rather than protection.

- Family members live nearby, sometimes intermarry (first cousins), and expect a great deal from one another regardless of practicality or ability to help.
- Loyalty to one's family takes precedence over personal needs. Cultural conflicts between American values and Arab values may cause significant conflicts for families.
- Sons are held responsible for supporting elderly parents. Elderly parents are almost always cared for within the home, typically until death. In the absence of the father, brothers are responsible for unmarried sisters.
- Although the Islamic right to marry up to four wives is sometimes exercised, particularly if the first wife is chronically ill or infertile, most marriages are monogamous and for life.
- Homosexuality is stigmatized. In some Arab countries, it is considered a crime, and participants may be killed. Fearing family disgrace and ostracism, gays and lesbians remain closeted. The health-care provider must not reveal sexual orientation to the family.

BIOCULTURAL ECOLOGY

- Most Arabs have dark or olive-colored skin, but some have blonde or auburn hair, blue eyes, and fair complexions. To assess pallor, cyanosis, and jaundice in dark-skinned people, examine the oral mucosa and conjunctiva.
- Infectious diseases such as tuberculosis, malaria, trachoma, typhus, hepatitis, typhoid fever, dysentery, and parasitic infestations are common with newer immigrants. Schistosomiasis (or bilharziasis) infects about one-fifth of Egyptians and has been called Egypt's primary health problem.
- In Jordan, where contagious diseases have declined sharply, emphasis has shifted to preventing accidental death and controlling noncommunicable diseases such as cancer, diabetes, hypertension, and heart disease. Glucose-6-phosphate dehydrogenase deficiency, sickle cell anemia, and the thalassemias are extremely common in the eastern Mediterranean.

- High consanguinity rates (roughly 30 percent of marriages in Iraq, Jordan, Kuwait, and Saudi Arabia) occur between first cousins and contribute to the prevalence of genetically determined disorders in Arab countries. Individuals are at increased risk to inherit familial Mediterranean fever, a disorder characterized by recurrent episodes of fever, peritonitis, or pleurisies, either alone or in some combination.
- Some individuals have difficulty metabolizing debrisoquine, antiarrhythmics, antidepressants, beta blockers, neuroleptics, and opioid agents.
- Closely assess the effectiveness of narcotics such as codeine and morphine.

HIGH-RISK HEALTH BEHAVIORS

- Smoking and nonuse of seat belts and helmets are major issues. Encourage use of seat belts and helmets, explaining state laws. Encourage cessation of smoking. Despite Islamic beliefs discouraging tobacco use, smoking remains deeply ingrained in the Arab culture: offering cigarettes is a sign of hospitality.
- Islamic prohibitions do appear to influence patterns of alcohol consumption and attitudes toward drug use.
- Women may be at high risk for domestic violence, especially new immigrants, because of the high rates of stress, poverty, poor spiritual and social support, and isolation from family members. Explain American abuse laws.
- Sedentary lifestyle and high fat intake among Arab Americans place them at higher risk for cardiovascular diseases.
- The rates of breast cancer screening, mammography, and cervical Pap smears are low because of modesty.

NUTRITION

- Although cooking and national dishes vary from country to country and seasonings from family to family, Arabic cooking shares many general characteristics. Spices and herbs include cinnamon, allspice, cloves, ginger, cumin, mint, parsley, bay leaves, garlic, and onions.

- Skewer cooking and slow simmering are typical modes of preparation. All countries have rice and wheat dishes, stuffed vegetables, nut-filled pastries, and fritters soaked in syrup. Dishes are garnished with raisins, pine nuts, pistachios, and almonds. Favorite fruits and vegetables include dates, figs, apricots, guava, mango, melon, papaya, bananas, citrus, carrots, tomatoes, cucumbers, parsley, mint, spinach, and grape leaves. Bread accompanies every meal and is viewed as a gift from God. Lamb and chicken are the most popular meats.
- Consumption of blood is forbidden; Muslims are required to cook meats and poultry until well done. Some Muslims refuse to eat meat that is not *halal* (slaughtered in an Islamic manner). Obtain halal meat from Arabic grocery stores or through Islamic centers or mosques.
- Muslims are prohibited from eating pork and pork products. Muslims are equally concerned about the ingredients and origins of mouthwashes, toothpastes, and medicines (e.g., alcohol-based syrups and elixirs) and insulin and capsules (gelatin coating) derived from pigs. However, if no substitutes are available, Muslims are permitted to use these preparations.
- Grains and legumes are often substituted for meats; fresh fruit and juices are especially popular, and olive oil is widely used.
- Food is eaten with the right hand because it is regarded as clean. When it is necessary to feed an Arab client in an in-patient facility, use the right hand, regardless of the dominant hand.
- Eating and drinking at the same time is viewed as unhealthy. Serve beverages after the meal is eaten.
- During Ramadan, the Muslim month of fasting, abstinence from eating, drinking (including water), smoking, and marital intercourse during daylight hours is required.
- Although the sick are not required to fast, many pious

Muslims insist on fasting while hospitalized. Adjust meal times and medications, including medications given by nonoral routes. Provide appointment times after sunset during Ramadan for individuals requiring injections (for example, allergy shots).

- Eating properly, consuming nutritious foods, and fasting are believed to cure disease. For some, illness is related to excessive eating, eating before a previously eaten meal is digested, eating nutritionally deficient food, mixing opposing types of foods (hot, cold, dry, moist), and consuming elaborately prepared foods.
- Gastrointestinal complaints are the most frequent reason for seeking care. Lactose intolerance is common. Eating yogurt and cheese, rather than drinking milk, may reduce symptoms in sensitive people.

PREGNANCY AND CHILDBEARING PRACTICES

- Fertility practices are influenced by traditional Bedouin values, which support tribal dominance and beliefs that "God decides family size." Procreation is regarded as the purpose of marriage; high fertility rates are favored.
- Sterility in a woman can lead to rejection and divorce. Approved methods for treating infertility are limited to artificial insemination using the husband's sperm and *in vitro* fertilization involving the fertilization of the wife's ovum by the husband's sperm.
- Many reversible forms of birth control are undesirable but not forbidden. They should be used when there is a threat to the mother's life, too frequent childbearing, risk of transmitting a genetic disease, or financial hardship.
- Irreversible forms of birth control such as vasectomy and tubal ligation are "absolutely unlawful" as is abortion, except when the mother's health is compromised by a pregnancy-induced disease or her life is threatened.
- Unwanted pregnancies are dealt with by hoping for a miscarriage "by an act of God" or by covertly arranging for an abortion.

- The pregnant woman is indulged and her cravings satisfied, lest she develop a birthmark in the shape of the particular food she craves. Girls are carried high; boys are carried low.
- Although pregnant women are excused from fasting during Ramadan, some Muslim women may be determined to fast. Labor and delivery are women's affairs.
- During labor, women openly express pain through facial expressions, verbalizations, and body movements. Nurses and medical staff may mistakenly diagnose Arab women as needing medical intervention and pain medications inappropriately.
- Care for the infant includes wrapping the stomach at birth, or as soon as possible thereafter, to prevent cold or wind from entering the baby's body.
- The call to prayer is recited in the Muslim newborn's ear.
- Male offspring are preferred.
- Male circumcision is almost a universal practice, and for Muslims it is a religious requirement.
- Mothers may be reluctant to bathe postpartum because of beliefs that air gets into the mother and causes illness.
- Many believe washing the breasts "thins the milk." Breast-feeding is often delayed until the second or third day after birth because of beliefs that the mother requires rest, that nursing at birth causes "colic" pain for the mother, and that "colostrum makes the baby dumb." Explain the importance of the immune properties of colostrum.
- Postpartum care foods, such as lentil soup, are offered to increase milk production, and tea is encouraged to flush and cleanse the body.

DEATH RITUALS

- Death is accepted as God's will. Muslim death rituals include turning the patient's bed to face the holy city of Mecca and reading from the Qur'an, particularly verses stressing hope and acceptance.

- After death, the deceased is washed three times by a Muslim of the same sex. The body is then wrapped, preferably in white material, and buried as soon as possible in a brick or cement-lined grave facing Mecca.
- Prayers for the deceased are recited at home, at the mosque, or at the cemetery.
- Women do not ordinarily attend the burial unless the deceased is a close relative or husband. Instead, they gather at the deceased's home and read the Qur'an.
- Death rituals for Arab Christians are similar to Christian practices in the rest of the world. Extended mourning periods may be practiced if the deceased is a young man, woman, or child. Although weeping is allowed, beating the cheeks or tearing garments is prohibited.
- For women, wearing black is considered appropriate for the entire period of mourning.
- Cremation is not practiced.
- Families do not generally approve of autopsy because of respect for the dead and feelings that the body should not be mutilated. However, Islam does allow forensic autopsies and autopsies for the sake of medical research and instruction.
- Organ donation and transplantation as well as administration of blood and blood products are acceptable.

SPIRITUALITY

- Most Arabs are Muslims. Islam is the religion of most Arab countries, and in Islam there is no separation of church and state; a certain amount of religious participation is obligatory.
- Islam has no priesthood. Islamic scholars or religious sheikhs, the most learned individuals in an Islamic community, assume the role of *imam*, or "leader of the prayer." The imam acts as a spiritual counselor.
- The major tenets of Islam are shown in Box 6–2.

Arab

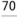

> ### BOX 6–2 • The Five Major Pillars, or Duties, of Islam
>
> - Declaration of faith
> - Prayer five times daily
> - Almsgiving
> - Fasting during Ramadan
> - Completion of a pilgrimage to Mecca

- Many Muslims believe in combining spiritual medicine, performing daily prayers, and reading or listening to the Qur'an with conventional medical treatment. Assist the patient and family in making accommodations for prayer.
- Prominent Christian groups include the Copts in Egypt, the Chaldeans in Iraq, and the Maronites. Contacting the local imam may be a helpful strategy for Muslims struggling with health-care decisions.
- School and work schedules revolve around Islamic holidays and weekly prayer. Because Muslims gather for communal prayer on Friday afternoons, the work week runs from Saturday through Thursday. Schedule appointments so that they can be completed before prayer time on Friday afternoon.
- The devout patient may request that his or her chair or bed be turned to face Mecca and that a basin of water be provided for ritual washing or ablution before praying. Provide hand-washing facilities along with other accommodations as needed.
- Providing for cleanliness is particularly important because the Muslim's prayer is not acceptable unless the body, clothing, and place of prayer are clean.
- Sometimes illness is considered punishment for one's sins. Others emphasize that sickness should not be viewed as punishment but rather as a trial or ordeal that brings about expiation of sins, which may strengthen character.

HEALTH-CARE PRACTICES

- Good health is considered the ability to fulfill one's roles.
- Diseases are attributed to an inadequate diet, shifts of hot and cold, exposure of one's stomach during sleep, emotional or spiritual distress, and envy or the "evil eye."
- Practices such as informed consent, self-care, advance directives, risk management, and preventive care are valued.
- Women are often reluctant to seek care because of cultural emphasis placed on modesty. Many fear that a diagnosed illness, such as cancer or psychiatric illness, may bring shame and influence their marriageability.
- Family members indulge the individual and assume the ill person's responsibilities. Although the patient may seem dependent and the family overly protective by American standards, family members' vigilance and "demanding behavior" should be interpreted as a measure of concern.
- Communicating a grave diagnosis is often viewed as cruel and tactless because it deprives clients of hope.
- Most expect physicians, because of their expertise, to select treatments. The client's role is to cooperate.
- The authority of physicians is seldom challenged or questioned. When treatment is successful, the physician's skill is recognized; adverse outcomes are attributed to God's will.
- Because many medications requiring a prescription in the United States are available over the counter in Arab countries, Arabs are accustomed to seeking medical advice from pharmacists.
- Witchcraft and magic, concerns about the powers of jealous people, the evil eye, and certain supernatural agents, such as the devil and jinn, are part of their religion.
- Those who envy the wealth, success, or beauty of others

Arab

- are believed to cause adversity by a gaze, which brings misfortune to the victim.
- Beautiful women, healthy-looking babies, and the rich are believed to be particularly susceptible to the evil eye. Thus, expressions of congratulations may be interpreted as envy.
- Protection from the evil eye is afforded by wearing amulets, such as blue beads, or figures involving the number five; reciting the Qur'an; or invoking the name of Allah. Do not remove amulets from the patient or from the bedside.
- Mental or emotional illnesses may be attributed to possession by evil jinn.
- Islamic medicine is based on the theory of four humors and the spiritual and physical remedies prescribed by the Prophet. Because illness is viewed as an imbalance between the humors—black bile, blood, phlegm, and yellow bile—and the primary attributes of dryness, heat, cold, and moisture, therapy involves treating with the disease's opposite: thus, a hot disease requires a cold remedy.
- Although methods such as cupping, cautery, and phlebotomy may be used, treatment with special prayers or simple foods such as dates, honey, salt, and olive oil is preferred.
- Preoperative instructions are thought to cause needless anxiety, hypochondriasis, and complications. Determine the need for preoperative teaching on an individual basis.
- Most regard pain as unpleasant and something to be controlled, anticipating immediate postoperative relief.
- Although expressive, emotional, and vocal responses to pain are usually reserved for the immediate family, under circumstances such as childbirth and illnesses accompanied by spasms, Arabs express pain freely.
- The tendency of Arabs to be more expressive with their family and more restrained in the presence of health professionals may lead to conflicting perceptions

regarding the adequacy of pain relief. Whereas the nurse may assess pain relief as adequate, family members may demand that their relative receive additional analgesia. Complete a thorough physical assessment for anticipating pain medication requirements.

- Mental illness is a major social stigma. Psychiatric symptoms may be denied or attributed to "bad nerves" or evil spirits.
- When individuals suffering from mental distress seek medical care, they are likely to present with a variety of vague complaints, such as abdominal pain, lassitude, anorexia, and shortness of breath. Patients often expect and may insist on somatic treatment, at least "vitamins and tonics."
- When mental illness is accepted as a diagnosis, treatment with medications, rather than counseling, is preferred. Hospitalization is resisted because such placement is viewed as abandonment.
- Because of social stigma, the disabled are often kept from public view.
- Medical treatments that require surgery, removal of causative agents, or eradication by intravenous treatments are valued more than therapies aimed at health promotion or disease prevention.

HEALTH-CARE PRACTITIONERS

- Many individuals find interacting with a health-care professional of the opposite sex quite embarrassing and stressful.
- Discomfort may be expressed by refusal to discuss personal information and by a reluctance to disrobe for physical assessments and hygiene. Women may refuse to be seen by male health care providers. Provide a same-sex caregiver whenever possible, especially with intimate care.
- Knowledge held by a doctor is thought to convey authority and power.
- Most clients who lack English communication skills prefer an Arabic-speaking physician.

References

Kulwicki, A. D. (2003). People of Arab heritage. In L. Purnell and B. Paulanka (Eds.), *Transcultural health care: A culturally competent approach* (2nd ed., pp. 90–106). Philadelphia: F. A. Davis Company.

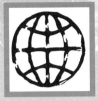

CHAPTER 7

People of Bosnian Heritage

Overview and Heritage

This profile provides an overview of some of the cultural and health issues of concern to Bosnian Muslim migrants and refugees in the United States. This description may not apply to all Bosnian Muslims because individual characteristics vary according to the primary and secondary characteristics of culture as presented in Chapter 1. Data describing this population are subject to considerable error because of the dislocations caused by military action and ethnic cleansing. The population of Bosnia-Herzegovina is estimated at 4 million. There are more than 1.2 million Bosnian immigrants and refugees worldwide, not all of whom are in the United States.

In the late 1960s, the government of the Socialist Federal Republic of Yugoslavia recognized the Bosnian Muslims as a distinct "nation" with an ethnic identity separate from the Serbians and the Croatians in Bosnia-Herzegovina. In 1991, Bosnia-Herzegovina declared independence; the ensuing civil war involved atrocities such as rape, torture, and murder as ethnic communities fought each other for the right to self-

75

determination. The United States sponsored peace talks in Dayton, Ohio, in 1995, which led to an agreement that called for a Muslim, Croat, and Bosnian identity-sharing power. In 1999, the Serbian segment failed to honor this working agreement. This and further governmental corruption and mismanagement of $5 million in humanitarian aid resulted in continued instability, ethnic attacks, and scattered land mines.

Recent Bosnian immigrants have migrated under special humanitarian provisions to escape fighting in the civil war. To avoid confusion with the religious term *Muslim*, an adherent of Islam, *Bosniak* or *Bosniac* has replaced Muslim as an ethnic term. The Federation of Bosnia and Herzegovina makes up a triangular-shaped republic of 17,741 square miles on the Balkan Peninsula. Sarajevo, the capital, is the largest city. The Bosnian region in the north is forested mountains; Herzegovina in the south is rugged, flat farmland. Life expectancy for males is 69.3 years and 74.9 years for females. Bosnian refugees include well-educated professionals, farm owners, skilled workers such as welders and mechanics, truck drivers, and other blue-collar workers. Their qualifications and skills may not be recognized in the United States, causing lower social status. Many are unable to find suitable jobs, especially when first entering the United States. Bosnian Muslims have identified their refugee stigma as a concern.

COMMUNICATIONS

- The primary language is Serbian, although a Bosnian language closely related to Serbo-Croatian is acknowledged. Those who come from war-torn areas may find it difficult to trust health-care providers and interpreters. When interpretation is needed, discuss the ethnicity of the interpreter as well as the language desired. Provide an interpreter with the same ethnic background, if possible.
- Physical touch between men and women is not shown outside the home. Provide a same-gender health-care provider for intimate care. If it is necessary for a male health-care provider to be alone in a room with a female patient, leave the door open.

- Females maintain eye contact with other women but not with men.
- Asking many questions, taking notes, and completing forms may increase the clients' sense of apprehension. Too many questions or unfamiliar gestures may be seen as disrespectful and interfere with a good health-care provider relationship. Take notes during assessments, and complete required forms out of view of the client.
- Traditional and older clients expect formality in greetings. Call the person by name with the appropriate title, Mr., Mrs., Miss, Ms., or Dr. Males should not extend the hand in greeting to a woman unless she extends her hand first.

FAMILY ROLES AND ORGANIZATION

- In Bosnia-Herzegovina, traditional life for Muslims involved arranged marriages, bride price, and a strong demarcation of male and female roles. A woman's role was restricted to the household, although for some urban dwellers there may have been a more relaxed approach. Many migrant families have not followed religious practices strictly; women frequently share the same status as men. This process may cause intergenerational conflict and marital disharmony. Accept diversity among Muslim families' decision-making practices and gender roles.
- Traditional women cover their entire bodies except for their faces, hands, feet, and hair when in public or with men other than their husband or brothers. The head covering is called a *hijab*. Some traditional men avoid shaking hands with women and do not look them directly in the eye. Whenever possible, provide a same-sex health-care provider.
- The home is the domain of women; outside the home is the domain of men, although there is variation with acculturation and education in the United States.
- All family members are expected to care for the elderly at home. The suggestion of a nursing home may be interpreted as insulting to the family honor.

Bosnian

- Babies and children commonly sleep in the same bed or same room with parents until the age of 2 years. Infants may be given food supplements, such as carrots or potatoes with milk, at 3 months of age. Toilet training may commence early at 6 months of age. Children are not pampered for fear of their becoming "softies."
- Traditionally, sons are given preference over daughters.
- Women are expected to remain virgins until marriage; otherwise, great shame may come to the family.
- Parents of a disabled child may feel shame and isolate themselves from the rest of the community, thus not taking advantage of available social services. Children may have unexplained behavioral problems, such as a fear of stairs or bedwetting, related to previous traumatic experiences in Bosnia.

BIOCULTURAL ECOLOGY

- Coloring varies from white to olive-toned skin; blue to brown eyes; and blond, brown, or black hair.
- Those coming from refugee camps and other difficult circumstances may have a higher incidence of tuberculosis. Others test positive because of the use of BCG in their home country. Approximately 7 percent of newer immigrants have intestinal parasites; there are high rates of respiratory illnesses and diseases. Screen all newer immigrants for tuberculosis and parasitic diseases.
- Tooth decay is endemic at all ages; ongoing dental care is a priority. Help clients access dental care.
- Many women were raped before coming to the United States, resulting in sexually transmitted diseases (STDs) and unwanted pregnancies. Given the high value placed on virginity and fidelity, a diagnosis of an STD or HIV/AIDS can be devastating to the client or family. Even to suggest a test for STDs can appear inappropriate or offensive. Statistics on STDs and HIV/AIDS do not exist for Bosnians in the United States or in Bosnia. When it is necessary to screen for STDs,

explain the need carefully, and do not reveal that testing
has occurred with other family members.
- Childhood immunizations rates in Bosnia approach
83 percent.

HIGH-RISK HEALTH BEHAVIORS

- Even though tobacco use is prohibited among strict
Muslims, 48 percent smoke. Encourage clients to
decrease or stop smoking; a reminder about the Islamic
prohibition on tobacco use may be helpful.
- Exercising for health is uncommon, and many,
especially women, tend to be overweight. Negotiate an
acceptable weight with clients using culturally
acceptable foods and preparation practices.

NUTRITION

- Under Islam, only *halal* meat can be consumed. For
meat to be halal, the animal must undergo ritual
slaughter by a Muslim, ensuring that no blood remains.
Pork, pork products, and alcohol are forbidden. Ask
clients if they follow Islamic rules. Help clients identify
foods that have animal shortenings or pork products,
such as gelatin, marshmallows, and other confections.
Avoid prescribing medicines with alcohol such as cough
suppressants and drops. Obtain halal meats from a
Muslim supplier of meats, or have the client's family
bring food from home.
- Most individuals eat or pass food only with the right
hand. The left hand is considered dirty because it is
used for toileting. Feed patients only with your right
hand.
- Fasting is required during the holy month of Ramadan,
as well as on other occasions. No foods or beverages
are consumed between sunrise and sunset. The ill are
not required to fast, but the devout may be reluctant to
break their fasting. Adjust medication administration
times and meals to accommodate fasting from sunup to
sundown.

Bosnian

PREGNANCY AND CHILDBEARING PRACTICES

- The law legalizing abortion and implementing family planning passed in former Yugoslavia in 1952 is still in effect in Bosnia-Herzegovina. This law has helped eliminate illegal, i.e., criminal, abortions. Women are used to a system in which abortion is used more often than the pill. The pill is unpopular due to its perceived side effects and fear that it may cause cancer. Women in the United States may not understand how to obtain an abortion or access fertility information. Help clients identify acceptable methods of fertility control and how and where to access services.
- Most pregnant women seek prenatal care and follow advice precisely unless it conflicts with Islamic laws. Discuss all recommendations with the client to determine if they are compatible with Islam.
- Many women prefer natural childbirth, although some accept medication during labor. During delivery, ensure that only the perineum should be exposed.
- Men are usually not present in the delivery room; rather, the laboring woman's mother, sisters, or other female family members are present. Determine the role of the husband and female family members well before the delivery occurs.
- Most mothers breast-feed for at least 6 months and some for 18 months. The mother and newborn avoid crowds for 30 to 40 days after delivery. Both boys and girls may be circumcised. Explain that female circumcision is illegal in the United States.

DEATH RITUALS

- When death is imminent, the patient should face Mecca. Family members gather around the person and recite prayers from the Qur'an. Arrange furniture, if necessary, for the bed to face Mecca. Make arrangements for the family to recite prayers at the bedside.
- Death is the transition from this life to the next. The body must not be touched with bare hands by a non-

Muslim and is entrusted with the family for proper and respectful disposition, including ritualistic washing, positioning of limbs, and wrapping in three shrouds. Help family obtain a Muslim to perform death rites.

- Prolonging life by artificial means is not encouraged. Although one is required to seek treatment for illness, do-not-resuscitate orders are desirable when treatment appears futile. Hospice care in the home is recommended. Help family obtain hospice care in the home.
- Suicide is forbidden; it may carry a stigma for the family when it does happen.
- Voluntary permission for autopsy is usually denied. When required by law, autopsy is permissible. Carefully explain the legal requirements for autopsy.
- After burial of the deceased, people gather at the home of the deceased or at a mosque to say additional prayers; this death rite may be repeated several times over the next 40 days and yearly thereafter.
- Women traditionally wear black from 30 days to a year, depending on their relationship to the deceased. Many men and women are stoic during bereavement, whereas others may wail uncontrollably, although Islamic law does not advocate this.

SPIRITUALITY

- Islam is the major religion (40 percent) in Bosnia-Herzegovina, but other religions include Orthodox Christianity, Roman Catholicism, Protestantism, Judaism, and Jehovah's Witness. Muslims, whether Sunni, Shi'ites, Khawarij, or Sufis, practice the Five Pillars of Islam (meaning submission to the will of God), which guide their way of life; these are listed in Box 7–1.
- During Ramadan, fasting is required between sunrise and sunset for 30 days. The date of Ramadan differs each year and is based on the lunar calendar. Barram is a religious holiday when men visit friends for 3 days; on the fourth day, women visit friends.

Bosnian

BOX 7–1 • Five Pillars of Islam

- Faith, which is shown by the proclamation of the Unity of God by saying "There is no God but Allah; Mohammed is the Messenger of Allah."
- Prayer, facing Mecca, is performed at dawn, noon, midafternoon, sunset, and nightfall.
- Almsgiving is encouraged to assist the poor and to support religious organizations.
- Fasting occurs to fulfill religious obligations, to wipe out previous sins, and to appreciate the hunger of the poor. (See Ramadan under Nutrition)
- A pilgrimage to Mecca *(hadj)* once in a lifetime is encouraged if the means are available.

- One must be in a pure state to pray, forbidding menstruating women to pray or touch the Qur'an. Once menstruation is complete, a ritual washing occurs before entering a mosque, praying, or participating in Ramadan. Help clients with cleansing rituals before praying.

HEALTH-CARE PRACTICES

- Under the laws of Islam, people are required to practice illness and disease prevention and to seek care when ill. Requiring running water for washing reinforces the high value placed on cleanliness. If patients are unable to shower or go to the bathroom to wash their hands, provide a pitcher of water (and a basin) to assist with this hygiene.
- Most individuals accept pain stoically in the presence of the health-care provider. The family, however, may request pain medication for the patient demonstrating the slightest sign of discomfort. Make a complete assessment before administering pain medication.
- The sick person is encouraged to communicate about suffering. The relatives give moral and physical support.

Treatment is often not considered complete without medication.

- Health-care providers are expected to give high significance to discussions of symptoms and complaints. Give detailed explanations of tests and procedures.
- Being admitted to a hospital brings fear that the illness is very serious or terminal. Hospital admittance may also be related, especially with people from rural areas, to the reluctance of a husband to expose his wife to the outside world.
- Traditional remedies include teas, humus, onion, cumin, mints, henna, herbs, dates, grasses, and ointments, which are used for colds, sore throats, fever, and other illnesses. Coughs may be relieved by the inhalation of the steam from chamomile tea with a linen cloth over the patient's head. Honey and pollen may be taken to ensure longevity. Incorporate nonharmful traditional practices into allopathic care when feasible.
- The Qur'an mentions the *evil eye* and tells people how to protect themselves from it and treat it. Talismans for protection are culturally specific and vary among countries and families within the same country. Common talismans include blue beads, which are hung on walls at the entrances to homes or on the person. Do not remove talismans unless the patient gives explicit permission to do so.
- Many individuals may be reluctant to seek dental care because in some regions of Bosnia dental care was painful. Provide support for the first visit to overcome fear induced by past dental treatment.
- Many individuals who have recently entered the United States are poor with low educational levels from rural areas. For them, health care has not been a priority. Earlier immigrants to the United States were from city environments and were well educated.
- Many Bosnians are embarrassed when they must use Medicaid, and thus they may be hesitant to seek health care. Be aware of the possible embarrassment that charity implies, and present Medicaid in a way that makes them feel comfortable.

Bosnian

- Many new immigrants do not own vehicles or have the funds to travel to a health-care provider. Help refugees find specialists for their physical and psychological health. Provide transportation if possible.
- Trust is a major issue for many. In Bosnia, in order to get health care, one must provide a bribe to receive treatment.
- Regardless of international law, women who have been raped are still not recognized as victims in Bosnia. At best, they are regarded as tarnished, at worst as "fallen women" who somehow invited their own misfortune. Many women who had been raped in prison camps in northwest Bosnia were evacuated to third countries via Croatia. Some mothers abandoned newborn children who resulted from rape.
- The effects of displacement, witnessing horrific events, and in some cases the effects of torture and rape may present as a post-traumatic stress disorder that many tend to keep hidden. However, this can contribute to marital problems, domestic violence, alcoholism, and attempted suicide. Some clients may suffer survivor guilt and worry about those left behind in Bosnia.
- There is a stigma associated with mental illness. Psychological distress is often expressed in somatic symptoms, particularly gastrointestinal or respiratory symptoms. Even when mental illness is recognized, health-seeking behavior is often limited by language proficiency and knowledge of services. Some view medication as the only treatment, thus rejecting psychotherapy, group therapy, or occupational therapy.
- Unemployment, for men particularly, may be associated with a depressive illness. Family honor is important, and unemployed males may feel isolated from community social life. Alcohol may be used to compensate for feelings of inadequacy and loneliness.
- Blood donation and transfusion and organ donation and transplantations are acceptable and are considered acts of piety.

HEALTH-CARE PRACTITIONERS

- Islamic recommendations in priority order for health-care providers are (1) Muslim physician/health-care provider of the same sex, (2) a physician/health-care provider of the same sex, (3) a Muslim physician/health-care provider of the opposite sex, and (4) a physician/health-care provider of the opposite sex. In times of emergency, opposite-gender health-care providers are generally acceptable.
- Most individuals prefer an older provider with recognized degrees and a position denoting authority in the health-care system. Male health-care providers should not ask females to undress more than absolutely necessary and should always have a female, preferably a family member, present during the examination.
- Many Muslim women prefer to see only female health-care providers and refuse gynecological examinations by males. This may also extend to male interpreters being present during consultations. Provide a same-gender interpreter if possible.
- Women do not readily discuss medical or health-care information with providers. Distrust from inequities in Bosnia may potentiate this practice. Ask only questions required for a diagnosis, and explain the reason for each question.

References

CIA World Factbook (2002). *World population data sheet.* Washington, DC: Population Reference Bureau. Retrieved September 1, 2003, from www.ciesin.org

The Koran. (1999). NY: Penguin Books.

Time Almanac. (2003). Retrieved September 1, 2003, from http://www.infoplease.com/.

Transcultural aspects of perinatal health: A resource guide. (2002). Tampa, FL: National Perinatal Association.

UNICEF; *CIA World Factbook 2002*; World Health Organization. Geneva: WHO. Retrieved September 1, 2003, from http://www.who.int/whosis/mort/html

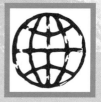

People of Brazilian Heritage

Overview and Heritage

Brazil, the largest country in South America, is 2,695 miles long from the north to the south and 2691 miles wide from the east to the west. The landmass is 3,286,487 square miles, or approximately 400,000 square miles less than that of the United States, excluding Alaska. The overall population is approximately 172,860,000. The capital of Brazil is the very modern interior jungle city of Brasilia, which has 1.8 million inhabitants. São Paulo, with a population of 18 million, and Rio de Janeiro, with a population of more than 10.6 million, are the largest cities in Brazil. All South American countries except Chile and Ecuador border Brazil.

To the east and northeast, Brazil is bordered by the Atlantic coastline, which is more than 3,600 miles long. Brazil is extremely diverse in topography. The sparsely populated tropical Amazon valley has little variation in temperatures throughout the year, whereas the southern districts have distinct summers and winters. The coastal plains have high temperatures and high humidity. The remainder of the country consists of high plateaus traversed with low mountain ranges where the climate varies with little or no rain for most of the year.

There is virtually no literature on Brazilian health conditions, practices, and beliefs. However, an abundance of literature and sites are available depicting the objective culture of the various groups in Brazil, including arts, music, dance, and cuisine. Brazilian heritage is rich in its mixture of Portuguese, French, Dutch, German, Italian, Japanese, Chinese, African, Arab, and native Brazilian Indians. The diversity of the population in Brazil reflects the diversity among Brazilians in the United States as well as the primary and secondary characteristics of culture as described in Chapter 1. Above all, Brazilians do not consider themselves Hispanics, despite similarities in their ethnic features.

Common knowledge among Brazilians living in the United States is that most of them are *escondidos* (hidden), or officially referred to as undocumented aliens. Most Brazilians in the United States are concentrated in communities around Boston; New York; Newark, New Jersey; and Miami. Smaller groups exist in Los Angeles, Detroit, and other locales. Larger Brazilian settlements in the United States have their own churches, spiritualists, beauty shops, travel services, and support services. The exact number of Brazilians living in the United States is unknown. Many Brazilians subsist in urban slums without privacy and think only of earning enough money to return home. They frequently leave children, wives, and family behind to become slaves of work in any type of situation. There are relatively few second- and third-generation Brazilians where both the mother and father have immigrated to the United States. Like other immigrants, many Brazilians are underemployed after immigrating, often giving up their professions to earn money as illegal domestic workers, waiters, cab drivers, and other low-paying positions. Immigrants often move to large cities where many networks help find "under-the-table" wages.

COMMUNICATIONS

- Portuguese is the official language of Brazil and continues to dominate the Brazilian communities. In the

United States, Brazilian Portuguese is different from its mother language in the meaning of certain words, accents, and dialects. Dialects vary among Brazilians. Language is frequently a barrier to accessing health care. Obtain an interpreter for Brazilians when necessary.

- Many Brazilians continue to be of "proper" old-world orientation where true feelings are not divulged for fear of hurting the receiver of the communication. Everything is said to be *tudo bom* (great), almost in a stoic sense. However, in the intimate circle of family and compatriots, the sharing of thoughts and feelings is common. Health-care providers must establish trust before attempting to obtain sensitive information in the health history.

- Young adult and adolescent Brazilians in the United States are generally more acculturated because of their desire and need to assimilate into the new culture. Among this group, there is more intragenerational than intergenerational communication when it comes to sharing thoughts and feelings.

- Most Brazilians use touch and eye contact. Women kiss each other on both cheeks when they meet and when they say good-bye. At times, women and men kiss in the same manner. Men shake each other's hands and slap each other on the back with the other hand. This gesture frequently ends in an embrace. Children are kissed, and there is much touching. The kissing of a child frequently includes the combination of a "kiss and smell."

- Spatial distancing is close. Facial expressions and symbolic gestures are commonplace. Do not take offense if Brazilians stand closer than you are accustomed when dealing with other clients.

- Most Brazilians in America are future-oriented. In general, they are not punctual and tend to arrive "a bit" late—from minutes to hours—especially for social occasions. Everyone seems to know the behavior of tardiness and plans around it. However, those in professional circles are punctual. Carefully explain the importance of being on time for health-care appointments.

- Brazilian names are lengthy, but the modern trend is to use only the first and last names. Traditionally, names appear as first name, mother's family name, and father's family name. "Junior" is added to a name if the son has been named after the father and *Neto* if the son has been named after the grandfather (third generation). When a woman marries, she may opt to drop her mother's maiden name and her father's name, or she may keep them both. At times *de, da/do, das/dos* is added to a name to denote "of" and seems to be done out of tradition. No rigid protocol is apparent. Children who have no father are often given the mother's maiden name to which *da Silva* is added, denoting that the line of paternity is unclear. Ask the client his/her full name and the name that is used for legal purposes.
- In day-to-day relationships, people are called by their first name or *Seu, Senhor* (more respectful) preceding the first name of a man, or *Dona* preceding the first name of a woman. Mothers, grandmothers, or respected strangers are referred to as *A Senhora*, and fathers, grandfathers, and respected men are called *O Senhor*. Doctors are addressed as *Doutor* or *Doutora*, and professors are addressed as *Professor or Professora*. The latter two are followed by the first name. Address Brazilian clients formally with Mr., Mrs., Ms., or appropriate title until told to do otherwise.

FAMILY ROLES AND ORGANIZATION

- Brazilian society is one of *machismo*, with the middle and upper classes being patriarchal in structure. However, as women assert their equality, more egalitarian relationships are becoming evident. Among middle and upper socioeconomic classes that were traditionally patriarchal, more egalitarian roles are beginning to develop. Lower socioeconomic households tend to be more matriarchal in nature. Be sure to identify the family decision-maker.

Brazilian

- Children are important to Brazilian families. In the event that a mother and child face deportation from the United States to Brazil, the baby is generally accepted into the family and often raised by the maternal grandmother. It is not uncommon for a wealthier family member to raise the child of a poorer relative. However, these children often enter the family in a second-class capacity.

- The elderly live with one of their children, and nursing home placement is uncommon. The elderly are respected, seen as the family counselors, and are always addressed as *O Senhor* or *A Senhora*. The elderly are included in family activities and usually accompany their children's families on vacation. The extended family is very important where a *jeitinho* (knack) is always procured for employing relatives in any type of service, from the government to a bank, or for helping a relative get into a special university or school. Include the elders and extended family in health-care decision-making.

- Godparents are a very important family extension. Poor families frequently ask their *patron* and *patrona* (employer and wife) to be godparents to their child. Godparent responsibilities include clothing, schooling, and caring for the children in case of the parents' death. The godmother is called *comadre* by the mother. *Compadre* is used in reference to the godfather.

- Although historically common in the lower socioeconomic classes, middle-class households with a single-female parent are becoming increasingly common among Brazilians in the United States. In middle-class families, the "no father" status is obscured by the child receiving the same middle and last names as the mother.

- Social status is very important in the Brazilian society, demonstrated in the titles that people use with each other and the practice of listing both parents' surnames. Class separation is maintained discretely by literacy status.

- Brazilians, especially from the south and southeast of Brazil, have become more accepting of gay and lesbian relationships. For many, same-sex relationships carry a stigma. Do not disclose same-sex relationships to family members or to others.

BIOCULTURAL ECOLOGY

- The "typical" Brazilian is a *moreno* with brown skin and eyes and black or brown hair. However, individuals from the southern states of Brazil may have blond hair and blue eyes.
- Specific diseases related to the regional topography and climate of Brazil include malaria, dengue fever, cholera, meningitis, rabies, trypanosomiasis, yellow fever, schistosomiasis, typhoid fever, Hansen's disease, hepatitis, and tuberculosis are present in various parts of Brazil. Because intestinal worms are common in Brazilian immigrants, parasitic diseases should be considered during health assessments.
- Interviews have substantiated that the incidence of gastrointestinal diseases increases when Brazilians first move to the United States. Changes in eating habits from the Brazilian long and ample midday dinner to American fast foods have left Brazilians in America with gastric complaints. A genetic tendency toward lactose intolerance can contribute to some of these gastric problems. Interviewees also report an increased incidence of allergies, especially in children of Brazilian immigrants.
- An endemic disease following Brazilians to the United States, and for which documentation is found, is AIDS. A seropositive person with a CD4 count under 200 can apply for voluntary entry into the United States under a law that allows individuals with terminal diseases to remain in the United States if the country of origin does not offer adequate treatment. This law apparently overrides the one that denies entrance to confirmed individuals who test positive for HIV. The law provides

Brazilian

a monthly stipend to pay for rent and food for those who cannot work. At the end of the year, a person may reapply to the Department of Justice for continuation of his or her visa. However, once the person is denied renewal, he or she must leave and may not return to the United States. For this reason, many undocumented people with AIDS prefer to remain underground so they may return to Brazil to see their loved ones and later return to the United States for further treatment. Refer clients as needed to social services to help them obtain needed services.

HIGH-RISK HEALTH BEHAVIORS

- Because Brazilian immigrants frequently settle in Brazilian enclaves in large cities in the United States, they are subject to the same risk factors as any socially vulnerable urban sub-population. The greatest risks are violence, drugs, and crime. Adolescents run the risk of resolving their adolescent identity crises by either banding together or joining gangs. School officials can help decrease violence and crime among Brazilians by instituting after-school program such as dance, music, sports, and other programs for teens.
- Smoking is a high-risk behavior among Brazilians living in the United States. Among men, drinking hard liquor is also prevalent. Accessibility and use of street drugs and an individual's desperate search for quick money are other identifiable high-risk behaviors and often involve living in crowded ghetto conditions where rent is inexpensive. Although many immigrants are aware of the ill effects of smoking and recreational drugs, loneliness and frustration are deterrents to stopping these habits. Encourage smoking cessation and moderation in alcohol consumption. Help clients find community support groups to decrease loneliness and smoking cessation programs.
- The undocumented status of Brazilian immigrants places them at a high risk for nonassimilation into the culture of the community in which they live.

NUTRITION

- Food is important in the celebration of all rites among Brazilians. Food and its counterpart, hunger, are often viewed as symbols that determine social relations. Food has symbolic content, is used as a reward or punishment, and establishes and maintains social relations.
- The mainstay of the Brazilian American's diet continues to be rice, beans, and farina. Roast beef, fresh chicken, and seafood are sought when they are not too expensive.
- *Cafe de manha* (breakfast) typically consists of bread with *cafe com leite* (half coffee and half hot milk). Sometimes *cuscus* (dry cornmeal mush) is served with milk. Fruit, fruit juices, and scrambled eggs, with or without sliced hot dogs, are common special breakfast fares among middle-class families. Sometimes sweet potatoes and yams grace a breakfast table.
- *O almoco* (dinner) is eaten at noon. This heavy meal, consisting of beans, rice, and farina, often includes *puree* (mashed potatoes) and *macarrao* (pasta). Desserts such as *pudim de leite* (custard), various cornmeal pastries, fruit, and *doce* (a sweet paste made by boiling sugar and fruit or fruit pulp) are common. A typical vegetable salad consists of finely cubed carrots, potatoes, and *shushu* (summer squash–like plant). A fruit salad with finely cubed fruits is also common.
- Brazilians in America have become vitamin- and health-food–conscious. Although this luxury is often not available to those who have immigrated for fast money, legal residents generally become health-food consumers. The preference, especially among young Brazilian women, is to rely on vitamins instead of food consumption to help them remain thin.
- Fruit juices are expensive, and special foods that are common to the Brazilian diet are hard to procure in the United States. Food limitations are imposed by expense and inaccessibility of Brazilian mainstay foods. However, many Brazilian communities in the United States have ethnic markets and restaurants. Large-chain

Brazilian

supermarkets often carry a section of ethnic foods, some of which are reasonably priced. Help clients identify low-cost nutritious, cultural foods.

PREGNANCY AND CHILDBEARING PRACTICES

- Although Brazil is predominantly a Catholic country, birth control is taught and used. Women are encouraged by their physicians or clinic personnel to have tubal ligations to prevent unwanted pregnancies. Frequently, unwanted pregnancies and abortions are, in the end, left in God's hands. Immigrants in the United States generally practice birth control so pregnancy will not interfere with their reasons for coming to the United States. Thus, fertility practices among immigrant Brazilians are a matter of convenience with a traditional fatalistic overtone. Help women identify acceptable methods of fertility control.

- Herbal teas are used for bringing on late menstrual periods and for stimulating natural abortions. At times, single women try to become pregnant to facilitate their chance of remaining permanently in the United States. This opportunity is greatly enhanced if the child is born here and has been able to attend school.

- Pregnant women are encouraged not to do heavy work and not to swim. Taboos also warn against having sexual relations during pregnancy.

- Some foods are to be avoided, and specific foods are recommended during pregnancy. Taboos generally vary according to geographic region, socioeconomic class, and ethnic background. Determine taboo and acceptable food choices for pregnant women.

- Many Brazilian mothers prefer to give their babies powdered dry milk in place of breast-feeding. Women wish to regain their figures as soon as possible. Some women often feel that their milk is *fraca* (weak). Breast-feeding is linked to a social stigma that a mother who breast-feeds may often be thought of as abandoned or sexually unattractive. Provide factual information on the nutritious effects of breast-feeding.

- A postpartum woman eats chicken soup to help her body return to normal. She is also advised not to eat spicy foods or *repadura* (a molasses candy) and not to drink *garapa* (sugar water) or *caldo de cana* (sugar cane juice) if she breast-feeds her infant. Support postpartum women's nonharmful food choices and practices.

DEATH RITUALS

- The death of a baby or an infant, historically, has been and continues to be treated joyfully and without much sadness, for the child has died pure and is regarded as an angel.
- If financially possible, the families of Brazilians who die in the United States personally accompany the body to Brazil for burial in the family vault. If family members cannot come to the United States, relatives meet at the airport upon the body's arrival in Brazil.
- Responses to death and grief depend on the family. The fatalistic expression, "It was God's will," helps the grieving process among the rich and the poor.
- Older people wear black for various amounts of time depending on their relationship with the family member. Frequently, the final portrait is hung in the family *chaper* or near the family altar, and prayers are recited. An eternal light burns.
- Relatives are honored on the anniversaries of their death, both at home and at masses. Often, the family places an obituary of remembrance with or without a picture of the deceased in the local newspaper on the anniversary of the death. Support bereavement practices within their cultural context.

SPIRITUALITY

- Although 90 percent of all Brazilians are Catholic, various Protestant sects are making inroads into the Brazilian culture. A few incorporate Indian animism, African cults, Afro-Catholic syncretism, and Kardecism, a spiritualist religion embracing Eastern mysticism.

Brazilian

- Aside from the *curandeiros* (folk healers), special healers exorcise and pray for the wellness of their clients. Saints are asked for help, and people wear medals or little pouches of special powders around their necks. Accept a wide range of religious practices among Brazilians.
- The meaning of life is found in religion, economy, fatalism, and reality. For some, life is *uma luta* (a battle). For others, life is an almost hedonistic attitude.
- The greatest source of strength for Brazilians is their immediate and extended families. Include family in health-care decisions.

HEALTH-CARE PRACTICES

- Most Brazilians do not talk about their illnesses unless the illnesses are very serious. Generally, illness is discussed only within the family. Many Brazilians feel that talking about an illness such as cancer negatively influences their condition. Do not disclose the patient's health condition to others. Accept that some patients may not want to talk about their illness.
- Because many Brazilians tend to shun hospitals, when they are hospitalized their families accompany them and stay around the clock. The patient is often brought food from home. The family is the nucleus of responsibility for health care and is eager to participate in care. Include the family in care of the patient whether in the hospital, long-term-care facility, or at home.
- Brazilians residing in the United States are legally required to have health insurance. However, many often cannot afford to pay for medical care and thereby revert to self-care.
- Brazilians are known for their self-medication practices. Antibiotic, neuroleptic, antiemetic, and most other prescription drugs are easily obtained over the counter in Brazilian pharmacies. Once in the United States, it becomes difficult to obtain the many drugs readily available in Brazil. Customarily, incoming Brazilians bring medicines requested by their friends and thus

maintain the circulation of medications not available to Brazilians living in the United States. Encourage patients to fully disclose the use of all medications and treatments so they do not conflict with prescription medicines.

- Because Brazilians tend to self-medicate, the procurement of necessary health care is often avoided or delayed. Consulting with someone who has the condition or with friends who know someone who has a similar condition may be the first step taken. A trip to the local pharmacist may be the second. A third response may be a desperate telephone call to Brazil asking for a particular medicine.

- The Brazilian culture is rich in folk practices and depends on geographic region, ethnic background, socioeconomic factors, and generation. Many Brazilians prefer to use homeopathic medicines and herbs. Traditional and homeopathic pharmacies are supplemented by *remedios populares* (folk medicines) and *remedios caseiros* (home medicines). A list of herbal remedies and formulas for home remedies can be accessed online at http://www.valeredenet.com Folk remedies and traditional health-care practices are intermeshed when a serious illness may be best treated by traditional caretakers. Some take homeopathic *bolinhas* (little white balls) prepared specifically for certain ailments.

- At times, support services for legal and undocumented Brazilians are hard to find for those who do not have language skills or the self-esteem to become assimilated into the culture of their newly found environments. Language is a major problem for these immigrants. They neglect to learn English and prefer to get by in their enclave community, which may be detrimental to health assessment. Help clients find legal assistance through social services. Obtain an interpreter when necessary.

- Another barrier to health care for Brazilians in the United States is cost. This, combined with lack of knowledge about the health-care system and facilities,

Brazilian

impedes both legal and illegal residents. Refer patients in financial need to social services departments.

- Brazilians generally do not like to talk about pain. However, once the emotional barrier is removed, they feel relieved to be able to discuss their discomfort. Many pain-relieving medicines are available without a prescription in Brazil. Frequently a person requiring these on a regular basis can request that friends or friends of friends bring a supply from Brazil. Explain the facts about pain medicine, and encourage disclosure of all pain medicine and treatments being used.

- Most Brazilians do not work if they are seriously ill. Sickness is a neutral role and is considered socially exempt. This role is free of guilt, blame, and responsibility. Sickness is often seen as something that just happens.

- Among the lower socioeconomic groups, the term *nervios* refers to an all-incorporating illness. *Nervios* is the ever-present folk diagnosis that identifies the weakness, craziness, and anger associated principally with hunger.

- Better-educated Brazilians accept blood transfusions, organ donation, and organ transplantation. As in the United States and other parts of the world, acceptance depends on religious credence and individual preference.

HEALTH-CARE PRACTITIONERS

- The folk-health field has many types of health-care practitioners. *Curandeiros* are divinely gifted; *rezadeiras* (praying women) help exorcise illnesses; card readers can predict fortunes; *espiritualistas* are able to summon souls and spirits; *conselheiros* are counselors or advisors; and *catimbozeiros* are sorcerers. Additionally, the *mae* or *pai de santo* are head priestesses or priests from the African-Brazilian Umbanda or Xango religion. All have the power to heal their believers. Encourage clients to disclose the use of folk healers and treatments prescribed. Incorporate nonharmful practices into prescriptions.

- Brazilians in the United States tend to respect physicians and nurses. Medical education is prestigious and highly sought by aspiring university students.

References

Lonely Planet. (2003). Retrieved December 24, 2003, from www.LonelyPlanet.com

Purnell, L. (2003). People of Brazilian heritage. In L. Purnell and B. Paulanka (Eds.), *Transcultural health care: A culturally competent approach* (2nd ed., chapter on CD). Philadelphia: F.A. Davis Company.

Scheper-Hughes, N. (1992). *Death without weeping: The violence of everyday life in Brazil.* Berkeley: University of California Press.

Talismans for health. (2003). Retrieved December 24, 2003, from http://www.hmr.com.br/default.asp

Time Almanac. (2002). Boston: Time Inc.

Brazilian

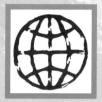

People of Chinese Heritage

Overview and Heritage

China's population of 1.3 billion people is dispersed over 3.7 million square miles, with cultural values differing according to geographic location as well as other primary and secondary characteristics of culture (see Chapter 1). Ninety-two percent of the population is Han; the remaining 8 percent is a mixture of 56 different nationalities, religions, and ethnic groups. Therefore, the information in this chapter should serve simply as a beginning for understanding Chinese people, not as a definitive profile. Chinese people who live in the "Chinatowns" in the United States maintain many of their cultural and social beliefs and values and insist that health-care providers respect these values and beliefs with their prescribed interventions. Chinese in the United States comprise the largest subgroup, exceeding 1.6 million people, among Asians/Pacific Islanders. The largest communities are in California, New York, Hawaii, and Texas.

A university education is highly valued; however, few have the opportunity to achieve this life goal because of limited enrollment opportunities. Often, young adults come to

Western countries to attend universities seeking more advanced prestigious educations. Many newer immigrants are professionals from Hong Kong who moved to Canada, the United States, and other Western countries to avoid the repatriation in 1997. This group usually has family connections or close friends in these countries.

Ideals based on the teachings of Confucius play an important part in their values and beliefs. These ideals emphasize the importance of accountability to family and neighbors and reinforce the idea that all relationships embody power and rule. Other important values are filial piety, industry, patriotism, deference to those in hierarchal status positions, tolerance of others, loyalty to superiors, respect for rites and social rituals, knowledge, benevolent authority, thrift, patience, courtesy, and respect for tradition.

COMMUNICATIONS

- The official language of China is Mandarin (*pu tong hua*), which is spoken by about 70 percent of the population, but there are other major, distinct dialects such as Cantonese, Fujianese, Shanghainese, Toishanese, and Hunanese. The dialects are so different that often two groups cannot understand one another verbally. However, the written language is the same throughout the country. It consists of over 50,000 characters (about 5,000 common ones); thus, most children are at least 10 to 12 years old before they can read the newspaper. If unable to obtain a dialect-specific interpreter, the interpreter should try writing the question.
- Most Chinese people speak in a moderate to low voice and consider Americans to be loud. Be cautious about tone of voice when interacting with Chinese clients.
- When asked whether they understand what was just said, the Chinese invariably answer yes to avoid loss of face.
- Negative queries are difficult to understand. Place instructions in a specific order, such as "First, at nine o'clock every morning get the medicine bottle. Second, take two tablets out of the bottle. Third, get your hot

water. Fourth, swallow the pills with the water." Do not use complex sentences with "ands" and "buts." Have clients demonstrate instructions to ensure that they are understood.

- Despite their reputation for not openly displaying emotion with strangers, among family and friends they are open and demonstrative. The Chinese share information freely once a trusting relationship has developed.

- Most individuals maintain a formal distance with each other, which is a form of respect. Health-care providers should touch clients only minimally. When touching is necessary, provide an explanation.

- Many Chinese people are uncomfortable with face-to-face communications, especially when there is direct eye contact. Most prefer to sit next to others. Arrange seating to promote positive communication.

- In formal business situations or greeting people with high rank, body movements may be limited. Watch for cues of expression.

- Titles are important to Chinese people. The family name is stated first and then the given name. Calling an individual by any name except his/her family name is impolite. If a person's family name is Li and the given name is Ruiming, then the proper form of address is Li Ruiming.

- Women do not use their husband's name after they get married. Therefore, unless the woman is from Hong Kong or Taiwan or has lived in a Western country for a long time, do not assume that her last name is the same as her husband's. Her family name comes first, followed by her given names and finally by her title. Many take an English name as an additional given name because Chinese names are often difficult for Westerners to pronounce. It is better to address them as "Miss Millie" or "Mr. Jonathan" rather than simply by their English name. Some give permission to use only the English name. In addition, some switch the order of their names to be the same as those of Westerners, with the family name last. This practice can be confusing. Address clients by their whole name or by their family name and title. Ask persons how they wish to be addressed.

FAMILY ROLES AND ORGANIZATION

- Kinship has traditionally been organized around the male lines. Each family maintains a recognized head, who has great authority and assumes all major responsibilities for the family. In recent times, some men include housework, cooking, and cleaning as their responsibilities when their spouses work. Most believe that the family is most important and, thus, each family member assumes changes in roles to achieve this harmony.
- Children are highly valued in China because of the government's mandate that each married couple may only have one child. However, in some rural areas if the first-born child is female, the couple may obtain permission to have a second child to continue the family line and provide labor. Resources are lavished on the child. Independence is not fostered. The entire family makes decisions for the child even into young adulthood.
- Children born in Western countries tend to adopt the Western culture easily while their parents and grandparents tend to maintain their traditional Chinese culture in varying degrees. Adolescents maintain their respect for elders even when they disagree with them. Teenagers value a strong and happy family life and seldom do things that jeopardize that unanimity. Adolescents question affairs of life and make great efforts to see at least two sides of every issue. Few teens earn money because they are expected to study hard and help the family with daily chores.
- Children feel pressure to succeed to help improve the future of the family; thus, most children and adolescents value studying over playing and peer relationships. Children are taught to curb their expression of feelings

because individuals who do not stand out are successful. However, children are becoming more outspoken as they read more and watch television and movies.

- The perception of family is developed through the concept of relationships. Each person is identified in relation to others in the family. The individual is not lost, just defined differently from individuals in Western cultures.

- Young men and women enter the workforce immediately after high school if they are unable to continue their education. Many continue to live with their parents and contribute to the family even after marriage (in their 20s) and the birth of a child (in their 30s).

- Extended families are important. Children may live with their grandparents or aunts and uncles so individual family members can obtain a better education or reduce financial burdens.

- Teenage pregnancy is not common among the Chinese, but it is increasing among Chinese in America.

- Older people are venerated and viewed as very wise. Children are expected to care for their parents; in China, law mandates this. When Chinese immigrants need additional assistance, call on local Chinese organizations to obtain help.

- Maintaining reputation is very important and is accomplished by adhering to the rules of society. True equality does not exist in the Chinese mind; if more than one person is in power, then consensus is important. If the person in power is not present at decision-making meetings, barriers are raised, and any decisions made are negated unless the person in power agrees. Ensure that the family spokesperson is in attendance at patient conferences.

- The word for privacy has a negative connotation and means something underhanded, secret, and furtive. People grow up in crowded conditions; they live and work in small areas, and their value of group support does not place a high value on privacy. Offer to make arrangements for the family to remain with the patient 24 hours a day if needed.

- The Chinese may ask many personal questions about salary, life at home, age, and children. Refusal to answer personal questions is accepted as long as it is done with care and feeling. The one subject that is taboo is sex and anything related to sex. This may create a barrier for a Western health-care provider who is trying to assess a Chinese client with sexual problems. Approach issues of sexuality tactfully and indirectly.
- Same-sex relationships are not condoned. In many provinces, they are illegal and punishable by death. Do not disclose same-sex relationships.

BIOCULTURAL ECOLOGY

- Skin color among Chinese is varied. Many have skin color with pink undertones; some have a yellow tone, and others are very dark. Hair is generally black and straight, but some have naturally curly hair. Most men do not have much facial or chest hair.
- Mongolian spots—dark bluish spots over the lower back and buttocks—are present in about 80 percent of infants.
- Bilirubin levels are usually higher in Chinese newborns, with the highest levels occurring on the fifth or sixth day after birth.
- The ulna is longer than the radius. Hip measurements are significantly smaller: females are 4.14 centimeters smaller, and males are 7.6 centimeters smaller than Westerners (Seidel et al., 1994). Not only is overall bone length shorter, but bone density is also less. An increased incidence of lactose intolerance when milk and milk products are consumed results in diarrhea, indigestion, and bloating. Provide instruction on adequate calcium consumption to prevent osteoporosis and fractures.
- Thalassemia affects people in one of two ways. One form is evidenced by a smaller but increased number of red blood cells and does not usually affect one's health status; the other form is evidenced as anemia followed by an early death. A sex-linked genetic disease common

Chinese

in the Chinese is glucose-6-phosphate dehydrogenase deficiency, an enzyme deficiency affecting the person's red blood cells, resulting in anemia. Assess clients for genetic conditions before medications are prescribed.

- Many immigrants have an increased incidence of hepatitis B and tuberculosis. The Rh-negative blood group is rare.

- Poor metabolism of mephenytoin occurs in 15 to 20 percent of Chinese. Sensitivity to beta blockers, such as propranolol, is evidenced by a decrease in overall blood levels accompanied by a more profound response. Atropine sensitivity is evidenced by an increased heart rate. Increased responses to antidepressants and neuroleptics occur at lower doses. Analgesics have been found to cause increased gastrointestinal side effects, despite a decreased sensitivity to them. Chinese people generally have an increased sensitivity to the effects of alcohol (Levy, 1993). Carefully monitor Chinese clients on medications such as propranolol, atropine, antidepressants, and neuroleptics.

- Women have a 20 percent higher rate of pancreatic cancer and higher rates of suicide after the age of 45 years, and all Chinese people have higher death rates related to diabetes than white ethnic groups.

HIGH-RISK HEALTH BEHAVIORS

- Smoking is a high-risk behavior for many men and teenagers. Most women do not smoke, but recently the numbers for Chinese women who smoke are increasing, especially after immigration to the United States. Tobacco use is a major problem and results in an increased incidence of lung disease. Screen newer immigrants for smoking-related health conditions.

NUTRITION

- Food habits are important, and food is offered to guests at any time of the day or night. Foods served at meals have a specific order, with focus on a balance for a healthy body.

- The typical diet is difficult to describe because each region in China has its own traditional diet. Traditional Chinese medicine frequently uses food and food derivatives to prevent and cure diseases and illnesses and to increase strength in weak and older people.
- Peanuts and soybeans are popular. Common grains include wheat, sorghum, and maize (a type of corn). Rice is usually steamed but can be fried with eggs, vegetables, and meats as well. Many Chinese people eat beans or noodles instead of rice. Meat choices include pork (the most common), chicken, beef, duck, shrimp, fish, scallops, and mussels. Tofu, an excellent source of protein, is a staple of the Chinese diet and is fried, boiled, or served cold like ice cream. Bean products are another source of protein. Many desserts or sweets are prepared with red beans.
- Fruits and vegetables may be peeled and eaten raw. Vegetables are lightly stir-fried in oil with salt and spice. Salt, oil, and oil products are important parts of the Chinese diet. Their healthy selection of green vegetables limits the incidence of calcium deficiencies.
- Drinks with dinner include tea, soft drinks, juice, and beer. Foreign-born and older people may not like ice in their drinks. Ask clients if they want ice in their drinks.
- Foods that are considered *yin* and *yang* prevent sudden imbalances and indigestion. A balanced diet is considered essential for physical and emotional harmony. Provide special instructions regarding risk factors associated with diets that are high in fats and salt.
- Chopsticks should never be stuck in the food upright because that is considered bad luck.

PREGNANCY AND CHILDBEARING PRACTICES

- Most Chinese families see pregnancy as positive and important in the immediate and extended family. Pregnancy is seen as women's business, although men are beginning to demonstrate an active interest in pregnancy and the welfare of the mother and baby. Women are very modest and may insist on a female

Chinese

midwife or obstetrician. Some agree to use a male physician when an emergency arises. Respect different views on involving men in pregnancy issues and selecting appropriate procedures.

- Pregnant women usually increase meat in their diets because their blood needs to be stronger for the fetus. Pregnant women may avoid shellfish during the first trimester because it causes allergies. Some may be unwilling to take iron because they believe that it makes the delivery more difficult.
- Traditional postpartum care includes 1 month of recovery, with the mother eating foods that decrease the yin (cold) energy. Ask what foods the mother plans to eat postpartum, and dispel myths.
- Many mothers do not expose themselves to the cold air and do not go outside or bathe for the first month postpartum because cold air can enter the body and cause health problems. Some postpartum women wear many layers of clothes and are covered from head to toe, even in the summer, to keep the air away from their bodies.
- Drinking and touching cold water are taboo for women in the postpartum period.
- Raw fruits and vegetables are avoided because they are considered "cold" foods. They must be cooked and be warm. Mothers eat five to six meals a day with high-nutritional ingredients including rice, soups, and seven to eight eggs. Brown sugar is commonly used because it helps rebuild blood loss. Drinking rice wine is encouraged to increase the mother's breast-milk production. Caution mothers that rice wine may prolong the postpartum bleeding time.

DEATH RITUALS

- Death is viewed as a part of the natural cycle of life; some believe that something good happens to them after they die.
- Death and bereavement traditions are centered on ancestor worship, a form of paying respect. Many believe that their spirits will never rest unless living

descendants provide care for the grave and worship the memory of the deceased.

- The dead are honored by placing food, money for the person's spirit, or articles made of paper around the coffin.
- The belief that the Chinese greet death with stoicism and fatalism is a myth.
- The number 4 is considered unlucky because it is pronounced like the Chinese word for death; this is similar to the bad luck associated with the number 13 in many Western societies. The color white is associated with death and is also considered bad luck. Black is a bad-luck color. Red is the ultimate good-luck color. Mourners are recognized by black armbands on their left arm and white strips of cloth tied around their heads.
- The purchase of life insurance may be avoided because of a fear that it is inviting death.

SPIRITUALITY

- The main formal religions in China are Buddhism, Catholicism, Protestantism, Taoism, and Islam. Prayer is generally a source of comfort. Some Chinese people do not acknowledge a religion such as Buddhism, but if they go to a shrine they burn incense and offer prayers. As immigration increases, many who practice Christian religions have become more visible.
- "Life forces" are sources of strength. These forces come from within the individual, the environment, and the past and the future of the individual and society.
- The individual may use meditation, exercise, massage, and prayer. Drugs, herbs, food, good air, and artistic expression may also be used. Good-luck charms are cherished, and traditional and nontraditional medicines are used.
- The family is usually a source of strength. Individuals draw on family resources and are expected to provide resources to strengthen the family. Resources may be defined as financial, emotional, physical, mental, or

spiritual. Calling on ancestors to provide strength as a resource requires giving back to the ancestors when necessary.
- The interconnectedness of life provides a source of strength for individuals from before birth to death and beyond.

HEALTH-CARE PRACTICES

- While many Chinese people have made the transition to Western medicine, others maintain their roots in traditional Chinese medicine, and still others practice both types of medicine. Younger people usually do not hesitate to seek health-care providers when necessary unless they believe that it does not work for them; then they use traditional Chinese medicine.
- Older people may try traditional Chinese medicine first and only seek Western medicine when traditional medicine does not seem to work. Even after seeking Western medical care, older people may continue to practice traditional Chinese medicine in some form. Some clients may not tell health-care providers about other forms of treatment they have been using because they are conscious of saving face. Ask clients in a nonjudgmental manner if they are using traditional Chinese medicine. Impress upon them the importance of disclosing all treatments because some may have antagonistic effects.
- Many individuals offer their knowledge about treatments and their medicines to friends and family members. Inquire about this practice when making assessments, setting goals, and evaluating the results of treatments.
- Traditional Chinese medical treatments are discussed in Box 9–1.
- The Chinese tend to describe their pain in terms of more diverse body symptoms, whereas Westerners tend to describe pain locally. The Western description includes words like "stabbing" and "localized," whereas the Chinese describe pain as "dull" and more "diffuse."

BOX 9–1 • Traditional Chinese Medical Treatments

Chinese

- Traditional Chinese medicine has many facets, including the five basic substances (*qi,* energy; *xue,* blood; *jing,* essence; *shen,* spirit; and *jing ye,* body fluids); the pulses and vessels for the flow of energetic forces (*mai*); the energy pathways (*jing*); the channels and collaterals, including the 14 meridians for acupuncture, moxibustion, and massage (*jing luo*); the organ systems (*zang fu*); and the tissues of the bones, tendons, flesh, blood vessels, and skin. The scope of traditional Chinese medicine is vast and should be studied carefully by professionals who provide health care to Chinese clients.
- Acupuncture and moxibustion are used in many treatments. Acupuncture is the insertion of needles into precise points along the channel system of flow of the *qi* called the 14 meridians. The system has over 400 points. Many of the same points can be used in applying pressure (acupressure) and massage (acumassage) to achieve relief from imbalances in the system. The same systems approach is used to produce localized anesthesia.
- Moxibustion is the application of heat from different sources to various points. For example, one source, such as garlic, is placed on the distal end of the needle after it is inserted through the skin, and the garlic is set on fire. Sometimes the substance is burned directly over the point without a needle insertion. Localized erythema occurs with the heat from the burning substance, and the medicine is absorbed through the skin.
- Cupping is another common practice. A heated cup or glass jar is put on the skin creating a vacuum, which causes the skin to be drawn into the cup. The heat that is generated is used to treat joint pain.

(Continued)

BOX 9–1 • Traditional Chinese Medical Treatments *(Continued)*

- Herbal therapy is integral to traditional Chinese medicine. Herbs fall into four categories of energy (cold, hot, warm, and cool), five categories of taste (sour, bitter, sweet, pungent, and salty), and a neutral category. Different methods are used to administer the herbs, including drinking and eating, applying topically, and wearing on the body.

They tend to use explanations of pain from the traditional Chinese influence of imbalances in the yin and yang combined with location and cause. Chinese cope with pain by applying oils and massage, using warmth, sleeping on the area of pain, relaxation, and aspirin.

- The balance between yin and yang is used to explain mental as well as physical health. Because a stigma is associated with having a family member who is mentally ill, many families initially seek the help of a folk healer. Many Chinese still view mental and physical disabilities as a part of life that should be hidden. Traditionally, an ill person is viewed as passive and accepting of illness. Illness is expected as a part of the life cycle.
- Many individuals feel uncomfortable touching their own bodies, which may be problematic when they need to provide their own health care; for example, breast self-examinations. People of the same sex may use touch if they are close friends or family. Men and women do not touch each other, and even couples that have been married for a long time do not show physical affection in public. Most women feel uncomfortable being touched by male health-care providers and tend to seek female providers. Always ask permission, and explain the necessity for touching clients during examinations and treatments.

- Families may be reluctant to allow autopsies because of their fear of being "cut up." Most accept blood transfusions, organ donations, and organ transplants.

HEALTH-CARE PRACTITIONERS

- Traditional Chinese medicine practitioners are shown great respect by the Chinese. In many instances, they are shown equal, if not more, respect than Western practitioners.
- Some distrust Western practitioners because of the pain and invasiveness of their treatments.
- Older health-care providers receive more respect than younger providers, and men usually receive more respect than women. Physicians receive the highest respect, followed closely by nurses with a university education. Other nurses with limited education are next in the hierarchy.
- If individual Chinese clients disagree with the health-care provider, they may not follow instructions. Moreover, they may not verbally confront the health-care provider because they fear that either they or the provider will suffer a loss of face.

References

Seidel, H., Ball, J., Dains, J., & Benedict, W.(1994). *Quick reference to cultural assessment*. St. Louis: Mosby.

Wang, Y. (2003). People of Chinese heritage. In L. Purnell and B. Paulanka (Eds.), *Transcultural health care: A culturally competent approach* (2nd ed., pp. 106–121). Philadelphia: F. A. Davis Company.

Chinese

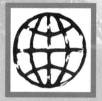

People of Cuban Heritage

Overview and Heritage

The Republic of Cuba, located 90 miles south of Key West, Florida, is a multiracial society with a population of 11,000,000 people of primarily Spanish and African origins; other ethnocultural groups include Chinese, Haitians, and Eastern Europeans. Spain, the United States, and the Soviet Union significantly influence Cuba's history and culture. Mistrust of government has reinforced a strong personalistic tradition and sense of national identity evolving from family and interpersonal relationships. This has resulted in an exile ideology and opposition to Fidel Castro, which characterizes the Cuban American's political stance. Desire for personal freedom, hope of refuge, political exile, and promise of economic opportunities prompted migration. Cubans in the United States take great pride in their heritage and tend to be conservative, Republican, and anticommunist. Many possess a strong ethnic identity, speak Spanish, and adhere to traditional Cuban values and practices. Their highest concentration is in Florida, although significant numbers live in New Jersey,

New York, Illinois, and California. The Catholic Church has influenced educational achievement, resulting in a high proportion of Cuban Americans who are self-employed or who work in wholesale and retail trade, banking and credit agencies, insurance, real estate, finance, and executive, administrative, and professional as well as technical positions.

COMMUNICATIONS

- Many live and transact business in Spanish-speaking enclaves. While the second generation speaks Spanish, many converse with friends or peers in "Spanglish," a mixture of Spanish and English. The highly educated are more likely to speak English at home. Assistance with required forms in the U.S. health-care system is needed by the less acculturated.
- Many value *simpatía* and *personalismo* in their interactions with others. *Simpatía,* the need for smooth interpersonal relationships, is characterized by courtesy, respect, and the absence of criticism or confrontation. *Personalismo,* the importance of intimate interpersonal relationships, is valued over impersonal bureaucratic relationships.
- *Choteo*, a lighthearted attitude, with teasing, bantering, and exaggerating, is often observed in their communications with others. Conversations are characterized by animated facial expressions, direct eye contact, hand gestures, and gesticulations. Voices tend to be loud, and the rate of speech is fast. Do not interpret these behaviors as family discord.
- Touching, handshakes, and hugs are acceptable among family, friends, and acquaintances and may be used to express gratitude to the caregiver. Touch is common between people of the same gender; older men and women rarely touch in public. Explain the essential necessity for touching private body areas during a physical examination.
- Most tend to emphasize current issues and problems rather than future ones. *Hora cubana* (Cuban time) refers to a flexible period that stretches 1 to 2 hours

beyond designated clock time. When setting up appointments, assess clients' level of acculturation with respect to time. One may need to explain the necessity of arriving on time for appointments.

- Cubans use two surnames representing the mother and father's family names. Married women may also add the husband's name. Thus, ask which name is used for legal purposes. When addressing clients, especially the elderly, formal rather than familiar forms of speech should be used unless told otherwise (i.e., Señor [Mr.], Señora [Mrs.], or Señorita [Miss]).

FAMILY ROLES AND ORGANIZATION

- Traditional family structure is patriarchal, characterized by a dominant and assertive male and a passive, dependent female. Traditionally, Cuban wives stay at home, manage the household, and care for children, whereas husbands are expected to work, provide financially, and make major decisions for the family. *La casa* (the house), the province of the woman, and *la calle* (the street), the domain of the man, demonstrate the distinction in gender roles and should be respected.
- Honor is attained by fulfilling family obligations and treating others with *respeto* (respect). *Vergüenza*, a consciousness of public opinion and the judgment of the entire community, is considered more important for women than for men. Machismo dictates that men display physical strength, bravery, and virility and be the spokesperson, even though they might not make the decisions.
- *La familia* (the family, nuclear and extended, including godparents) is the most important source of emotional and physical support. Multigenerational (3 to 4 generations) households are common, including a high proportion of people 65 years and older who live with their relatives. Family, the most important social unit, is involved in all decisions. Specifically, ask who makes which decisions for the family. Verbal consent for invasive procedures from family members as well as

from next of kin is often required. Extended family members are often good resources for home care.

- According to U.S. standards, Cuban parents tend to pamper and overprotect their children. Children are expected to study, respect their parents, and follow *el buen camino* (the straight and narrow). Boys are expected to learn a trade or prepare for work and to stay away from vices. Girls are expected "to remain honor-able while single," to prepare for marriage, to avoid the opposite sex, and not to go out without a chaperone. When a daughter reaches 15 years, a *quinceaneras*, or elaborate 15th birthday party, is typically held to celebrate this rite of passage for the daughter. Adolescents may undergo an identity crisis and reject their heritage, causing parents to feel their authority is being challenged. Explain American child abuse laws, taking into consideration the culturally complex definition of what may be considered child abuse.

- Personal relationships, known as *compadrazgo*, are typical, with heavier reliance for help on family and personal relationships than on government or organizations.

- Traditional families seldom discuss sex openly; initiating these discussions with health teaching may be welcome.

- Little information is available on homosexuality. Same-sex behaviors among men may be regarded as a sign of virility and power rather than homosexual behavior. The gay lifestyle is contradictory to the machismo orientation of this culture. Same-sex couples may be alienated from their families. Given the stigma associated with homosexuality in this culture, a matter-of-fact, nonjudgmental approach must be used when questioning clients regarding sexual orientation or sexual practices. Do not disclose same-sex relationships to family members.

BIOCULTURAL ECOLOGY

- More than 80 percent are white, and only 5 percent are black with physical features similar to those of African Americans. Because of their European ancestry, most have skin, hair, and eye colors that vary from light to dark. To assess for cyanosis and jaundice in individuals with dark skin, it is essential to assess the color of the sclera and conjunctiva, palms of the hands, soles of the feet, and buccal mucosa and tongue rather than relying on skin tone.

- Cuban Americans tend to have lower incidences of diabetes mellitus, obesity, and hypertension than other Hispanic groups or whites. Because of their diet, which is high in sugar, many exhibit a high prevalence of tooth loss, filled teeth, gingival inflammations, and periodontitis.
- Specific information related to drug metabolism is limited; however, in general, many require lower doses of antidepressants and experience greater side effects than non-Hispanic white populations.

HIGH-RISK HEALTH BEHAVIORS

- Cuban Americans tend to exhibit a higher incidence of smoking than other Hispanic or European groups. Encourage smoking cessation.
- Alcohol use is greater among males than females and among younger versus older groups. When assessing alcohol consumption, determine the amount consumed during holidays and celebrations, not just on a daily basis.
- Violent deaths account for high mortality rates among adolescents and young adults. Suicide rates also exceed those of the white non-Hispanic population.
- Use of preventive services depends on accessibility, which, in turn, is significantly influenced by education, annual income, and age.

NUTRITION

- Food allows families to reaffirm kinship ties, promotes a sense of community, and perpetuates customs and heritage. Rejecting food that is offered may be perceived as rejecting the person who is offering the food.

- Staple foods include root crops like yams, yuca, malanga, and boniato; plantains; and grains. Many dishes are prepared with olive oil, garlic, tomato sauce, vinegar, wine, lime juice *(sofrito)*, and spices. Meat is usually marinated in lemon, lime, sour orange, or grapefruit juice before cooking. Health-care providers should determine food preparation practices as well as customary foods consumed. Fats or flavorings used for cooking can add significant calories to meals. All major food groups are well represented in the Cuban diet; however, fiber content and leafy green vegetables may be lacking (Fig. 10–1). Lactose intolerance is common among most Hispanic groups.

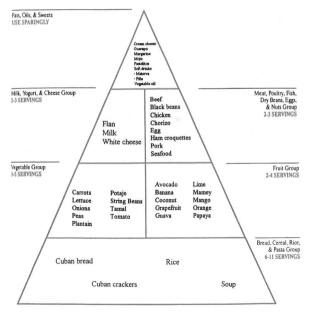

FIGURE 10–1. The Food Guide Pyramid for Cubans. (From *Hispanic Americans in Florida: An overview of their food habits*, by A. Rodriguez, 1995.)

- A leisurely noon meal (*almuerzo*) and a late evening dinner (*comida*), sometimes as late as 10 or 11 PM, are often customary. Meal times should be determined, and medication schedules should be adjusted accordingly.
- Being overweight is seen as positive, healthy, and sexually attractive. Clients should be coparticipants in deciding an acceptable weight. Counsel clients about the differences between being overweight and obese and the health hazards associated with obesity. Incorporate clients' traditional and preferred food choices into nutritional health planning.

Figure 10–1 depicts the food guide pyramid for Cubans. Popular Cuban American foods include the following:

Entrees and side dishes:

roast pork	*lechon*	fried pork chunks	*masas de puero*
sirloin steak	*palomilla*	shredded beef	*ropa vieja*
pot roast	*boliche*	roasted chicken	*pollo asado*
ripe plantains	*platanos maduros*	green plantains	*platanos verdes*
fried green plantains	*tostones* or *mariquita*		

Deserts:

custard	*flan*	egg pudding	*natilla*
rice pudding	*arroz con leche*	coconut pudding	*pudín de coco*
bread pudding	*pudín de pan*		

Beverages:

sugar cane juice	*guarapo*	iced coconut milk	*coco frio*
Cuban soft drinks	*batidos*	Sangria, or beer	*Materva*
strong coffee	*café cubano*		

PREGNANCY AND CHILDBEARING PRACTICES

- Cuban women's fertility rate is lower than that of other Hispanic American women. Cuba's current reproductive rate is among the lowest in the developing world. Even before the revolution, Cuba had the lowest birthrate in Latin America. This low fertility rate has been attributed to the fact that many women are in the workforce. Preterm births and neonatal and post-neonatal deaths are lower among Cuban American women than among other Hispanic American groups. Women are less likely to use oral contraceptives than other Hispanic American women. **Explain that condoms not only help prevent pregnancy but also decrease the incidence of SIDA (HIV) and other sexually transmitted diseases. Determine on an individual basis the methods of birth control acceptable to each client.**

- Prenatal care is higher than among other Hispanic and white non-Hispanics. **Stress that medical evaluations during pregnancy are necessary to help ensure the health of the mother and baby. When language barriers exist, use videos and literature in Spanish for teaching.** Mothers tend to use advice about child health given by their spouses, mothers, mothers-in-law, and clerks and pharmacists.

- Childbirth is a time for celebration, with family members and friends congregating in the hospital. Traditionally, men have not attended the births of their children, but younger, more acculturated, fathers are frequently present. **Respect the cultural beliefs of families if fathers are not wanted or do not wish to be in the delivery room.**

- During the postpartum period, ambulation, exposure to cold, and bare feet place the mother at risk for infection. Family members and relatives often care for the mother and baby for about 4 weeks postpartum. Most women consider breast-feeding better than bottle feeding; approximately half choose to breast-feed. **Mothers tend to wean infants from the breast and introduce solid foods at a young age, but bottle weaning**

Cuban

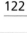

Cuban Dietary and Folk Beliefs and Practices About Pregnancy

- Women eat for two during pregnancy.
- Morning sickness is cured by eating coffee grounds.
- Eating a lot of fruit ensures that the baby will be born with a smooth complexion.
- Wearing necklaces during pregnancy causes the umbilical cord to be wrapped around the baby's neck.
- Raising one's arms over the head while pregnant may cause the umbilical cord to wrap around the infant's neck.
- **(Respect nonharmful cultural beliefs when pre-scribing care with regard to nutrition. Assess which foods are eaten or avoided during pregnancy in order to provide a culturally appropriate nutritional plan.)**

often occurs at a median age of 4 months, fostering their beliefs that "a fat child is a healthy child" and that breast-feeding may contribute to a deformity or asymmetry of the breasts.
- Cutting the infant's hair or nails in the first 3 months is believed to cause blindness and deafness. Do not cut the baby's hair or nails without asking permission.

DEATH RITUALS

- In death, as in life, the support of the extended family network is paramount. Bereavement is expressed openly as loud crying, with other physical manifestations of grief. Death is often seen as a part of life and some, especially men, may approach death stoically. Recognize that the lack of an open display of emotion may not imply indifference to the dying or deceased.
- The dying person is typically attended by a large gathering of relatives and friends. In Catholic families, individual and group prayers are held for the dying to provide a peaceful passage to the hereafter. Religious

artifacts such as rosary beads, crucifixes, or *estampitas* (little statues of saints) are placed in the dying person's room. For adherents of *Santería,* death rites may include animal sacrifice, chants, and ceremonial gestures. Summon appropriate clergy to perform appropriate death rites. A place should be found for family members to gather during this time, preferably close to the dying person.

- Candles are lighted after death to illuminate the path of the spirit to the afterlife. When candles with open flames are not permitted, electric candles are usually acceptable. Remain open-minded and responsive to physical and psychosocial needs of the dying and the bereaved, and accord them the utmost respect and privacy.
- A *velorio* (wake) lasts 2 to 3 days and is usually held at a funeral parlor or in the home where friends and relatives gather to support the bereaved family. Burial in a cemetery is common practice, although some may choose cremation.
- The deceased are customarily remembered and honored on their birthdays or death anniversaries by lighting candles, offering prayers or masses, bringing flowers to the grave, or gathering with family members at the grave site.

SPIRITUALITY

- Approximately 85 percent of Cuban Americans are Roman Catholic; the remaining 15 percent are Protestants, Jews, and believers in African Cuban Santería. Roman Catholicism is personalistic and characterized by devotion and intimate, confiding relationships with the Virgin Mary, Jesus, and the saints. Catholic practices must be assessed on an individual basis. Religious beliefs and practices must be viewed in an open, sincere, and nonjudgmental manner by including specific information regarding the type of religion practiced. In the inpatient setting, privacy is important if clients and families need to perform certain rituals or prayers. A visit from a priest, rabbi, or *santero* may promote a sense of psychological support and spiritual well-being.

- Significant religious holidays include *Noche Buena* (Christmas Eve), Christmas, *Los Tres Reyes Magos* (Three Kings Day), and the festivals of the *La Caridad del Cobre* and Santa Barbara.
- *Santería* or *Regla de Ocha* is a 300-year-old African Cuban religious system that combines Roman Catholic elements with ancient Yoruba tribal beliefs. Followers of Santería believe in the magical and medicinal properties of flowers, herbs, weeds, twigs, and leaves. Sweet herbs such as *manzanilla, verbena*, and *mejorana* are used for attracting good luck, love, money, and prosperity. Bitter herbs such as *apasote, zarzaparilla*, and *yerba bruja* are used to banish evil and negative energies. Santería is viewed as a link to the past and is used to cope with physical and emotional problems. By law, as long as standards of safety and sanitation are maintained, families must be allowed space and privacy to be able to engage in specific religious ceremonies and rituals.
- Physical complaints may be diagnosed and treated by a physician, whereas the *santero* may assist in balancing and neutralizing the various aspects of the illness. Deeply held religious beliefs provide guidance and strength during the long and difficult process of migration and adaptation and continue to play an important role in their day-to-day lives.
- Belief in a higher power is evident in practices used to maintain health and well-being or cure illness, such as using magical herbs, special prayers or chants, ritual cleansing, and sacrificial offerings. Many tend to be fatalistic, believing that they lack control over circumstances influencing their lives. Fatalistic beliefs do not mean that the client is not willing to engage in preventive practices.

HEALTH-CARE PRACTICES

- African Cubans may seek biomedical care for organic diseases but consult a *santero* for spiritual or emotional crises. Conditions such as *decensos* (fainting spells) or *barrenillos* (obsessions) may be treated solely by a *santero* or simultaneously with a physician.

- Many tend to seek help only in response to crisis situations. **Visits to health-care providers must be used for health teaching and promotion.**

- Many Cuban Americans rely on the family as the primary source of health advice. Older women provide traditional home remedies such as herbal teas or mixtures to relieve mild or moderate symptoms or cure common ailments. **Include the entire family in health promotion and health teaching to increase compliance with health prescriptions. Because health often means simply the absence of pain, explain the importance of preventive measures and health promotion activities.**

- Older Cuban Americans were socialized into a strong health ideology and successful primary care system while still in Cuba. Use of preventive services in the United States is generally determined more by access to care than by acculturation.

- Many Cuban Americans use traditional medicinal plants in the form of teas, potions, salves, or poultices. In Cuban communities, stores called *botanicas* sell herbs, ointments, oils, powders, incenses, and religious figurines to relieve maladies, bring luck, drive away evil spirits, or break curses. Santería necklaces and animals used for ritual sacrifice are often available at *botanicas*. **Determine which medicinal products are harmful and which will cause no harm. Nonharmful practices should be incorporated into the plan of care. Ascertain if clients are using over-the-counter medicine or sharing prescriptions of others, and explain the hazards of overuse of these medications as well as using medicines that were originally prescribed for other family members.** According to Estape (1995), cultural approaches used to treat common ailments are shown in the following box.

- Language is the greatest barrier to health care. Additional barriers include red tape and transportation problems, cost of services, and inconvenient hours. **Obtain interpreters when necessary.**

Cuban

Cuban Cultural Treatment for Ailments

Herbal tea	_Ailment_
Cosimiento de anis (anise)	Stomachaches, flatulence, baby colic; anxiety
Cosimiento de limon con miel de abeja (lemon and honey)	Cough and respiratory congestion
Cosimiento de apasote (pumpkin seed)	Gastrointestinal worms
Cosimiento de canela (cinnamon)	Cough, respiratory congestion, menstrual cramps
Cosimiento de manzanilla (chamomile)	Stomachaches
Cosimiento de naranja agria (sour orange)	Cough and respiratory congestion
Cosimiento de savila (aloe vera)	Stomachaches
Cosimiento de tilo (linden leaves)	Anxiety
Cosimiento de yerba buena (spearmint leaves)	Stomachaches, anxiety

Fruit or Vegetable	_Ailment_
Chayote (vegetable)	Anxiety
Zanaoría (carrots)	Visual problems
Toronja y ajo (grapefruit and garlic)	Elevated blood pressure
Papaya y toronja, y pina (papaya, grapefruit, and pineapple)	Gastrointestinal parasites
Remolacha (beets)	Influenza, anemia
Cascara de mandarina (fruit)	Cough

Home Remedies	***Ailment***
Agua con sal (salt water)	Sore throat
Agua de coco (coconut water)	Kidney problems and infections
Agua raja (turpentine)	Sore muscle and joint pain
Bicarbonato, limon y agua (baking soda, lemon, and water)	Upset stomach or heartburn
Cebo de carnero (fat of lamb)	Applied directly on skin for contusions and swelling
Mantequilla (butter)	Applied directly on burns to soothe pain
Clara de huevos (egg white)	Applied directly to scalp to promote hair growth

Amulets

Azabache is a black stone placed on infants and children as a bracelet or pin to protect them from the "evil eye."

La manito de coral, symbolic of the hand of God protecting a person, may also be worn as a necklace or bracelet.

Los ojitos de Santa Lucía, or the eyes of Saint Lucy, may be hung on a bracelet or necklace for prevention of blindness and protection from the evil eye.

- Many immigrants may suffer from loneliness, depression, anger, anxiety, insecurity, and health problems. According to Bernal (1994), assessment should include the following:

    1. How long the family has lived in the United States and the reasons for migration
    2. Extent of connectedness to the culture of origin
    3. Family developmental conflicts and dysfunctional family development patterns

- Physical, emotional, and financial resources available for caring for sick clients either at home or in care facilities must be determined.

Cuban

- Dependency is a culturally acceptable sick role that allows the extended family network to assume the chores and tasks of the sick person. Help is sought in response to crisis situations, pain, and discomfort and is often a signal of a physical disturbance that warrants consultation with a traditional or biomedical healer. Pain is expressed with verbal complaints, moaning, crying, and groaning that may or may not signify a need for pain medication. Individual assessments for clients with pain are needed to determine clients' perceptions of causes, remedies, and possible coping behaviors. Explaining that pain medications promote healing may encourage better acceptance of pain medications.
- Blood transfusions and organ donations are usually acceptable. Dispel myths related to organ donation, blood transfusions, and organ transplantation. Assistance from a priest or other clergy may be helpful.

HEALTH-CARE PRACTITIONERS

- Both traditional and biomedical care are acceptable. Folk remedies may be used at home, but if the condition persists, folklore practitioners such as *santeros* and biomedical practitioners may be used either simultaneously or successively. *Santeros* may prescribe treatment or perform rituals to enable ill people to recover by invoking supernatural deities to intervene to help make them well. It is essential to ask clients if they are using folk practitioners, their reasons for using them, and the treatments that have been prescribed. Collaborating with folk healers and practitioners may increase compliance with health prescriptions.

References

Bernal, G. (1994). Cuban families. In M. Uriarte-Gaston and J. Canas-Martinez (Eds.), *Cubans in the United States* (pp. 135–156). Boston: Center for the Study of the Cuban Community.

Estape, E. (1995). *The Cuban culture: Folk remedies and magicoreligious beliefs*. Unpublished manuscript. Miami, FL: Florida International University.

Thomas, J. T., & DeSantis, L. (1995). Feeding and weaning practices of Cuban and Haitian immigrant mothers. *Journal of Transcultural Nursing, 6*(2), 34–42.

Time almanac. (2001). Boston: Time Inc.

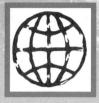

People of Egyptian Heritage

Overview and Heritage

Egypt has a land mass of 386,900 square miles ($1\frac{1}{2}$ times the size of Texas) and a population of more than 68 million people. Over 95 percent of the land is barren desert, with 90 percent of the population living on 3 percent of the total land area, the Nile Valley and Delta. The capital, Cairo, has more than 14 million people, followed in population by Alexandria, with 3,380,000 people. Except for a few hills outside Cairo, Egypt has a flat terrain on both sides of the southern Nile Valley and the Sinai Peninsula. The Nile River, a main artery for Egypt and an orientation point for its terrain, runs through the center of the country from south to north to the Mediterranean Sea. The Nile, considered Egypt's lifeline, provides water and supports agriculture.

The Egyptian people have a strong sense of identity with their country and demonstrate pride in coming from such an old civilization. Egyptian history is inextricably connected to the Nile River and dates back to about 4000 BC. The ancient Egyptians were the first to believe in life after death, in mummifying bodies, and in building elaborate tombs to preserve and protect these bodies for the afterlife. Egyptians also developed the plow, a system of writing, and medical skills such as surgical operations. The Arab conquest of Egypt around 641 AD spread the Islamic and Arabic culture among the Egyptians and has lasted to this day. This long history and the diversity of populations have influenced the value systems, beliefs, and explanatory frameworks Egyptians use in their daily lives.

Many Egyptians immigrated to the United States in an attempt to escape economic stagnation during President Gamal Abdel Nasser's regime of failed economic policies. After the 1952 military revolution, Egyptians immigrated in two main waves. The first wave consisted of graduate students who came to the United States to obtain advanced degrees. After the defeat of the Egyptian army by the Israelis in 1967, many of these students, believing the totalitarian military regime of Egypt did not offer hope for economic recovery, changed their status to immigrant. The second wave of immigration resulted from the heightened mass dissatisfaction, hopelessness, and anger toward the government after the 1967 war. A lenient government policy made it easy and safe for anyone who wanted to leave the country, resulting in the largest exodus from Egypt in modern history. Included in this wave were many Coptic and other Egyptian Christians. Egyptians in the second wave were more diverse in their educational backgrounds, although most of them were college graduates. Second-wave immigrants worked as engineers, physicians, dentists, accountants, and technicians; however, some with college degrees initially accepted employment as gas station attendants, cab drivers, security guards, and other blue-collar positions to ensure employment. After improving their language skills and obtaining degrees from American universities, many obtained professional positions. Many of the less successful from this group returned to their home country or plan for such a return.

More than 1 million people of Egyptian ancestry live in the United States. The highest concentrations are in New York, Los Angeles, Washington, DC, Chicago, and San Francisco. Egyptians prefer to work in large urban areas and usually

Egyptian

choose suburban areas for living. However, they do not live in large and concentrated numbers in any single geographic area. Because of their relatively recent arrival, limited scholarly literature is available about their health-care beliefs and practices. Egyptians have immigrated under many different circumstances. Their beliefs and practices vary according to the primary and secondary characteristics of culture as presented in Chapter 1.

COMMUNICATIONS

- The dominant language of Egyptians is Arabic, a Semitic language, understood by all Arab nationals who hear it in popular Egyptian movies, songs, and television programs. The written Arabic language is the same in all Arab countries, but spoken Arabic is dialectical and does not necessarily follow proper Arabic grammar.
- For Egyptians in the United States, English is the language of communication in business and contact with American society. Most speak a mixture of Arabic and English, switch with great ease from one language to another, and sometimes speak a mixture of Arabic, English, and French. In discussing subjects such as politics or religious issues, the level of excitement heightens, and the tone of speech is sharpened so an outside observer may mistakenly characterize exchanges as chaotic or angry. **Do not assume that sharpened speech patterns and increased voice volume demonstrate anger.**
- Respect is expected when speaking with those who are older or in higher social positions. Respect is demonstrated in Arabic by differentiation in the words used to address those who are equal in age or position and those who are older in age or higher in position (see the discussion for the format of names discussed below). Politeness, *adab,* is related to what is appropriate, expected, and socially sanctioned. Truth and reality may be sacrificed for what is appropriate and polite. Sharing negative news directly or asking for things directly is

not polite. A poor prognosis of an illness is not immediately shared. Slowly and deliberately introduce and
share a poor prognosis in stages.
- Significant value is related to the status of insiders and
outsiders and the private and public spheres. Private
spheres are reserved for immediate family, some members of the extended family, and friends who are elevated to the status of family. The public sphere includes
acquain-tances, public officials, and the rest of the
world and may include completely different communications and versions of the same events or incidents.
- Egyptians tend to be in touch with their inner feelings
and are highly expressive of them. Egyptians tend to
share problems and the most minute details about their
lives with their trusted circle of insiders. However,
because they are externally oriented, they tend to look
outside for explanations of their feelings rather than
focus on their own actions.
- Nonverbal communication patterns are vivid. Because
their personal space tends to be small, Egyptians stand
and sit very close to each other. In spite of their preference for closeness, women and men use personal space
during interactions differently. Do not take offense if
Egyptians stand closer to you than you are accustomed.
- Women tend to keep male friends as far away as male
strangers. Distance is kept as a sign of uncertainty in
the relationship. They tend to touch each other
frequently and easily, and touch is both reflexive and
deliberative. For example, they tend to touch others
while speaking to solicit attention, concentration, and
emphasis.
- Men, whether strangers or acquaintances, touch each
other. Similarly, it is acceptable for women to touch
each other.
- Traditionally, it is unacceptable for women and men to
touch each other unless they are close family members.
Touch between the sexes is accepted in private and only
between husbands and wives, parents and children, and
adult brothers and sisters. Devout Muslim men and
women do not touch each other; even a handshake is

Egyptian

not practiced. In these situations, a nod of the head substitutes for a physical greeting.

- Family members and friends of the same gender always hug and kiss on both cheeks. Friends of different sexes normally shake hands. Among Christians and westernized Egyptians and Egyptian Americans, greetings usually include formal courteous hugs and kisses on the cheeks. Strangers or nonfamily members do not touch each other except for a handshake. If they are close family members, for example a brother and sister, they can greet each other with a hug and a kiss.

- Egyptians speak with their mouth, face, and hands, with their entire body communicating the meaning of their language. Their facial expressions are mirrors of their internal processes and reflections of their inner evaluations of their situations. A momentary wide-eyed gaze to a child means "stop it now." A wink to an adult means "watch what you are saying."

- Dissatisfaction is demonstrated by intentionally looking "through" the person or by avoiding eye contact. Egyptians think of those who do not maintain eye contact or who have shifty eye contact as people who should not be trusted. Among the more traditional, women and men who are strangers may avoid eye contact out of modesty and respect for religious rules. Do not assume that lack of eye contact means that the person is not listening, does not care, or is not telling the truth. Children are taught not to *tebarrak* (stare), which denotes disrespect for those who are older or higher in status.

- Egyptians tend to be congenial and personable, injecting humor to lighten stressful encounters or business meetings. Some exaggerate and overly assert judgments of events and situations.

- Older Egyptians cherish the past, whereas younger Egyptians live in the present, with its decreased availability of options, and in the future, with its potential, realizing that acquisition of goods comes with a high price tag.

- In Egypt, social time takes a high priority, and

engagements are not concluded because of other scheduled appointments; therefore, guests are expected to arrive 1 to 2 hours late. However, they are punctual for business engagements and meetings.

- Both male and female children are given a first name; the father's first name is used as the middle name; the last name is the family name. A person is called formally by the first name, such as Mr. William.
- Respect for individuals is demonstrated in the use of titles, which vary by social position. Older people should never be called by their first name without an adjective or title. The accepted U.S. custom of addressing clients by their first name may be insulting to Egyptians. Always address an older person as Mr., Mrs., Ms., or a title that denotes a profession, such as engineer, doctor, physician, or a doctoral degree.

FAMILY ROLES AND ORGANIZATION

- Men are formally considered the head of the household. The demands of life on immigrants and nuclear families promote sharing responsibilities and decision-making. Although men are considered the major breadwinners, they may, however, participate in shopping, in cleaning, and in activities related to entertaining with their wives. Many Egyptian men tend to control family budgets, which causes many interpersonal conflicts and much distress for women.
- In order to preserve traditional roles that contribute to a more egalitarian family organization, family roles change considerably after immigration. The absence of an extended family results in greater fluidity in roles and participation in all family matters.
- Social status is gained through professional accomplishments, financial success, and involvement in Egyptian community affairs.
- Children are central to Egyptian families; they are treasured in the present and viewed as security for their parents' future. During their early years, they are expected to be studious and goal-oriented, respectful,

Egyptian

and loyal to the family. Children are not permitted to use foul language or swear in the home or in front of parents, although this is true to a lesser extent in the United States. Answering back to parents is not condoned and is considered rude and disrespectful.

- When children become adults, they are expected to take care of their elderly parents. However, second-generation Egyptians tend to blend with other Americans. Their sense of responsibility toward their parents is a topic of major concern.

- Religious beliefs and teachings forbid premarital sex and adultery for both Egyptian Muslims and Christians. As girls reach puberty and questions of dating, courting, and prom night arrive, some parents cannot cope with the freedom allowed within American society. They worry more about the consequences of dating and their daughters getting pregnant and fleeing the home than about raising a healthy and well-adjusted young woman. In the extreme, a few families send their daughters with their mothers back to Egypt to complete their education through college under more restrictive conditions or to get married. The greatest calamity that may happen in an Egyptian household is to have a daughter lose her virginity before marriage. This fear stems from a potential lack of marriageability of the daughter, loss of face for the father, and gossip within the community. Therefore, parents monitor their daughters' relationships and whereabouts carefully.

- Similar restrictions are placed on teenage sons, although they are allowed more freedom and more autonomy in decision-making. Most parents prefer that their sons not date and discourage their sons from sexual activities. However, if sons disobey the rules of the household, the incident is not regarded as gravely. **Encourage open communication in the family to allow children to see restrictions as temporary.**

- Raising children who are considered *moaddabeen* by Egyptian standards is important. A child who is *moaddab* is one who respects parents, defers to them for decisions, is mindful of elderly people, does not drink or indulge in immoral acts, listens to parents' advice, and does not answer back during conflict.

- Without extended families in the United States, Egyptian are at a loss for help in resolving family issues, which increases their vulnerability, isolation, and stress. The option of going to counselors or health-care professionals for advice is rarely exercised. Preserving family secrets and honor is more important than external support.

- Egyptian children are expected to marry Egyptians. However, because many second-generation Egyptian Americans do not reside in areas with an abundance of Egyptians, cross-cultural marriages are becoming more commonplace.

- As Egyptians grow older, they are treated with gentleness and are never made to believe that their usefulness is limited because of retirement. Their children and extended families are obligated to care for them. The elderly do less by choice and expect more services, respect, and reverence from family members and subordinates.

- Women gain status with age and with childbearing. Elderly women, however, are expected to care for the elderly men in the family. Many elders have a morbid fear of being forced to move into a nursing home. Many consider returning to their home country to avoid the humiliation of aging in America with the potential loss of home, family care, respect, and loneliness. Consider alternative ways to support this community and enhance their self-care activities to help them avoid feelings of loneliness and a sense of abandonment in old age. Where mosques or Middle Eastern Orthodox churches exist, these organizations are used to promote social gatherings. In the absence of such organizations, Egyptian cultural clubs promote meetings, discussions, and sharing news from the homeland.

- The divorce rate among Egyptian immigrants is low. Divorce is not considered a stigma but an unfortunate situation and one in which the children pay the greatest price. In cases of divorce in which one parent raises the

Egyptian

children, the Egyptian community supports the single parent, including his or her own parent(s).

- Communal and same-sex families are a concept that does not exist in Egyptian societies. Same-sex relationships are rarely disclosed. To be gay or lesbian is considered immoral and is not accepted by any Arab or Middle Eastern religions. To discover a gay son or lesbian daughter is akin to a catastrophic event for Egyptian Americans. Do not disclose same-sex relationships to family members or others.

BIOCULTURAL ECOLOGY

- Most Egyptians have olive skin tones; some are fair-skinned; and others are dark-skinned. Northern Egyptians exhibit a fairer complexion than most other Egyptians. Southern Egyptians (Nubians) are generally black, with very fine facial features. Upper Egyptians have a darker complexion. The average height of Egyptian men is about 5'10", and women have an average height of 5'4".
- Several risk factors are peculiar to life along the banks of the Nile. Egyptians suffer from a host of parasitic diseases. The most common is schistosomiasis, *bilharzias,* which leads to cirrhosis, liver failure, portal hypertension, esophageal varices, bladder cancer, and renal failure. Filariasis is another challenging parasitic disease endemic to Egyptians. Trachoma and other acute eye infections affect both rural and urban populations. Other infectious diseases include typhoid and paraty-phoid fevers, which are more frequent in urban than in rural areas. Streptococcal disease and rheumatic fevers are frequent among children, and tuberculosis continues to be a major problem in Egypt. Question Egyptians who have positive tuberculin tests about a history of bacille Calmette-Guérin vaccination. Screen recent Egyptian immigrants for health conditions common in their home country, such as schistosomiasis, filariasis, and trachoma.
- Modern diseases such as obesity, hypertension, and

lower back pain affect a high percentage of Egyptians. Similarly, cardiovascular diseases resulting from stress, obesity, lack of exercise, and hypertension are increasing.

- Egyptians are at a genetic risk for thalassemias, which can be detected from a molecular genetic standpoint through carrier screening and prenatal diagnosis. Screen Egyptians for thalassemias.
- Some evidence indicates that Egyptians are poor metabolizers of beta blockers. Closely monitor drug interventions with clients on beta blockers.

HIGH-RISK HEALTH BEHAVIORS

- Smoking does not appear to be a major risk factor for Egyptian Americans. The few who do smoke, smoke heavily and are unwilling to quit. Assist clients in finding smoking cessation programs.
- Use of illegal drugs is minimal in this community. Although some Egyptian Americans may overindulge in alcohol, the teachings of Islam prohibit its use. Many who drink alcohol tend to do so socially and in limited quantities.
- Although exercise and fitness are regularly included in the curricula of schools and colleges, exercise is not part of the daily lives among Egyptians in America. Explain the factual scientific basis of the health benefits of exercise.
- Overeating food delicacies that are high in fat, sodium, and sugar; sedentary lifestyles; and an entertainment style based on eating contribute to obesity and immobility. Include dietary assessment as part of the intake interview.
- Egyptians are at risk for stomach and intestinal problems, which include heartburn, flatulence, constipation, hemorrhoids, and fecal impaction. These conditions result from limited roughage, lack of fluids, and rapid consumption of food. Another factor contributing to constipation may be their expectations and the meaning they attach to regularity that prompts them to push and

Egyptian

strain to force a bowel movement prematurely. **Encourage fluids and a diet high in roughage to help combat constipation.**

- It takes Egyptian immigrants a number of years in America to learn to respect traffic rules, wear seat belts, and drive cautiously. **Explain legal requirements for the use of seat belts and helmets.**

- Pap smears and mammograms tend to be new preventive health practices for Egyptians. Pap smears for unmarried women are discouraged and are considered totally unacceptable in unmarried females due to the value of virginity until marriage. Gynecologic examinations are given only to married women, usually during the check-up for a first pregnancy. **Education about the importance of mammograms and Pap tests promotes compliance with regular check-ups.**

NUTRITION

- Food is an important component of Egyptian social life. Food is associated with generosity and giving. Offering and accepting food are indicative of friendship. Egyptians entertain lavishly and enjoy good food, which represents nurturing. The more food a person eats, the greater the potential expectation for health. Thus, children tend to be overfed. Food is also associated with the ability of the head of the family to provide for family members. Therefore, parents take pride in the amount and the quality of food they bring to their families.

- Egyptians prefer not to drink water or fluids with meals because they believe that fluid displaces the volume that could be used for food, decreasing their appetite for solid nutrients. Some believe that fluids dilute the stomach "juices," making digestion difficult and causing indigestion.

- Preferred meats are lamb, chicken, beef, and veal. Favorite vegetables are peas, green beans, cauliflower, and molokhia, a green vegetable that is cooked like soup. Most Egyptians consider meat dishes as main dishes, complemented by vegetables and rice.

- Rice, a main staple, adorns dinner or lunch tables on a daily basis even when potatoes are served. Tomato-based red sauces are popular, and some pasta and vegetable dishes are dressed with rich white sauces such as bechamel. Egyptians use lentils, fava beans, and bulgur in their cooking. Whole-wheat bread is preferred.

- Egyptians acquired a taste for tea from their years under British rule. They drink strong tea with hot milk or mint leaves with several teaspoons of sugar several times a day. Those who prefer tea without milk drink it with mint leaves. Egyptians also drink coffee, a habit acquired from Turkish rule. The coffee is thick, strong, and served in small demitasse cups, with or without sugar. Egyptians also consume a large quantity of soft drinks. Encourage the use of less sugar in tea and coffee and the use of low-calorie soft drinks.

- Hostesses insist on giving guests excessive amounts of food and act insulted if guests refuse the food. Those who understand the ritual may insist on refusal or may take the food and not eat it. Completely emptying the plate may be seen as an indication that the guest did not have enough to eat. Leaving some food on the plate is more polite than refusing it.

- Whether in Egypt or in America, devout Muslims do not consume pork or drink alcohol. Egyptians do not mix hot and cold or sweet and sour foods at the same meal. For example, the accepted habit in America of eating ice cream as dessert with coffee is a foreign concept for Egyptians. Some Egyptians grew up believing that mixing fish and milk may cause digestive problems or behavioral problems and thus are generally not combined. Some individuals may drink milk with yeast to increase their intake of vitamin B complex.

- Egyptian Christians fast for a varied number of days for several major religious celebrations. For them, fasting constitutes not eating any animal products.

- Many rituals are revived during the month of Ramadan,

Egyptian

the 9th of 12 Islamic months that follow the lunar calendar. Therefore, Ramadan does not coincide with a particular month in the Christian calendar; instead, it rotates and can fall on any of the Christian calendar months. Ramadan rituals are based on the teaching of the *Qur'an* (Koran), which calls for a month of fasting to experience the plight of the poor and the underprivileged. Fasting during Ramadan precludes taking anything by mouth or intravenously and abstaining from sexual activities. Adjust medication schedules to accommodate fasting.

- Most Egyptian Muslims eat only well-cooked meat and do not touch rare meat. They prefer kosher meat, trusting the Jewish dietary restrictions and food preparation practices. In the absence of kosher meat, they use meat obtained at regular supermarkets.

PREGNANCY AND CHILDBEARING PRACTICES

- Although Egyptians in America may practice family planning and birth control, these practices are not used before conceiving the first child. A couple is not complete until they have a child; they are usually under stress, fearing marriage instability caused by lack of childbearing, until they conceive their first baby. Even if the husband is the cause of delayed or permanent infertility, women are threatened by the potential of divorce and are expected to conceive within their first year of marriage. Pregnancy brings women a sense of security and their husbands' and in-laws' respect. Giving birth, particularly to a son, considerably strengthens the status and power of women. After the first child, fertility control methods include birth control pills, condoms, and early withdrawal. Women take an active role in limiting pregnancies; they are willing to use any method of birth control to achieve and maintain a small family size.
- Pregnancy gives women permission to decrease their responsibilities. Women are expected to curtail physical activities during pregnancy for fear of miscarriage.

Women are also advised to eat more because they are feeding two. Some women have *waham* (strong cravings) for certain foods. It is believed that if these foods are not consumed, babies may be born with the imprint of the needed foods.

- Women invariably request that a female family member accompany the birthing mother. When a woman goes into labor with only her husband in attendance, it is considered an emergency. Acculturated Egyptian men want to be included in the birthing experience, which may offend Egyptian newcomers.

- The cold and hot theory for health and illness may prevent women from bathing during the postpartum period. Bathing or hair-washing could expose them to colds and chills. Egyptian Americans respond well to a sound rationale for bathing in a hot tub or taking a shower that dispels beliefs about the potential for infection.

- The postpartum period lasts 40 days, during which new mothers are expected to rest, eat well, be confined to the house with their babies, and not engage in any sexual activities. They are usually cared for by family members and are not expected to have any demands put on them. Chicken and chicken soup help women during their postpartum transition.

DEATH RITUALS

- Most Egyptians react vigorously and dramatically to the loss of a family member, expressing their grief outwardly. Wailing and public crying occur on first learning of death. This public reaction is an expected demonstration of their grief for the deceased. Health-care workers should accept alternative grieving practices.

- Death is considered inevitable, although any loss brings shock and despair. Older people speak calmly about their own impending death. Egyptians with a strong religious foundation do not fear the nearness of death; instead, they consider it a journey to another world that

Egyptian

is believed to be better. Egyptian Muslims and Christians believe in an afterlife and expect rewards for good deeds accomplished in their first life. They anticipate reuniting with those who preceded them.

- For Egyptian immigrants, the Islamic burial rituals are carried out in designated cemeteries. Among Muslims, Islam calls for burial of the deceased as soon as possible. The burial ritual includes cleaning the body and wrapping it in a white cotton wrap. Verses from the Qur'an are read, and a special prayer is recited at the mosque before the body is buried underground in a simple tomb. On the night of the burial, friends and family gather to give their condolences and respect to the grieving family. Some Muslim families insist on having the deceased buried in Egypt, which is a very costly process involving approval from both countries and transporting the deceased in a special casket.

- Forty days after the burial, another mourning ritual takes place in the home of the deceased's family. Family members listen while passages from the Qur'an are read by a religious man to console the family. Thereafter, a similar ritual takes place on the anniversary of the death.

SPIRITUALITY

- Prayers, even for the nondevout Muslim or Christian, are significant during times of illness. Egyptians may bring the Qur'an or their Bible to their hospital beds and usually put it under the pillow or on the bedside table. Prayers may be recited by the individual, in groups for Muslims, or in religious settings such as mosques or churches. Families and friends pray for each other, invoking good health, cure of illness, and peace. Prayers during holidays are enjoyed, particularly in groups and in religious settings.

- Muslims who can afford the expense and are in good health make the pilgrimage to Mecca sometime during their lifetime. The journey is thought to provide Muslims with a source of inner fulfillment.

- Most Egyptians talk about their religious teachings during episodes of illness. They derive comfort, strength, and meaning from verses in the Qur'an and of prophets. Family members use these verses to remind them that they are at the mercy and under the control of God and that God may have a particular reason for their suffering. To lose hope may mean they are losing faith in God and His abilities.
- The Qur'an and the sayings of Mohammed, the prophet of Islam, have made a major contribution to Muslim health care. In particular, preventive health care is embodied in many of Mohammed's prophetic sayings. Cleanliness and hygiene are essential to practicing Muslims. A number of elaborate prayer rituals are also related to health care and prevention of illness. For example, before praying, Muslims must engage in a purification ritual, which consists of washing every exposed body part. Prayer, required five times daily, consists of elaborate bending and kneeling movements in systematic ways, increasing a person's range of movements, limbering stretches, and meditative poses. Religion and prayers are believed to provide protection from illnesses. Make arrangements for Muslims to pray.

HEALTH-CARE PRACTICES

- Egyptian health care is influenced by Greek, or *unani,* medicine, and by humoral systems. The principles behind the humoral system are based on dividing many aspects of life into four: the year into four seasons; matter into fire, air, earth, and water; the body into black phlegm, black bile, yellow bile, and blood; and the environment into hot, cold, moist, and dry. Diseases follow these humors with treatments based on opposite humors. Egyptians believe that cold and moist environments cause illnesses by changing from cold to hot or vice versa; the opposite humor is used for treating the illness.
- Egyptians believe that suddenly being presented with bad news without preparation causes illness. Although a

Egyptian

person's mental and physical health is intricately interwoven, treatment sought from the health-care system is focused on physical or biomedical treatment. **Deliver news about a serious illness gradually and in stages.**

- Family or religious people usually handle mental health problems outside the health-care system. Egyptians tend to manifest symptoms of mental health problems somatically. Therefore, they seek medical care to deal with the physical manifestations of mental conditions.

- Most Egyptians in America join an HMO or have private medical insurance. Even though they may refuse to have life insurance (Islam does not condone insurance), they realize the importance of quality health care.

- Egyptians experiencing a health problem consult family members and friends before visiting a trusted health-care professional. Once in the health-care system, they prefer immediate, personalized attention. They value tests and prescriptions for their illnesses and follow medical regimens and prescriptions carefully, particularly if they consist of oral medications, injections, or both. However, they tend to be skeptical of treatments such as weight reduction, exercise, and diet restrictions. The family of a client expects and prefers to be involved in all health-care decisions. **Include the nuclear family in health-care decision-making.**

- Their focus on human relations and interpersonal contact makes it difficult for Egyptians to encounter changing staff and assignments during treatments. They believe they have a better chance of receiving quality care if trusting relationships are formed. **Assign the same health-care provider whenever possible to establish trust.**

- Egyptians practice self-medication and tend to share medications freely. They use Western medications as well as home remedies such as herbs, hot compresses, and hot fluids and foods. Many Egyptians keep a medicine cabinet filled with antibiotics, tranquilizers, sleeping pills, and pain medications. They also believe that vitamins given intramuscularly and intravenously are more effective than vitamins taken in pills. Some common herbal and home remedies are boiled mint leaves for a stomachache; boiled cumin for gas; boiled caraway for coughs; and hot pads for aches, pains, and boils. **Encourage full disclosure of all treatments such as over-the-counter-medicines, medicines brought by friends from Egypt, herbs, and home treatments that are being used.**

- Regulation of prescription drugs in the United States restricts the use of prescriptions, prompting some Egyptians in America to get their supply of medications from their home country or friends.

- According to Islam, illnesses are caused by lack of hygiene, exposure to diseases, or environmental conditions, although it is up to God who gets sick and who does not.

- People are expected to care for themselves and work at preventing illnesses when possible. In addition, beliefs related to the healing powers of shrines and holy men or saints and the counter powers of the *Jenn* (devil) and *arwah* (evil spirits) influence health care. Thus, ceremonies are designed to eliminate the devastating powers of the *Jenn*; among them are the famous *zar* ceremony and the *hegab*. The *zar* ceremony includes gathering friends and relatives around a sick person, with loud music playing and drums beating to increase the frenzy of dance and movement. The energy of the group and their solidarity help eliminate the bad spirits from the body, taking with them the illness or the handicapping condition. *Zar* is rarely practiced among Egyptians in America. A person who is trying to get rid of an illness wears the *hegab*, an amulet with sayings from the Qur'an. Some also use the *amal*, which is designed to bring bad luck or illness to an unloved person. Egyptians believe the "evil eye" is responsible for personal calamities. The evil eye is cast by those who have blue eyes, by those who tend to speak of an admired person or object in a boastful manner, or by

Egyptian

the mere description of beauty, wealth, or health without saying some verses from the Qur'an or Bible. These verses protect the person from losing whatever good they possess. Some use blue beads or religious verses inscribed on charms to protect them or their children from the evil eye. Children are particularly at risk for the evil eye and need more protection than adults.

- Barriers to health care among Egyptians in America are related to economics, work demands, and full schedules. Another barrier is the difference in explaining health problems. The extent of specificity required in the U.S. health-care system, the narrative storytelling nature of Egyptians, and the contextual way in which Egyptians view a situation all contribute to a frustrating experience for both the immigrant and the health-care professional.

- Egyptians avoid pain at all costs by seeking prompt interventions. They tend to be verbally and nonverbally expressive about pain. Although they tend to be more constrained in front of health-care professionals or other "strangers," they are quite expressive in front of family members, using grunting, pushing, screaming, or guttural sounds or gasping for air. The absence of these responses in front of health-care professionals makes verification of the intensity of pain difficult.

- Egyptians present a more generalized description of pain, regardless of whether it is localized. They usually describe general weakness, dizziness, or overall tension and stress associated with pain. They also use metaphors reflecting humoral medicine such as earth, rocks, fire, heat, and cold to describe their pain. Perform a complete pain assessment before administering pain medications.

- Psychosomatic interventions are more effective than psychologically-based interventions such as counseling or psychoanalysis. Although Egyptians may seek therapy and counseling, they prefer to seek the advice of family members or trusted friends rather than strangers. They also do not like to refer to treatments as psychotherapy or analysis.

- Although there is public sympathy and acceptance of the disabled, families still tend to be protective and shield them from public display. Families assume responsibility for the care of their disabled members, not expecting help or services from society. Egyptians, however, tend to hide their disabled family members from others for fear of evoking reactions of pity. However, they are open with health-care professionals in the hope of receiving better health care.
- Egyptians have a general belief that chronic illnesses can be controlled by the scientific sophistication of Western medicine. Less regard is held for complementary therapies, and the demand is greater for scientifically supported remedies, regardless of their intrusiveness. Egyptians tend to be hopeful, persistent, and optimistic about their prognoses. Therefore, they may shop around for health care that promises a better prognosis.
- Rehabilitation programs that include drastic changes in lifestyles are less appealing if the programs are not scientifically supported. Explain the scientific basis of rehabilitation programs.
- Egyptian families take care of their sick members. Promotion of self-care is viewed with suspicion, and sick people are not expected to participate in programs to enhance their self-care capabilities. Rather, they are expected to preserve their energy for healing. Attempts to engage Egyptian clients in self-care by promoting responsibility for daily care, for example, by keeping a colostomy incision clean, are resisted and perceived as a request to decrease the work of the nurse and the other staff.
- Sick people are also relieved from making major health-care decisions; their families make all these decisions for them. Explain the necessity of self-care activities that promote healing and recovery, and include the family caregivers in planning care.
- Egyptians have no taboos against blood transfusions or organ transplants. All measures needed to heal, cure, or prolong life are welcomed. Their trust and respect for the health-care system and health-care professionals

Egyptian

facilitate their decision-making. They are hesitant, however, to pledge their own organs to others or to permit an autopsy because of their belief in the afterlife.

HEALTH-CARE PRACTITIONERS

- In general, Egyptians have a positive perception of the American health-care system. They believe that physicians and nurses are experts and are caring and responsive to the needs of their community. Using the services of acupuncturists, podiatrists, chiropractors, and physical therapists is foreign to those not integrated into the American culture.

- For some, the meticulous diagnostic approaches practiced by American physicians may be misinterpreted. Accustomed to Egyptian physicians whose clinical judgments and skills have been developed within a system that lacks adequate resources for meticulous diagnoses, some may misperceive an American physician's thoroughness as a lack of experience or appropriate knowledge. Therefore, they may shop for physicians whose clinical judgments are congruent with their cultural expectations of a prompt and firm diagnosis. Others may view the laborious and involved diagnostic process, which uses many resources and tests, as an indication of the gravity of the diagnosis.

- First- and second-wave Egyptian Americans may not consider gender as an important criterion in the selection of their health-care providers. Third-wave immigrants may prefer same-gender health-care providers, although this preference may be mitigated by their respect for Western medicine. In addition to religious fundamentalism, modesty may influence the desire for same-sex health-care providers. For some, sharing the intimate details of their health history is enhanced if the health-care provider is the same gender. Some may also view older female physicians as more experienced and therefore more trustworthy than younger female physicians. **Provide a same-sex health-care provider whenever possible.**

- Physicians are highly respected. Egyptians prefer physicians affiliated with large, respected organizations because they believe them to be more experienced. For some, the physician's age, years of experience, and position in the organization may indicate better qualifications.
- Egyptians' contacts in the homeland with nurses who are knowledgeable and expert in their fields have been minimal. Consequently, their expectations of nurses are usually far below their experiences in the U.S. health-care system. They view American nurses as well educated and well qualified and are grateful for their expertise and for their attention.

References

Gay Egypt. (2003). Retrieved December 25, 2003, from www.gayegypt.com

Hattar-Pollara, M., Meleis, A.I., & Naguib, H. (2000). A study of the spousal role of Egyptian women in clerical jobs. *Health Care for Women International, 21*(4), 305–317.

Levy, R. (1993). Ethnic and racial differences in response to medicines: Preserving individualized therapy in managed programmes. *Pharmaceutical Medicine, 7,* 139–165.

Lonely Planet. (2001). *http://www.lonelyplanet.com*

Meleis, A.I. (2002). Egyptians. In P. St. Hill, J. Lipson, and A. Meleis (Eds.), *Caring for women cross-culturally: A portable guide.* Philadelphia: F. A. Davis Company.

Meleis, A.I., & Sorrell, L. (1981). Arab American women and their birth experiences. *American Journal of Maternal Child Nursing, 6,* 171–176.

Purnell, L. (2003). People of Egyptian heritage. In L. Purnell and B. Paulanka (Eds.), *Transcultural health care: A culturally competent approach,* (2nd ed., chapter on CD). Philadelphia: F.A. Davis Company.

Reizian, A.E., & Meleis, A.I. (1987). Arab Americans' perceptions of and responses to pain. *Critical Care Nurse, 6*(6), 30–37.

Time Almanac. (2001). Boston: Time Inc.

Egyptian

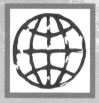

CHAPTER 12

European American Heritage

Overview and Heritage

The term *dominant American culture* in this chapter refers to the middle-class values of citizens of the mainland United States. The United States, the world's oldest constitutional democracy, comprises 3.5 million square miles and includes a population of nearly 284 million people. The word "American" is used for residents of the United States. The dominant American culture evolved from that of early immigrants, primarily from Northern European countries. Today, the United States includes immigrants or descendents of immigrants from almost every nation and culture of the world.

Americans value individualism, free speech, freedom of choice, independence, self-reliance, confidence, "doing" rather than "being," egalitarian relationships, nonhierarchal status of individuals, achievement status over ascribed status, volunteerism, friendliness, openness, futuristic temporality, and ability to control the environment. Many emphasize material possessions and physical comfort. The extent to which people conform to this dominant culture depends on the primary and secondary characteristics of culture discussed in Chapter 1.

COMMUNICATIONS

- The official language is English, but accents vary throughout the United States and are usually understandable to all. Having well-developed verbal skills is considered important.
- Voice volume is loud compared with many other world cultures.
- The rate of speech varies depending on location within the United States, with people from the South generally speaking slower than people in the Northeast.
- Many individuals readily disclose personal information about themselves. Personal sharing is encouraged in a wide variety of topics, but not religion.
- People of the same sex (especially men) or opposite sex do not generally touch each other unless they are relatives or close friends. Health-care providers should recognize that low-touch culture of the United States is reinforced by sexual harassment guidelines and policies.
- Regardless of class or social standing of the conversants, Americans maintain direct eye contact without staring.
- Men and women extend the right hand when greeting someone for the first time.
- Most Americans are future-oriented but try to balance the past with the present. Punctuality is valued in both business and social settings.
- Usual name format is given name, middle name (optional), and family name. People usually refer to each other by the given name. However, in the health-care setting, use Mr., Mrs., Miss, Ms., or appropriate title on first meeting someone and until told to do otherwise.

FAMILY ROLES AND ORGANIZATION

- A value is placed on egalitarian relationships and decision-making, although great variations exist within families. Women may have careers, and men often assist with child care, household chores, and cooking responsibilities.

- Great value is placed on children, and many laws help protect children.
- Autonomy is encouraged in children and teenagers. Children and teenagers are encouraged to have friends of the same and opposite genders.
- Teenagers are expected to refrain from premarital sex, smoking, recreational drug use, and alcohol use until they leave home. Most teenagers move out of their parents' home when their education is completed or when they turn age 18 years.
- Social attitudes toward homosexual activity vary widely and sometimes carry a stigma. **Health-care providers must be very careful not to disclose clients' same-sex relationships to family members.**

BIOCULTURAL ECOLOGY

- The leading causes of death in Americans are heart disease, cancer, chronic obstructive lung disease, unintentional injury, diabetes, and HIV.
- Nearly 1 million people in the United States are HIV-positive or have AIDS, with the highest concentrations in large urban areas.
- Illnesses and diseases, with an increased incidence in white ethnic groups in the United States, include appendicitis, diverticular disease, colon cancer, hemorrhoids, varicose veins, cystic fibrosis, rosacea, osteoporosis and osteoarthritis, and phenylketonuria.

HIGH-RISK HEALTH BEHAVIORS

- Cigarette-smoking has been declining in the United States. Higher socioeconomic groups are more likely to drink but also more likely to drink without problems. **Encourage responsible drinking and smoking cessation.**
- High-risk sexual behavior continues with the continuing

incidence of STD and HIV infections. **Encourage health screening and preventive behaviors such as condoms and safer-sex practices.**

- Many laws have been enacted, although they vary from state to state, requiring automobile seat belts, child restraints, and helmets for bicycle and motorcycle riders. **Encourage use of seat belts, child restraints, and helmets.**

NUTRITION

- The typical diet is high in fats and cholesterol and low in fiber. **Encourage low-fat, low-cholesterol, and high-fiber diets using the USDA food pyramid. See Figure 12–1.**

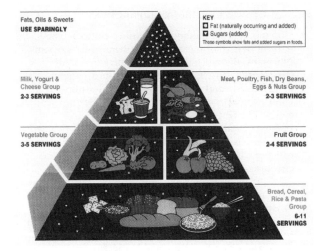

FIGURE 12–1. Food Guide Pyramid: A Guide to Daily Food Choices. (Source: U.S. Department of Agriculture/U.S. Department of Health and Human Services.) Available at http://www.nal.usda.gov/fnic/Fpyr/guide.pdf

- Given the varied topography of the United States, there are no food shortages for a healthy diet. Teach clients about healthy foods and preparation practices.
- Meal times and food choices vary according to ethnic background, the region of the country, urban versus rural residents, and weekdays versus weekends.
- Breakfast is usually consumed between 6:00 AM and 9:00 AM, depending on the person's work schedule.
- The noontime meal, typically consumed by 1:00 PM, is called lunch in urban areas and dinner in rural areas.
- The evening meal, dinner in urban areas or supper in rural areas, is served between 6:00 PM and 9:00 PM and is usually the largest meal of the day.
- Determine meal times, and adjust medications accordingly.

PREGNANCY AND CHILDBEARING PRACTICES

- Commonly used methods of fertility control include natural ovulation methods, birth control pills, foams, Norplant, the morning-after pill, intrauterine devices, condoms, abortion, and sterilization procedures such as vasectomy and tubal ligations. Sterilization in the United States is strictly voluntary, but abortion remains a controversial issue.
- Pregnant women are expected to seek preventive care, eat a well-balanced diet, and get adequate rest in order to have a healthy pregnancy and baby. Women are encouraged to breast-feed. Discourage smoking, drinking alcohol, consuming large amounts of caffeine, and taking recreational drugs.
- Prospective fathers are encouraged to take prenatal classes with expectant mothers and provide a supportive role in the delivery process. Fathers who do not want to participate should not be made to feel guilty.
- Respect cultural beliefs associated with pregnancy and the birthing process.
- Integrate nonharmful cultural practices into preventive teaching and interventions.

Possible Restrictive Beliefs for Pregnant Women

- Pregnant women should refrain from being around loud noises for prolonged times.
- Wearing an opal ring during pregnancy can harm the baby.
- Eating strawberries or being frightened by a snake causes birthmarks.
- Congenital anomalies can occur if the mother sees or experiences a tragedy during her pregnancy.
- Nursing mothers should eat a bland diet to avoid upsetting the baby.
- The infant should wear a band around the abdomen to prevent the umbilicus from protruding and becoming herniated.
- A coin, key, or other metal object should be put on the umbilicus to flatten it.
- Cutting a baby's hair before baptism can cause blindness.
- If the pregnant woman raises her hands over her head while pregnant, it may cause the cord to wrap around the baby's neck.
- Moving heavy items can cause a pregnant woman's "insides" to fall out.
- Children born with physical or mental abnormalities are punishment from God for acts of the parents.

DEATH RITUALS

- Death and responses to death are difficult topics for many Americans to verbalize.
- The dying person should not be left alone. Make accommodations for a family member to be with the dying person at all times.
- Health-care personnel are expected to care for the family as much as for the patient during this time.
- Most people are buried or cremated within 3 days of death; extenuating circumstances may lengthen this period to accommodate family and friends who must

travel a long distance to attend a funeral or memorial service. The family decides if the deceased will have an open or closed casket.

- More people are choosing to remain at home and participate in a hospice for end-of-life care to have their comfort needs met. **One requirement for hospice care is that the patient must sign documents indicating that he or she does not want extensive life-saving measures performed.** Although women may be more expressive than men, most Americans demonstrate their grief conservatively. Generally, tears are shed, but loud wailing and uncontrollable sobbing rarely occur.

SPIRITUALITY

- Dominant religions in the United States are those of the Judeo-Christian faiths and include Catholicism, Protestantism, and Judaism. However, there are many other recognized religions that are consistent with religious freedom, the reason that many people immigrated to the United States. Although church and state

Bereavement Support Strategies

- **Being physically present**
- **Acknowledging the patient's pain**
- **Encouraging a reality orientation**
- **Openly acknowledging the family's right to grieve**
- **Recognizing varied behavioral responses to grief**
- **Assisting the client and family to express their feelings**
- **Encouraging interpersonal relationships**
- **Promoting interest in a new life**
- **Making referrals to other resources such as a priest, minister, rabbi, or pastoral care person, with the patient's or family's permission**

are separate, many public events and ceremonies still open with a prayer.

- Inquire if the person wants to see a member of the clergy.
- In times of illness, many people say prayers. Ask clients if they need anything to say prayers.
- Do not remove religious symbols or statues as they provide solace to the person. Removing them may increase or cause anxiety.

HEALTH-CARE PRACTICES

- The United States is undergoing a paradigm shift from curative and restorative medical practices and sophisticated technological care to health promotion and wellness, illness and disease prevention, and increased personal responsibility. Most believe that individuals, families, and the community have the ability to influence health. Many view good health as a divine gift from God.
- Advance directives are an important part of medical care, which allows patients to specify their wishes concerning life and death decisions before entering an inpatient facility. These directives also designate the name of a family member or significant other to speak for the patient and make decisions when or if the patient is unable to do so. Some patients have a living will that outlines their wishes in terms of life-sustaining procedures in the event of a terminal illness or a fatal accident. Each inpatient facility has these forms available and will ask the patient what his or her wishes are. Patients may sign these forms at the hospital or elect to bring their own forms.
- Even when a client is covered by health insurance, an insurance company representative may need to approve health visits and validate specific procedures, medicines, and treatments for which it will pay. Those who cannot afford insurance should be referred to a social worker to help them obtain the necessary treatments.
- As an adjunct to biomedical treatments, many people

European

use acupuncture, acupressure, acumassage, herbal therapies, massage therapy, aromatherapy, and other complementary treatments. An awareness of combined practices when treating or providing health education to individuals and families helps ensure that therapies do not conflict with each other, intensify the treatment regimen, or cause an overdose. Inquire about all therapies being used, such as foods, teas, herbal remedies, nonfood substances, over-the-counter medications, and medications prescribed or loaned by others. Often, traditional, folk, and magicoreligious practices are and should be incorporated into the plan of care for clients. To help prevent contradictory or exacerbated effects of prescription medication and treatment regimens, ask clients about self-medicating practices.

- Pain is the "fifth vital sign." Patients should be made comfortable and not have to tolerate high levels of pain. Offer and encourage pain medication, and explain that it will help the healing process.
- In 1992, the Americans with Disabilities Act went into effect, protecting handicapped individuals from discrimination. Rehabilitation and occupational health services focus on returning individuals with handicaps to productive lifestyles in society as soon as possible.
- Traditional practice calls for fully disclosing health conditions to clients/patients, who then disclose the information to the family.
- Most Americans favor organ donation and transplantation and blood or blood products transfusions. Jehovah's Witnesses do not receive blood or blood products. Assist clients in obtaining a religious leader to support them in making decisions regarding organ donation or transplantation if requested.

HEALTH-CARE PRACTITIONERS

- Most people combine biomedical health-care practices with traditional practices, folk healers, and magicoreligious healers.

- Standard practice is to assign staff to patients regardless of gender differences. Recognize and respect differences in gender relationships when providing care. Respect clients' modesty by providing adequate privacy and assigning same-sex caregivers whenever the patient requests.
- The advanced practice role of registered nurses is gaining respect as their numbers increase and the public sees them as equal or preferable to physicians and physician assistants. The public holds nurses in high regard.

References

Cardiovascular disease. Centers for Disease Control and Prevention. Retrieved July 3, 2003, from http://www.cdc.gov

Current and accurate cancer information. National Cancer Institute. Retrieved July 3, 2003, from http://www.cancernet.nci.nih.gov

Hanson, I., & Rogdman, E. (1996). The use of living wills at the end of life: A national study. *Archives of Internal Medicine, 156,* 1018–1022.

National Center for HIV, STD, and TB Prevention. Centers for Disease Control and Prevention. Retrieved July 3, 2003, from http://www.cdc.gov

Peele, S., & Brodsky, A. Alcohol and society. Retrieved July 3, 2003, from http://www.peele.net

Purnell L., & Paulanka, B. (Eds.). (2003) *Transcultural health care: A culturally competent approach* (2nd ed.). Philadelphia: F.A. Davis Company.

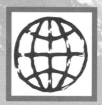

People of Filipino Heritage

Overview and Heritage

This chapter discusses the major cultural characteristics of Filipinos. Predominantly of Malayan ancestry, they have also been influenced by Spain and the neighboring Chinese, Japanese, East Indian, Indonesian, Malaysian, and Islamic cultures. The Philippine culture is distinct from its Asian neighbors largely because of major influences from the Spanish and American colonization. The Philippine archipelago consists of 7,107 islands located in southeastern Asia, east of Vietnam and slightly north of the equator. With a population of more than 83 million and a land mass of 115,830 square miles, the Philippine land mass is slightly larger than Arizona. The tropical climate is suitable for year-round agriculture and fishing, but it is affected by the seasonal northeast and southwest monsoons.

Following the Spanish-American War in 1898, the Philippines were ceded to the United States. Native speakers refer to the country as Filipinas or Pilipinas and use Philippine when speaking to outsiders or when writing in English. The issue of whether to use F or P when referring to the country, its people, or its national language is a matter of debate. There is no letter F in the indigenous **Tagalog** language. The national language is Filipino.

Filipino Americans are a diverse group whose regional variations influence the spoken dialect, food preferences, and traditions as well as the other primary and secondary characteristics of culture discussed in Chapter 1. Approximately 1.85 million Filipinos live in the United States and are concentrated in California, Hawaii, Illinois, New Jersey, New York, Washington, and Texas. Filipino immigration to the United States began in 1902, when the Philippines became an American territory. From 1909 until the 1920s, male Filipino laborers were recruited to work on Hawaiian plantations and in businesses on the West Coast. Since the passage of the 1965 Immigration Act, the Philippines has become the largest source of immigrants from Asia. Economic and educational opportunities and reunification with family members in the United States continue to be the primary motivating factors for emigration. Filipinos view educational achievement as a pathway to economic success, status, and prestige for the individual and the family.

COMMUNICATIONS

- Although more than 100 dialects are spoken in the Philippines, most Filipinos speak the national language, Filipino. English is used for business and legal transactions, and in school all instruction beyond the third grade is conducted in English. Business and social interactions commonly use a hybrid of Tagalog and English (Tag-Lish) in the same sentence. Tag-Lish is often used in health education.
- Nouns are used in place of the generic and gender-neutral pronouns *siya* (singular "he/she") and *sila* (plural "they/them"). Hence, it is customary for Filipinos to use "he" and "she" interchangeably in reference to the same individual.
- Communication is highly contextual. The individual is acculturated to attend to the context of the interaction and to adopt appropriate behaviors.

Filipino

- Most Filipinos are observant, displaying an intuitive feeling about the other person and the contextual environment during interactions. Meanings are embedded in nonverbal communication.
- The emphasis on maintaining smooth interpersonal relationships brings a consequent ambiguity in communication to prevent the risk of offending others. Filipinos may sacrifice clear communication to avoid stressful interpersonal conflicts and confrontations.
- Saying "no" to a superior may be considered disrespectful, which predisposes an ambiguous positive response.
- Focusing on action-oriented strategies may be seen as coercive.
- Saving face, a characteristic pattern of behavior employed to protect the integrity of both conversants, is a consequence of the cultural value placed on maintaining smooth interpersonal relations.
- During a teaching session, a Filipino client's nod may have several meanings, such as comprehension or agreement ("Yes, I hear you"; "Yes, we are interacting"; "Yes, I can see the instructions") or some other message that may be difficult for the client to disclose.
- Health-care workers should ask indirectly whether the Filipino client understands instructions and should have the person or family member do a return demonstration of a procedure or repeat an instruction rather than question his or her comprehension. Speak clearly and slowly. Allow time for a response to questions, giving time for translating the dialect into English.
- One may not disagree, talk loudly, or look directly at a person who is older or who occupies a higher position in the social hierarchy. Direct eye contact depends on the extent of acculturation, amount of time in the United States, age, and education. Some individuals may avoid prolonged eye contact with authority figures and older people as a form of respect. Older men may refrain from maintaining eye contact with young women because it may be interpreted as flirtation or a sexual advance.

- Most individuals are comfortable with silence and allow the other person to initiate verbal interaction as a sign of respect.
- Greater distance is observed when interacting with outsiders and people in positions of authority.
- Same-gender closeness and touching are normal behaviors. Young adults of the same gender may hold hands, put one arm over another's shoulder, or walk arm-in-arm.
- Most Filipinos have a relaxed temporal outlook. They have a healthy respect for the past, the ability to enjoy the present, and hope for the future. Past orientation is evident in their respect for elders, strong sense of gratitude, obligation to older generations, and honoring the memories of dead ancestors. Future orientation is manifested in the strong sense of family commitment to provide for the education of the young, parental participation in the care of their children and grandchildren, and a strong work ethic.
- Promptness for social events is determined situationally. "Filipino time" means arriving much later than the scheduled appointment, which can be from one to several hours.
- The kinship system is extended bilineally and is reflected in the format for names, giving the child identity with both parents.
- Children carry the surnames of their father and their mother. For example, Jose Romagos Lopez and Leticia Romagos Lopez are the children of Maria Romagos and Eduardo Lopez. The middle name or initial is the mother's maiden name. After marriage, Eduardo keeps the same name, whereas his sister's name becomes Leticia Lopez Lukban (her husband being Ernesto Lukban). The middle name is generally abbreviated as an initial. Nicknames symbolize affectionate regard for the person and are commonly used instead of the first name; hence, Nini, Baby, Bongbong. Address Filipino adults by their title or professional affiliation such as Mr., Mrs., Miss, Ms., doctor, or attorney.

Filipino

FAMILY ROLES AND ORGANIZATION

- In contemporary families, although the father is the acknowledged head of the household, authority is considered egalitarian. The mother plays an equal and often major role in decisions regarding health, children, and finances.
- Traditional female roles include caring for the sick and children, maintaining positive relationships with kin, and managing the home.
- Parents and older siblings are involved in the care and discipline of younger children.
- In extended-family households, older relatives and grandparents share much authority and responsibility for the care and discipline of younger members. Institutionalization of aged parents is tantamount to abandonment of filial obligation.
- Parents traditionally expect their children to pursue a college education, have economically productive careers, and raise a family.
- Dating at an early age is discouraged for young daughters. Sex education and sex are not discussed openly within the family.
- Traditional families desire that their daughters remain chaste before marriage. Pregnancy out of wedlock brings shame to the whole family.
- Conditions such as mental illness, divorce, terminal illness, criminal offenses, unwanted pregnancy, and HIV/AIDS are not readily shared with outsiders until trust is established. In times of illness, the extended family provides support and assistance.
- A family visit to the hospital may take on the semblance of a family reunion. Make arrangements for visitations by large numbers of family. Elicit help for visitor control from a respected family member.
- Homosexuality may be recognized but is often considered an aberrant behavior. Thus, to save face and decrease stigmatization for the family, it is not openly practiced or acknowledged. Do not disclose same-gender relationships to family members.

BIOCULTURAL ECOLOGY

- The typical Filipino may be of Malayan ancestry, with a brown complexion and a multiracial genetic background.
- The youthful features of Filipinos make it difficult to assess their age. Common Filipino physical features may include jet black to brunette or light brown hair, dark- to light-brown pupils with eyes set in almond-shaped eyelids, deep brown to very light tan skin tones, mildly flared nostrils, and slightly low to flat nose bridges.
- The high melanin content of the skin and mucosa may pose problems when assessing signs of jaundice, cyanosis, and pallor. **The usual manifestations of anemia (pallor and jaundice) should be assessed in the conjunctiva.**
- Filipinos range in height from under 5 feet to the height of average Americans.
- Approximately 40 percent have blood type B and a low incidence of the Rh-negative factor.
- A high incidence of glucose-6-phosphate dehydrogenase, thalassemias, lactose intolerance, and malabsorption may exist.
- Newborns may have Mongolian spots: bluish green discolorations on their buttocks that are physiological and that eventually disappear.
- Filipino people are at high risk for developing coronary heart disease, hypertension, diabetes at midlife and old age, hypercholesterolemia, renal stones, hyperuricemia, gout, and arthritis. Breast, cervical, prostate, thyroid, lung, and liver cancers are major threats to this population.
- Liver cancer tends to be diagnosed in the late stages of the disease and appears to be associated with the presence of the hepatitis B virus. Silent carriers of the virus are common among Asians, and its presence is detected only when other problems are being evaluated. **Routinely screen for hepatitis B virus among recent immigrants.**
- Asians require lower doses of central nervous system

Filipino

depressants such as haloperidol, have a lower tolerance for alcohol, and are more sensitive to the adverse effects of alcohol.

- Because of availability of over-the-counter antibiotics and lack of adequate medical monitoring of these drugs in the Philippines, Filipino immigrants may be insensitive to the effects of some anti-infectives.
- A positive reaction to tuberculin or to the Mantoux test is observed because of the practice of giving bacille Guérin-Calmette vaccinations in childhood. Chest x-rays and sputum cultures are recommended for screening and diagnosis of tuberculosis.

HIGH-RISK HEALTH BEHAVIORS

- Filipinos who are more acculturated have higher rates of alcohol abuse and increased smoking rates. Carefully explain the physical and psychological problems of alcohol abuse and tobacco use.
- Less educated Filipinos in the United States have increased rates of HIV/AIDS compared with other Asians/Pacific Islanders. Take every opportunity to include HIV/AIDS education in health teaching.
- The more recent immigrants in the United States frequently do not access health services until their illness is advanced because they are not aware of available services and may not have linguistic competence in the English language. Educate the Filipino community about the availability of services. Provide interpreters as necessary.

NUTRITION

- Food and meal patterns emphasize generosity, hospitality, and thoughtfulness, which support group cohesiveness. Spanish, Chinese, and American influences are integrated into contemporary cuisine.
- Foods may be sautéed, fried, or served with a sauce. Rice is a staple food and is eaten at every meal, either steamed, fried, or as a dessert.

- Except for babies and young children, milk is almost absent in the Filipino diet, partly due to lactose intolerance. Milk in desserts such as egg custard and ice cream seems to be tolerated.
- Cold drinks or foods such as orange juice or fresh tomatoes are not served for breakfast in order to prevent stomach upset.
- Dietary calcium is derived from green leafy vegetables and seafood.
- Households may keep potted medicinal plants that are used for common colds, stomach upsets, urinary tract infections, and other minor ailments.
- Daily consumption of garlic to combat hypertension is common. Ginger root is boiled and served as a beverage to relieve sore throats and promote digestion.
- Bitter melon is prepared and eaten as a vegetable and believed to prevent diabetes. Greens such as *malunggay* and *ampalaya* leaves are used in stews to regain stamina for someone believed to be anemic or run-down. Knowledge of indigenous food sources and meal patterns, nutritional content of Filipino foods and American food substitutes, and accessibility of traditional ingredients are important aspects of nutritional assessment and counseling.

PREGNANCY AND CHILDBEARING PRACTICES

- The only acceptable method of contraception is the rhythm method. Abortion is considered a sin. Recent Filipino immigrants who come from urban areas and who are more educated may be open to alternative methods of birth control.
- Many Filipino women are embarrassed to have male doctors perform vaginal examinations.
- The pregnant Filipino woman's network of family and community health advisers, whose opinions she respects, are important support for building trust and rapport in the client-provider relationship.

  Box 13–1 describes common beliefs about pregnancy.

BOX 13–1 • Prenatal Beliefs About Pregnancy

- Some women refuse to take vitamins because they are afraid that vitamins could deform the fetus.
- Some individuals believe that when pregnant women crave certain foods, the craving should be satisfied to avoid harm to the baby. They believe that if the mother craves dark-skinned fruit or dark-colored food, the infant's skin will be dark.
- Sudden fright or stress may harm the developing fetus.
- Eating blackberries will make the baby have black spots.
- Eating black plums will give the baby dark skin.
- Eating twin bananas will result in twins being born.
- Eating apples will give the baby red lips.
- When a woman's stomach is not round or the mother's face is blemished, the baby will be a boy.
- Going outside during a lunar eclipse is harmful to the baby.
- Going out in the morning dew is bad for the baby because evil spirits are present.
- Funerals are avoided because the spirit of the dead person may affect the baby.
- Wearing necklaces may cause the umbilical cord to wrap around the baby's neck.
- Sitting by a doorway will make the delivery difficult.
- Sitting by a window when it is dark may let evil spirits come to the pregnant woman.
- Sweeping at night may sweep away the good spirits.
- Knitting might tangle the baby's intestines at birth.
- Naming the baby before it is born or after a dead person is bad luck.

- Some women prefer to have their mothers rather than their husbands in the delivery room.
- Women who came from rural regions in the home country may prefer the squatting position for birthing.

- More rural women breast-feed their infants and for a much longer time than their urban counterparts.
- Common reasons for not breast-feeding are insufficient milk, mother working, nipple and breast problems, and mother's poor health.
- Supplementing breast-feeding with other liquids and foods occurs as early as 2 months.
- Beliefs about the postpartum period are included in Box 13–2.

BOX 13–2 • Postpartum Practices and Beliefs

- Mothers should eat plenty of hot soups (chicken with papaya) to promote milk production.
- Postpartum mothers should avoid exposure to cold and should use warm water to drink and bathe for a month.
- Showers are prohibited because they may cause arthritis. However, the woman's mother may give her a sponge bath with aromatic oils and herbs, or a *hilot*, traditional healer, may give an aromatic herbal steam bath followed by full body massage, including the abdominal muscles, to stimulate a physiological reaction that has both physical and psychological benefits.
- Eating sour or ice-cold foods may cause abdominal cramps for both the baby and mother.
- The mother and baby should not go out for a month except to visit a doctor.
- One should give money to charity or to the needy when a baby comes to your house for the first time.
- The baby's abdomen is wrapped with a cloth until the umbilical cord falls off to prevent an umbilical hernia.
- Garlic, salt, or a rosary is placed near the baby's crib to ward off evil spirits.
- Hanging the baby's placenta in a tree will make the baby a good climber.

Filipino

DEATH RITUALS

- Family members generally wish to provide the most intimate caregiving rituals for the patient regardless of the setting. Make arrangements for the family to participate in caregiving.
- Illness and death may be attributed to supernatural and magic or religious causes such as punishment from God, angry spirits, or sorcery.
- Religiosity and fatalism contribute to stoicism in the face of pain or distress as a way of accepting one's fate.
- Before the decision is made to inform the patient about his or her terminal condition, a discussion among family members should occur. They may request the doctor not to divulge the truth to protect the patient.
- The ethical principles of beneficence and malfeasance take precedence over patient autonomy.
- Planning for one's death is taboo and may be considered tempting fate. Hence, many traditional Filipinos are averse to discussing advance directives or living wills. Most believe in life after death.
- A priority for the family is to gather around the dying person and during the immediate period after death to pray for the soul of the departed. When death is imminent, contact a priest if the family is Catholic. Do not remove religious medallions, rosary beads, a scapular, or religious figures on the patient or at the bedside.
- After death, a wake may last from 3 days to 1 week (to wait for the arrival of kin from other states or countries).
- Women generally show emotions openly by crying, fainting, or wailing. Men are expected to be more stoic and grieve silently.
- Cremation is acceptable to avoid the spread of disease.
- On the first-year anniversary of death, family and friends are reunited in prayer to celebrate this memorable event.
- Most women wear black clothing for months or up to a year after the death. The one-year anniversary ends the ritual mourning.

SPIRITUALITY

- The dominant religious affiliations are Catholicism (the majority), Protestantism, Muslim, and Buddhism. Most seek medical care; they believe that part of the efficacy of a cure is in God's hands or by some mystical power.
- Novenas and prayers are often said on behalf of the sick person. Performance of religious obligations and sacraments and daily prayers are some of the ways health and peaceful death are achieved. Provide for spiritual needs of patients by making accommodations to their practicing beliefs.
- Strength comes from an intimate relationship with God, family, friends, neighbors, and nature.
- The concept of self is formed from the relationship with a divine being.

HEALTH-CARE PRACTICES

- Some Filipinos are fatalistic, tending to accept fate easily, especially when they feel they cannot change a situation.
- Decisions about when, where, and from whom to seek help are largely influenced by the intimate circle of family.
- Many individuals accept and adhere to medical recommendations but also use alternative sources of care suggested by trusted friends and family members, which include indigenous medical practices. Often, major decisions are delegated to the physician rather than to the patient or family taking an active collaborative role in decision-making.
  Stress that medications need to be taken as prescribed, medications are ordered specifically for each ailment, unused drugs should be discarded, and the use of medications by individuals other than the intended may have serious consequences.
- Care for the body through adequate sleep, rest, nutrition, and exercise is common practice.
- A high value is placed on personal cleanliness. Keeping

Filipino

oneself clean and free of unpleasant body odors is viewed as good for one's health and face-saving. To be slovenly and disorderly is to be shamelessly irresponsible. Aromatic baths are taken both for pleasure and to restore balance.

- Illness in infancy and childhood may be attributed to the "evil eye." Healing rituals may involve religion (prayers and exorcism), sacrifices to appease the spirits, use of herbs, and massage.
- Balance and moderation are embedded in the hot and cold theory of healing. Change should be introduced gradually. Sudden changes from hot to cold, from activity to inactivity, from fasting to overeating, and so forth, introduce undue bodily stresses that can cause illness.
- Some believe that after strenuous physical activity, a rest should precede a shower; otherwise the person could develop arthritis, and exposure to sudden cold drafts may induce colds, fever, rheumatism, pneumonia, or other respiratory ailments. Some individuals avoid hand-washing with cold water after ironing or heavy labor. Exposure to cold such as showers is avoided during menstruation and during the postpartum period.
- Some Filipinos do not seek care for illness until it is quite advanced.
- Many people accept minor ailments stoically and consider them natural imbalances that will run their normal course and disappear.
- Often patients do not complain of pain despite physiological indicators. Many view pain as part of living an honorable life and view this as an opportunity to reach a fuller spiritual life or to atone for past transgressions. Offer and, in fact, encourage pain relief interventions.
- Mental illness may be attributed to an external cause such as witchcraft, soul loss, or spirit intrusion.
- Minimal expressions of psychological and emotional discomfort may be observed. The discomfort in discussing negative emotions with outsiders may be

manifested by somatic complaints or ritualistic behaviors, such as praying. **Explore the underlying meaning of somatization (loss of appetite, inability to sleep), and observe client interactions with others for valuable information.**

- Many believe that mental illness is hereditary and that it carries a certain stigma.
- Family members tend to take care of emotional problems to minimize exposing the problems to outsiders. **Involving a trusted family member or friends, initiating contact with a Filipino mental health worker, especially a Filipino physician, may increase the likelihood of getting the person into a culturally compatible treatment program.**
- The birth of a developmentally disabled child may be viewed as God's gift, an opportunity to become a better person or family, a curse from some unknown "angry spirit," negligence while pregnant, or a family matter that should be kept private; institutionalization may not be readily accepted.
- Organ donation is not an option, except perhaps in cases in which a close family member is involved. Many Filipinos who follow Catholic traditions believe that keeping the body intact as much as possible until death is preparation for the afterlife.

HEALTH-CARE PRACTITIONERS

- Western medicine is familiar and acceptable to most. Some accept the efficacy of folk medicine and may consult both Western-trained and indigenous healers.
- Folk healers are less common in the United States, with the exceptions of the West Coast and Hawaii. When available, they contribute by facilitating cultural rapport between health-care providers and clients.
- The *hilot* (traditional healer) is often willing to be included in the counseling session and provide support for the patient's compliance with medical treatment. The *hilot* may provide a special prayer to be incorporated into the medically prescribed treatment plan to increase

the client's sense that all available resources are being used.

- Linguistically and ethnically congruent practitioners are preferred.
- A practitioner of the same gender and the same culture may encourage more Filipinos to take advantage of disease prevention services. Include a Filipino primary care provider whenever possible. A bilingual person is helpful to improve communication with older Filipinos.

References

Pacquiao, D. (2003). People of Filipino heritage. In L. Purnell and B. Paulanka, (Eds.). *Transcultural health care: A culturally competent approach* (2nd ed., pp. 138–160). Philadelphia, F.A. Davis Company.

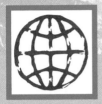

People of German Heritage

Overview and Heritage

The Federal Republic of Germany is one of the most densely populated countries in Europe, with a population of 82 million people. There are 58 million Germans in the United States. The first wave of German immigrants came to the United States for religious freedom and settled in the colonies along the eastern seaboard. The second wave arrived between 1840 and 1860 and was fleeing political persecution, poverty, and starvation. Many worked as indentured servants. The 1930s and 1940s saw a third wave because of the rise of fascism in Germany.

Germans have a deep respect for education. Credibility, social status, and level of employment are based on educational achievement. Germans receive a stronger education than Americans, with the German undergraduate degree being equal to the American master's degree. Because educational standards are high, smaller numbers of students enter the university system. To Germans, success means being employed, and education is the way to achieve this success.

COMMUNICATIONS

- German is the official language of the Federal Republic of Germany. There are many German dialects, making it difficult for some to understand each other. German is a low-contextual language, with a greater emphasis on verbal than nonverbal communication. A high degree of social approval is shown to people whose verbal skill in expressing ideas and feelings is precise, explicit, straightforward, and direct.

- Feelings are considered private and are often difficult to share. Sharing one's feelings with others often creates a sense of vulnerability or is looked on as evidence of weakness.

- The act of expressing fear, concern, happiness, or sorrow allows others a view of the personal and private self, creating a sense of discomfort and uneasiness. Therefore, philosophical discussions, hopes, and dreams are shared only with family members and close friends.

- Emotions are experienced intensely but are not always expressed among family or friends. "Being in control" includes harnessing one's emotions and not revealing them to others. Newer generations are more demonstrative in sharing their thoughts, ideas, and feelings with others. **Do not assume that just because a person may not express or display emotions the person does not care about his or her health or the situation.**

- Personal touch and displays of affection, such as hugging and kissing, vary. In families where the father plays a dominant role, little touching occurs between the father and children. This relationship may become more demonstrative as parents and children age. Affection between a mother and her children is more evident. In other families there is an outward expression of love from parents, grandparents, and extended family members; hugs and kisses are expected and often demanded as a "reaffirmation of love."

- Whereas close friends are often extended warmth through handshakes, brief embraces, and sometimes kisses, strangers are kept at arm's length and greeted formally; Germans generally are careful not to touch people who are not family or close friends.

- Most individuals place a high value on privacy. People may live side by side in a neighborhood and never develop a close friendship. Germans would never consider dropping in on another German neighbor, because this behavior is incongruent with their sense of order.
- Doors are used to protect privacy. A closed door requires a knock and an invitation to enter, regardless of whether the door is encountered in the home, business, or hospital. Even looking into a room from the outside is considered a visual intrusion.
- **Do not enter a patient's room without knocking on the door and requesting permission to enter.**
- Eye contact is maintained during conversations, but staring at strangers is considered rude.
- To focus on the present is to ensure the future. The past, however, is equally important, and Germans begin their discussions with background information, which always includes a history.
- Most individuals pride themselves on their punctuality. Being on time is an obsession. In the mind of a German, who is always on time, there are rarely good excuses for tardiness, delays, or incompetence that disturbs the "schedule" of events. **If the health-care provider is late with an appointment or treatment, provide a thorough explanation.**
- Traditionally, Germans keep social relations on a formal basis. Those in authority, older people, and subordinates are always addressed formally. Only family members and close friends address each other by their first names. Calling Germans by their first name may be considered a sign of disrespect or poor upbringing. Younger generations or the more acculturated may be less formal in their interactions. Because of cultural blending, health-care professionals will find that many clients vary widely in their observance of these rules of etiquette. **Greet clients formally unless told to do otherwise. Ask clients how they would like to be addressed.**

German

FAMILY ROLES AND ORGANIZATION

- Traditional families view the father as head of the household. In the United States, the husband and wife are more likely to make decisions mutually and share household duties.
- Older people are sought for their advice and counsel, although the advice may not always be followed. They are admired for maintaining their level of independence and their continued contributions to society. Many live alone or with aging spouses. Helping elderly parents or grandparents to remain in their own home is important to families. By providing a helping hand with home maintenance, shopping, and finances, the family is able to safeguard and prolong a state of independence, even when living hundreds of miles away. For those who grow dependent, moving in with children or residing in a retirement nursing home is a viable choice. **Include the extended family in decision-making. Consider using family members to assist with personal care and medical treatments when the need arises.**
- Prescriptive behaviors for children include using good table manners, being polite, doing what they are told, respecting their elders, sharing, paying attention in school, and doing their chores.
- Prescriptive behaviors for adolescents include staying away from bad influences, obeying the rules of the home, sitting like a lady, and wearing a robe over pajamas.
- Restrictive and taboo behaviors for children include talking back to adults, talking to strangers, touching another person's possessions, and getting into trouble. Restrictive and taboo behaviors for adolescents include smoking, using drugs, chewing gum in public, having guests when parents are not at home, going without a slip (girls), and having run-ins with the law.
- Family and lifelong friendships are highly valued. Concern for one's reputation is a strong value. One's family reputation is considered part of a person's identity and serves to preserve one's social position.

- When illness, dependence, and disability interfere and prevent family members from carrying out their roles, others assume decision-making responsibilities either temporarily or permanently.
- Pregnancy outside marriage results in overt or subtle disapproval. Because families are concerned about their reputations in the community, the presence of an unwed mother taints their reputation and may result in the family being ostracized by others. If marriage follows the pregnancy, less sanctioning occurs, but the fact that pregnancy existed before marriage creates a stigma for the woman, and sometimes for the child, that may last for the rest of their lives.
- Many middle-aged gays and lesbians may fear exposure because of the extreme discrimination homosexuals experienced in Nazi Germany. When encountering gays and lesbians who need support, a referral to one of the gay and lesbian religious groups may be helpful.

BIOCULTURAL ECOLOGY

- Germans range from tall, blond, and blue-eyed to short, stocky, dark-haired, and brown-eyed. Because many Germans have fair complexions, skin color changes and disease manifestations can easily be observed. For those with fair skin, prolonged exposure to the sun increases the risk for skin cancer. Counsel clients on exposure to sun, and recommend protection.
- Leading causes of death include heart disease, cancer, cerebrovascular disease, and accidents.
- In 1998, researchers localized the genetic cause for a syndrome of symptoms for a new form of myotonic muscular dystrophy. This new form of the disease, called DM2, appears to be most common in Americans of German descent (Mackle, 2001). Hereditary hemochromatosis, a toxic level of iron accumulation, can cause diabetes, chronic fatigue, liver disease, impotence, and even heart attacks. The disorder is due to a mutation in the HFE gene located on chromosome 6 and is more common among people of German descent.

German

- Sarcoidosis is found mostly in women between the ages of 20 and 40 years and occurs in all races, but people of German descent are at a higher risk. Sarcoidosis causes persistent cough or no symptoms. The cause is unknown; its diagnosis is often missed.
- Dupuytren's disease, a deformity of the hand in which the fingers are contracted toward the palm, is more common among Germans. Affecting mostly older males, the disease causes the synthesis of excessive amounts of collagen. The excess collagen is deposited in a ropelike fashion from the palm into the fingers, permanently fixing the fingers in a state of flexion. Peyronie's disease is often found in people with Dupuytren's disease. A benign plaque forms within the erectile tissue of the penis, which causes it to bend, resulting in reduced flexibility and causing pain during erection. This can prohibit sexual intercourse. The disease occurs mostly in middle-age men and often in men who are related.
- An increased incidence of cystic fibrosis (CF) is found among Hutterite German-speaking communal farmers living on the Great Plains of North America. Mutations in the Hutterite population, a genetic isolate with an average inbreeding coefficient of about 0.05, exhibit an increased prevalence of CF carriers. Maternal-child professionals can assist clients by encouraging genetic counseling to ensure early diagnosis of CF in their infants.

HIGH-RISK HEALTH BEHAVIORS

- Smoking and excessive alcohol consumption remain high-risk behaviors for most Germans. Encourage smoking cessation and limiting alcohol consumption to two drinks a day.
- Most individuals enjoy the outdoors, fresh air, and exercise. Sports are played for exercise and the pleasure of participating in group activities. Encourage water sports and other activities among elderly people, disabled people, mothers, and small children. Because Germans

are social joiners, encourage health club memberships for exercise.

NUTRITION

- Food is a symbol of celebration for Germans and is often equated with love. Children are rewarded for good behavior with food. Their infatuation with food can lead to overeating, resulting in obesity.
- Real cream and butter are used. Gravies, sauces, fried foods, rich pastries, and sausages are only a few of the culinary favorites that are high in fat content; meats are stewed, roasted, and marinated and are often served with gravies. Vegetables (fresh is preferred) are often served in a butter sauce. Foods are also fried in butter, bacon fat, lard, or margarine. Traditional food preparation methods use high-fat ingredients that add to nutritional risks. Garlic and onions are eaten daily to prevent heart disease.
- One-pot meals such as string beans and potatoes, cabbage and potatoes, chicken potpie, pork and sauer-kraut, stews, and soups are served as family meals. Casseroles are also popular. Foods prepared with vine-gar and sugar as flavorings are also favorites. Potato salad, cucumber salad, coleslaw, chow, pickled eggs, pickled cucumbers, cauliflower, tongue, and herring are common examples of favored foods prepared with these flavorings. Encourage reducing portion size, overcoming harmful food rituals, and reducing fat intake.
- Those who are ill receive egg custards, ginger ale, or tomato soup (without cream) to settle their stomach. Prune juice is given to relieve constipation. Soup from fresh tomato juice is used to treat a migraine headache.
- Ginger ale or 7-Up relieves indigestion and settles an upset stomach. After gastrointestinal illnesses, a recuper-ative diet is administered to the sick family member, beginning with sips of ginger ale over ice. If this is retained, hot tea and toast are offered. The last step is coddled eggs, a variation of scrambled eggs prepared

German

with margarine and a little milk. If these foods are tolerated, the sick person returns to the normal diet.

PREGNANCY AND CHILDBEARING PRACTICES

- Heterologous artificial insemination, use of contraceptive pills, and unnatural contraception are forbidden among strict Catholic Germans. Therapeutic or direct abortion is forbidden as the unjust taking of innocent life.
- Prescriptive practices during pregnancy include getting plenty of exercise and increasing the quantity of food to provide for the fetus. Restrictive practices during pregnancy include not stretching and not raising the arms above the head to minimize the risk of the cord wrapping around the baby's neck.
- A child born with the membrane (the amniotic sac, also knows as a "veil") over its head is believed to be a special child, a belief shared by many cultures.
- Prescriptive practices for the postpartum period include getting plenty of exercise and fresh air for the baby. If the mother is breast-feeding, she should eat foods that enhance the production of breast milk.

DEATH RITUALS

- Death is a transition to life with God. Because illness is sometimes perceived as a punishment, the duration and intensity of the dying process may be seen as a result of the quality of the life led by the person. Death is considered part of the life cycle, a natural conclusion to life. Individuals who embrace a set of religious beliefs may look forward to a life after death, often a better life.
- Careful selection of the clothes to be worn by the deceased and the flowers that represent the immediate family is important. Traditionally a 3-day period of mourning is reserved after the death of a family member.
- The body of the deceased is prepared and "laid out" in the home, where support from family and friends is

readily available. Neighbors come to do the chores and to sit with the family of the deceased until the burial. A short service is held in the home before the body is taken to the church, where family and friends can attend a funeral service. After the church services, the body is taken to the cemetery for burial. After a short graveside service, the minister invites everyone at the graveside service to go to the home of the deceased for food.

- The viewing provides an opportunity for family, friends, and acquaintances to view the body, offer their condolences, and extend their offers of assistance should the family need help in the future.
- Crying in public is permissible among some families, but in others the display of grief is private.
- A tradition of wearing black or dark clothing when attending a viewing or a funeral may be expected of both family and friends.

SPIRITUALITY

- Major religions include Roman Catholicism, Methodism, and Lutheranism. Other religions, such as Judaism, Islam, and Buddhism, have substantial membership. Recognize that individuals' decisions may vary from the formal position of their religious groups.
- Prayer is used to ask for healing, for effectiveness of treatments, for strength to deal with the symptoms of the illness, and for acceptance of the outcome of the course of the illness. Prayers are often recited at the bedside with all who are present joining hands, bowing their heads, and receiving the blessing from the clergy.
- Reading the Bible is an important spiritual activity. Most families have a family bible, which is passed down through the generations. It serves as spiritual comfort and as a reservoir of family historical data such as the dates of births, marriages, and deaths. Individual sources of strength are their beliefs in God and in nature, although they may not attend church on a regular basis.

German

- Family and other loved ones are also sources of support in difficult times. Home, family, friends, work, church, and education provide meaning in life for individuals of German heritage. Family loyalty, duty, and honor to the family are strong values.

HEALTH-CARE PRACTICES

- In traditional families, the mother usually ensures that children receive check-ups, get immunizations, and take vitamins. Women in the family often administer folk/home remedies and treatments. German Americans use a variety of over-the-counter drugs, believing that individuals are responsible for their own health.
- Common, natural folk medicines include roots, herbs, soups, poultices, and medicinal agents such as camphor, peppermint, and spirits of ammonia. Folk medicine includes "powwowing," use of special words, and wearing charms. **Ascertain if over-the-counter and folk remedies are being used so as to determine if there are contraindications with prescription medications.**
- Even when experiencing pain, many individuals continue to carry out their family and work roles. Many value being stoic when experiencing pain. **Health-care professionals may not be able to identify verbal or nonverbal clues about pain among Germans. Careful interviewing and astute observation must be used to accurately assess the level of pain they experience.**
- Mental illness may be viewed as a flaw, resulting in this group being slow to seek help because of the lack of acceptance and the stigma attached to needing help. Physical disabilities caused by injury are more acceptable than those caused by genetic problems.
- People's discomfort with expressing personal feelings to strangers may impede the counseling process and influence the counseling methods used. Most need to discuss the past without expressing their feelings. **Recognize that clients may not readily discuss feelings, especially during the initial counseling session.**

- Blood transfusions, organ donation, and organ transplants are acceptable medical interventions.

HEALTH-CARE PRACTITIONERS

- Health-care providers hold a relatively high status among Germans. This admiration stems from the love of education and respect for authority.
- Most individuals accept care from either gender. Some younger and older, more traditional women prefer intimate care from a same-sex health-care provider.

References

Mackle, B. (2001). New gene found for myotonia: Muscular dystrophy—unusual mutation involved. MDA News. Retrieved August 22, 2003, from www.mdaa.org/news/010803dm_mutation.html

Steckler, J. (2003). People of German ancestry. In L. Purnell and B. Paulanka (Eds.), *Transcultural health care: A culturally competent approach* (2nd ed., chapter on CD). Philadelphia: F.A. Davis Company.

Time Almanac, (2001). Boston: Time Almanac, Inc.

German

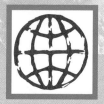

People of Greek Heritage

Overview and Heritage

This chapter presents two groups of people with Greek heritage. The first group refers to those or their ancestors who emigrated from Greece, the second group originated in Cyprus. Both groups share the same history and have a common language and religion. The Greek and Greek Cypriot diaspora is of considerable size and has spread to all continents and numerous countries. The largest Greek community outside Greece is in the United States, and the largest Greek Cypriot community outside Greece is in Britain.

Greece, a small country in southern Europe, enjoys a climate similar to that of southern California; covers slightly more than 50,000 square miles; and has a population of 10.6 million. The capital, Athens, has a population of 3 million. The land is very mountainous, with small patches of fertile land separated by hills, mountains, and the sea. The main crops are wheat, grapes, olives, cotton, and tobacco. Cyprus, located in the most eastern part of the Mediterranean Sea, is a small mountainous island with an area of 3,572 square miles (9,251 square kilometers). The capital is Nicosia. The population of 758,000 is more than 80 percent Greek Cypriot. The Greek Orthodox church stems from Cyprus. The characteristics of members of the Greek and Greek Cypriot communities vary considerably according to the time of immigration; rural, island, or urban residence; and other primary and secondary characteristics of culture as described in Chapter 1.

The core values of *philotimo* (honor and respect) and *endropi* (shame) are key when considering the experience of Greeks and Greek Cypriots. Although values of honor and shame are found in all societies, they attain immense importance among Mediterranean groups. Although *philotimo* is a characteristic of one's family, community, and nation, it most centrally implies concern for other human beings. *Philotimo* is a Greek's sense of honor and worth that is derived from one's self-image, one's reflected image (respect), and one's sense of pride. *Philotimo* is enhanced through courage, strength, fulfilling family obligations, competition with other people, hospitality, and appropriate behavior. Shame results from any conduct that is considered deviant. The system of honor and shame in the Mediterranean countries is derived from complementary differences of the sexes, the solidarity of the family, and a relationship of hostility and competition between unrelated or unconnected families.

COMMUNICATIONS

- Although all Greeks, whether in Greece, Cyprus, or the diaspora, use the same form of written language, there are regional and country variations in spoken Greek. Diasporic Greek communities regard the retention of the Greek language as an essential part of their identity; thus, much effort is expended encouraging second and subsequent generations to speak Greek. Many first-generation Greek Cypriots speak very little or no English. Obtain an interpreter when necessary; do not rely on family members, who may not fully disclose because of honor and shame.
- Greek and Greek Cypriot people tend to be expressive in both speech and gesturing. They use their hands frequently in gesturing while talking. They embrace family,

friends, and others to indicate solidarity. Whereas inner-most feelings, such as anxiety or depression, are often shielded from outsiders, anger is expressed freely, some-times to the discomfort of those from less expressive groups. Because Greeks and Greek Cypriots value warmth, expressiveness, and spontaneity, Northern Europeans are often viewed as "cold" and lacking in compassion.

- Eye contact is generally direct, and speaking and sitting distance is closer than that of European Americans. Do not take offense if patients stand closer to you than you are accustomed. Do not assume that prolonged eye contact is a sign of anger.

- Patients often appear to be compliant in the presence of the health-care worker, but this may be only superficial compliance, which is employed to ensure a smooth relationship. Stress the importance of letting the health-care provider know the patient's intentions on complying with health prescriptions.

- Greeks are oriented to the past as they are highly con-scious of the glories of ancient Greece. They are present-oriented with regard to *philotimo,* family life, and situations involving family members. However, they tend to be future-oriented with regard to educa-tional and occupational achievements. Greek Americans differentiate between "Greek time," which is used in family and social situations, and "American/clock time," which is used in business situations. Greek time emphasizes participating in activities until they reach a natural breaking point, whereas American/clock time emphasizes punctuality.

- For Greeks and Greek Cypriots, having a Greek name is an important sign of their heritage. Honorific titles might be given to members of the community who are elders or otherwise respected. Terms such as *Thia* (aunt), *Kyria* (Mrs.), or *giagia* (grandma) may be used. First names come either from the Bible, such as Maria and Petros (Peter), or from ancient Greek mythology and history, such as Eleni (Helen) and Alexandros (Alexander). Ideally, first daughters are named for the mother's mother and first sons for the father's father. Following tradition, middle names are the first name of the father; thus, all children of Stavros might carry his first name as their middle name. In health-care situations, it is not appropriate to call an elderly woman or man by the first name. The prefix Kyria or Kyrie should be used with the first name: for example, Kyria Maria or Kyrie Alexandre. Alternatively, the preferred mode of address is using the surname preceded by Mr., Mrs., or Ms.

FAMILY ROLES AND ORGANIZATION

- The father is considered the head of the household in Greek and Greek Cypriot families. The complexity of household dynamics is noted in the well-known folk saying, "The man is the head, but the wife is the neck that decides which way the head will turn." This acknowledges the primacy of fathers in the public sphere and the strong influence of women in the private sphere. In recent years, there has been increased recognition of a trend toward more equality in decision-making.

- The core values of *philotimo* and *endropi* set the pattern for the family and for the enactment of gender roles. The roles of husband and wife are characterized by mutual respect (a partnership). However, their relationship is less significant than that of the family as a unit. Fathers are responsible for providing for the family, whereas women are responsible for the management of the home and children. Protection of family members and maintenance of family solidarity tends to be foremost among their values. As a consequence, they are often friendly but somewhat superficial and distant with those considered "outsiders."

- Traditionally, the cleanliness and order of the home reflect the moral character of the woman.

- The family environment supports dependence and achievement. The family goals of achievement are directed toward and internalized by the children. Using a family conference is a useful tactic for teaching healthy behaviors and compliance with mutually acceptable health prescriptions.

- Children are included in most family social activities and tend not to be left with babysitters. The child is the recipient of intense affection, helpful interventions, and strong admiration. The child may be disciplined through teasing, which is thought to "toughen" children and make them highly conscious of public opinion. Accept alternative forms of childrearing as long as they are not psychologically or physically abusive.

- Greek children are expected to succeed in school. This attitude is fostered by an achievement orientation, high educational and occupational aspirations, a cohesive family unit that exhorts children to succeed, nationalistic identification with the cultural glories of ancient Greece, and private schools that teach the Greek language and culture.

- Adolescents, particularly young women, tend to reside with their parents until they get married. Unlike previous generations, spouse selection is left to the adolescent, with parental approval. Girls have considerably less freedom in dating than their brothers, and it is common for girls to be prohibited from dating until they are in the upper grades of high school. Adolescents in more traditional families may experience stress as the differences in family and peer values precipitate family conflict.

- Suppression of personal freedom by parents is a major risk factor for suicidal attempts in Greek and Greek Cypriot adolescent girls. Additional areas identified as high-stress for Greek adolescents include extreme dependence on the family, intense pressure for school achievement, and a lack of sexual education in the home. School nurses and counselors are in a good position to provide sex education and to discuss issues related to personal freedom.

- Prestige is connected to the idea that honor is collective rather than individual. Because a person loses honor if a family member acts improperly, the honor of each family member is a matter of concern for all family members. **Do not disclose "improper" behavior to family members or others.**

- Elders hold positions of respect; their stories, whether as pioneers, veterans, or hard-working business people, are well known throughout the community. Their notable deeds are heralded and documented in community histories, which are usually maintained by the Greek Orthodox churches in each local community.

- Families feel responsible to care for their parents in old age, and children are expected to take in widowed parents. Failure to do so results in a sense of dishonor for the son and guilt for the daughter. Treatment of the *giagia* (grandmother) and the *pappou* (grandfather) reflects the themes of closeness and respect emphasized in the family. Grandparents tend to participate fully in family activities. **Include grandparents in health teaching activities.**

- If the elder person is ill, living with the family is the first preference, followed by placement in a residential care facility. Although living alone is often the least preferred residential pattern, many elderly people are choosing to live alone with the support of family, friends, and health-care providers. **Help the family obtain needed support services for providing care to family members in the home setting.**

- Elderly Greek and Greek Cypriot widows and widowers, particularly those who speak little or no English, may experience social isolation if they do not have close contact with their children.

- Fictive kin, termed *koumbari* (coparents), serve as sponsors in either (or both) of two religious ceremonies: baptism and marriage. Ideally, the baptismal sponsor also serves as the sponsor of the child's marriage. The relationship of the sponsor is so important that families who are joined by this bond of fictive kinship are prohibited from intermarrying.

- The basis of social status and prestige is family *philotimo* and cohesiveness. However, social status is also received from attributes such as wealth, educational achievement, and achievements of its members. Honor is the social worth of the family as judged by the community.

- Greek and Greek Cypriot communities tend to be relatively conservative. As a consequence, alternative lifestyles encompassing premarital sex, divorce, and same-sex relationships are considered sources of concern for family members and the community. **Do not disclose matters of personal privacy to family members or others.**

BIOCULTURAL ECOLOGY

- Greeks and Greek Cypriots are most commonly of medium stature, shorter than northern Europeans, but taller than other populations of southern Europe. Although some Greeks have blue eyes and blond hair, usually from the northern provinces of Greece, most Greeks have dark hair and dark skin.
- Current causes of death among Greeks and Greek Cypriots are those of developed countries and include cancer, cardiovascular, and cerebrovascular diseases.
- Recent immigrants have high rates of typhoid and hepatitis A and B. **Assess recent immigrants for health conditions such as typhoid and hepatitis A and B.**
- Two important genetic conditions, thalassemia and glucose-6-phosphate dehydrogenase (G-6-PD), are seen in relatively high proportions among Greek populations.
- G-6-PD deficiency leads to hemolysis, which is generally well tolerated except under specific circumstances, including exercise, infections, and the presence of oxidant drugs such as primaquine, quinidine, thiazolsulfone, dapsone, furazolidone, nitrofural, naphthalene, toluidine blue, phenylhydrazine, and chloramphenicol. Even common medications such as aspirin can induce a hemolytic crisis. This threat is sufficiently severe that the World Health Organization recommends that all hospital populations in areas with high proportions of Greeks and Greek Cypriots be screened for G-6-PD deficiency before drug therapy. **Make clients aware that**

broad beans (fava beans) can induce hemolysis and an acute anemic crisis when ingested. Consider G-6-PD deficiency in Greek clients with unconjugated jaundice.

- Thalassemia is an inherited genetic disorder manifested by a slow production of or failure to synthesize hemoglobin A or B chains. Two main types are commonly known: thalassemia major (sometimes known as Cooley's anemia, homozygous or beta thalassemia major), and thalassemia minor (referred to as thalassemia trait or beta thalassemia minor). Thalassemia major, if untreated, results in death. Undiagnosed infants become pale, irritable, do not eat, suffer from recurrent fever, and fail to thrive. Eventually the liver, spleen, and heart are damaged as a result of the accumulation of iron contained in the red blood cells. Treatment includes regular blood transfusions, prevention of iron overload with deferoxamine, and bone marrow transplants. Most individuals with thalassemia minor are not aware of it unless they are tested for it. In recent years, prenatal screening programs in Greece, Cyprus, Britain, America, Canada, and Australia, where most of the diaspora resides, have drastically reduced the number of babies being born with thalassemia major. Most Greek and Greek Cypriot women choose to have an abortion if they are found to carry an affected fetus. Screen Greek clients for thalassemias, and advise them of genetic risks.

HIGH-RISK HEALTH BEHAVIORS

- Greeks in Greece, the United States, Canada, and Australia demonstrate less nontherapeutic drug use, alcoholism, and high-risk sexual behaviors than other groups in European or North American countries. These patterns are not due to an emphasis on health promotion but rather to a hyperawareness of the social consequences of these behaviors for the family.
- A commitment to honor and concern for the reputation and standing of the family are prime deterrents to many high-risk behaviors. Alcohol is most often considered a

food item and is consumed with meals. However, losing control by being "under the influence" engenders considerable gossip and social disgrace, focused not only on the individual but also on the family.

- Obesity among both sexes and smoking among men are high among Greeks. Although a high level of risk-taking appears to be part of survival, it is in fact perpetuated by the belief that "God will look after me" in that God will prevent anything untoward happening and that if anything should happen, God will heal and sustain the person.

- Greeks and Greek Cypriots tend to disregard standard health promotion behaviors. Safety measures for adults, such as seat belts and helmets, are often viewed as infringements on personal freedom and are frequently ignored, particularly by the older generation. Explain the legal aspects of seat belt and helmet laws, and encourage their use.

NUTRITION

- Greeks describe their culture as an "eating culture." Food is a centerpiece of everyday life as well as of social and ritual events.

- Fasting is an integral part of the Greek Orthodox religion. General fast days are Wednesdays and Fridays. During fasts, it is forbidden to eat meat, fish, and animal products such as eggs, cheese, and milk. At least 3 days of fasting must be observed by anyone wishing to take Holy Communion. Some first-generation Greeks and Greek Cypriots observe the four major fasting periods that include the Great Fast, Lent, for 7 weeks before Easter; the Fast of the Apostles, from Monday 8 days after Pentecost to June 28, the eve of the Feast of the Saints Peter and Paul; the Assumption fast, from August 1 to August 14; and the Christmas fast, from November 15 to December 14. Make accommodation for patients to fast if it is not contradictory to their health status. People with health conditions and small children are exempt from fasting.

- Greeks and Greek Cypriots base their diet on cereals, pulses, lentils, vegetables, fruits, olive oil, cheese, and milk. They are also relatively high consumers of sweets and snacks. For adults, dairy products are consumed in the form of yogurt or cheeses such as feta, kopanisti, kefaloteri, kasseri, and halloumi.
- The prevalence of lactose maldigestion in Greek adults is about 75 percent; however, milk intolerance rarely occurs in children. Acknowledge the presence of lactose intolerance, and help clients choose alternative sources of calcium.
- Fats are consumed in the form of olive oil, butter, and olives. Meats include chicken and lamb or, in the United States and Britain, beef adaptations. Eggs; lentils; and fish such as shrimp and other shellfish, whitefish, and anchovies are additional sources of protein.
- Vegetables such as potatoes, eggplant, courgettes (zucchini), spinach, garlic, onions, peas, artichokes, cucumbers, asparagus, cabbage, and cauliflower are common Greek food choices.
- Bread choices include pita, crescent rolls, and egg breads. Other foods include rice, tabouli, macaroni, and cracked wheat (bourgouri). Fruit preferences include grapes and currants, figs, prunes, oranges, lemons, melons, watermelons, peaches, and apricots.
- Common seasonings used by Greeks are anise, basil, cumin, cinnamon, citron, cloves, coriander, dill, fennel, ginger, garlic, lemon, marjoram, mint, mustard, nutmeg, oregano, parsley, rose, sage, sesame, thyme, vinegar, bay leaf, and honey.
- Beverages such as coffee, tea, chocolate milk, and wine are common choices.
- Several different special breads, pastries, and cakes are served at traditional ceremonies: New Year's bread, *vasilopita*; Easter pastries, *tsoureki* and *flaouna*; Christmas bread, *chistosomo*; *prosfora*, a traditional bread for funerals and remembrance ceremonies, which is served with *koliva*, a mixture of boiled wheat, almonds, pomegranate seeds, sesame seeds, and raisins;

and traditional small individual wedding cakes called
kourapiedes.
- Food choices and preparation practices should be
initiated on the intake assessment.

PREGNANCY AND CHILDBEARING PRACTICES

- In North America, Greeks have deliberately limited
family size so children can be adequately cared for and
educated. A wide variety of birth control measures, such
as intrauterine devices, birth control pills, and condoms
are preferred. The strong pro-life Greek Orthodox
church condemns birth control while silently accepting
the reality. Help clients identify acceptable birth control
methods.
- Abortion is absolutely condemned as an act of murder
except in circumstances that threaten the life of the
mother or when a young woman becomes pregnant as a
result of rape. In practice, a number of women, particularly those who are unmarried, have legal abortions
because of the negative consequences of having a baby
out of wedlock. Inflicting *endropi* on the family is
believed to be more severe than the consequences of
abortion. Do not disclose abortions to family or other
members of the community.
- Infertile couples experience mental stress, evidenced as
depression for women and anxiety for men. For these
couples, the reputation of the husband may be at risk
if the woman is unable to achieve her highest role.
Although adoption is rare among Greeks and Greek
Cypriots, it is becoming a more acceptable option for
couples who cannot conceive.
- Pregnancy is a time of great respect for women and a
time when women are given special considerations.
Proscriptions include not attending funerals or viewing
a corpse, refraining from sinful activity as a precaution
against infant deformity, and praying to St. Simeon.
- Pregnant women are encouraged to eat large quantities;
foods high in iron and protein are particularly
important. If a pregnant woman remarks that a food

Greek

smells good or if she has a craving for a particular food, it should be offered to her; otherwise the child may be "marked." This is the usual explanation for birthmarks. **Factually explain the potentially harmful effects on the fetus and mother of excessive weight gain during pregnancy.**

- After delivery, most traditional Greeks consider the mother ritually impure and particularly susceptible to illness for 40 days. During this time, she is admonished to stay at home and not attend church. At the end of the 40 days, the mother and child attend church and receive a ritual blessing. **Arrange for a visiting nurse if the mother is reluctant to see health-care providers in their offices.**

- For breast-feeding mothers, early showering is sometimes thought to result in the infant developing diarrhea and becoming allergic to milk. Newborns are generally breast-fed, and solids are not introduced early.

- When relatives visit an infant in the hospital, silver objects or coins may be placed in the crib for good luck. **Do not remove good luck charms from the infant's crib or bed.**

DEATH RITUALS

- Last rites are administered in the sacrament of Holy Communion given by a priest or occasionally by a deacon.

- A *klama* (wake) is held in the family home or, more commonly in North America today, in a funeral home. All relatives and friends are expected to attend for at least a brief time. Even people with whom the deceased had considerable strife are expected to attend. The wake ends when the priest arrives and offers prayers. Pictures and mirrors may be turned over. During the wake, women may sing dirges or chant. In some regions, people practice "screaming the dead," in which they cry a lament, the *miroloyi*. This ritual may involve screaming, lamenting, and sobbing by female kin.

- In Greece and Cyprus, the *kidia* (funeral) is held the

following day at the Orthodox church, with internment in a cemetery. After internment, family and friends gather for a meal of fish, symbolizing Christianity; wine, cheese, and olives in the family home or a restaurant.

- On the basis of the Orthodox belief in the physical resurrection of the body, Greeks and Greek Cypriots reject cremation. The extent of adherence to this precept varies in North America, but Greeks and Greek Cypriots in Britain do not practice cremation.
- Black is the color of mourning dress and is often worn by family members throughout the 40 days of mourning; for widows it may be worn longer. Formerly, a widow was expected to wear black and no jewelry or makeup for the rest of her life. While black armbands are still worn in Greece and Cyprus, that custom is virtually nonexistent in immigrant communities.
- After death, family and close relatives, who may stay at home, mourn for 40 days. Close male relatives do not shave as a mark of respect. A memorial service follows 40 days after burial and at 3 months, 6 months, and yearly thereafter. At the end of this service, *koliva* (boiled wheat with powdered sugar) is served to participants, and mourning is conducted with joyful reverence. Accept varied expressions of grief and rituals related to death and dying.

SPIRITUALITY

- Most Greeks in America are affiliated with the Greek Orthodox church, whereas Greeks and Greek Cypriots in Britain are affiliated with the Archdiocese of Thyateria and Great Britain. The central religious experience is the Sunday morning liturgy, which is a high church service with icons, incense, and singing or chanting by the choir.
- The Greek Orthodox religion emphasizes faith rather than specific tenets. The Greek faith does not emphasize Bible reading and study. Some parishioners attend church services weekly; others attend only a few times a year.

Greek

- Easter is considered the most important of holy days, and nearly all Greeks and Greek Cypriots in America and Britain attempt to honor the day.
- There is a strong belief in miracles, even among second and subsequent generations of Greeks and Greek Cypriots in America and Britain. Daily prayers may be offered to the saints. Women often consider faith an important factor in regaining health. Family members may make "bargains" with saints, such as promises to fast, be faithful, or make church donations if the saint acts on behalf of the ill family member. They may call on an individual's namesake or a saint believed to have special affinity with healing.
- For Greeks and Greek Cypriots, sources of strength are the family, the close network of extended family and friends, and the history of the glories of ancient Greece. The Greek concept of self consists of the interrelationship of the three values: self-respect, a sense of freedom, and the concept of the ideal person. The self emerges through relationships with other people but primarily from the family. Freedom is a central element in self-concept. Self-reliance, that is, nonreliance on people outside the family, is a virtue.
- Particularly in immigrant communities, the Greek Orthodox church serves as a base for spirituality, language, social and political organization, and an ongoing identity with Greece and Cyprus.
- A distinctive feature of the Greek Orthodox religion is the place it assigns to icons, such as paintings of saints, the Virgin Mary, and Christ. These icons are not religious art but have sacred significance as sources of connection to the spiritual world. Icons grace the walls and ceilings of churches and cathedrals and are also found in personal altars in homes. In the homes, holy vigil candles are often kept burning. To ensure safety and health, many begin each day by kissing the blessed icons and making the sign of the Greek cross.
- When a person is ill, the icon of the family saint or the Virgin Mary may be placed above the bed. Do not remove religious art or icons from the patient's bedside.

- Many Greeks and Greek Cypriots also may sprinkle their homes with holy water from Epiphany Day church services to protect the members of their household from evil.

HEALTH-CARE PRACTICES

- The amount of acceptance and use of biomedicine is highly related to one's level of education and generation of immigration. Although fourth-generation Greek Americans are highly traditional in many aspects of their lives, such as religion, language retention, and food preferences, they have not retained many of the folk beliefs and practices concerning health care.
- Greek immigrants tend to be anxious about health, to lack trust in health professionals, and to rely on family and community for advice and remedies. **Inquire about home treatments in a nonjudgmental manner.**
- To be healthy means to feel strong, joyful, and content; to be able to take care of oneself; and to be free from pain. Threats to health result from a lack of balance in life; departure from family; neglect of education or work; and failure to demonstrate right behaviors, such as respect toward parents, sharing with family, upholding religious precepts, and staying out too late.
- Problems are considered originating outside the individual's control and are attributed to God, the devil, spirits, and envy or malice of others. The gods may punish the nonreligious with illness, *asthenia,* or *arrostia*, but more often the forces of evil are believed to cause illness.
- The family generally assumes responsibility and care for a sick member and works to control interactions with health professionals. **Encourage empowerment, and help the family care for their family member.**
- Greeks are extremely reluctant to use welfare services or other forms of governmental assistance to meet their health-care needs. Reliance on public assistance might indicate that the sick person and family are not self-reliant. Greeks in America are also reluctant to rely on

Greek community organizations, such as the women's Philoptochos Society (Friends of the Poor), for support.

- First-generation Greek and Greek Cypriots in Britain use voluntary organizations to obtain information and advice in Greek and to receive help completing various documents that enable them to receive the financial and other benefits to which they are entitled. No stigma is attached to the utilization of Greek/Greek Cypriot community organizations in Britain because their function is not associated with the *philoptochos* movement, whose function is to help the poor.

- In Britain, the National Health Service provides free health care to all citizens. Greek Cypriots readily take their children to the family doctor and do not delay seeing the physician for their own health problems when these are severe enough to prevent them from going to work or from executing important family functions and roles.

- Men in particular tend to delay seeking medical help when they can self-care for something considered nonacute or when they suspect they may be suffering from something more serious such as cancer (Papadopoulos & Lees, 2002).

- Three traditional folk healing practices are particularly notable: those related to *matiasma* (bad eye or evil eye), *practika* (herbal remedies), and *vendousas* (cupping). *Matiasma* results from the envy or admiration of others. While the eye is able to harm a wide variety of things including inanimate objects, children are particularly susceptible to attack. Common symptoms include headache, chills, irritability, restlessness, and lethargy; in extreme cases, *matiasma* has resulted in death. Greeks employ a variety of preventive mechanisms to thwart the effects of envy or evil eye, including protective charms in the form of *phylactos*, amulets consisting of blessed wood or incense, or blue "eye" beads, which "reflect" the eye. **Do not remove protective charms from the patient or from the bedside.**

- When the diagnosis of *matiasma* is suspected, the most common method of detection consists of placing olive

Greek

oil in a glass of water. If the oil disperses, then the eye has been cast. Subsequent treatment consists of physical acts, such as making the sign of the Greek cross over the glass of water or reciting ritual prayers passed on in families by members of the opposite sex. In particularly severe cases, the Orthodox priest may recite special prayers of exorcism and use incense to fumigate the afflicted person.

- *Practika* are herbal and humoral treatments used for initial self-treatment. Chamomile, the most popular herb, is generally used in teas for gastric distress or abdominal pain, including infant colic and menstrual cramps. It is also used as an expectorant to treat colds.

- Liquors, such as anisette, ouzo, and *mestika*, are used primarily for colds, sore throats, and coughs and are consumed alone or in combination with tea, lemon, honey, or sugar, either alone or in some combination. Occasionally, liquors are used for treatment of *nevra* (nerves). Raw garlic is used as prevention for colds, and cooked garlic is used for blood pressure and heart disease. Encourage clients to fully disclose the use of complementary and alternative practices.

- *Vendousas*, a healing practice, is used as a treatment for colds, high blood pressure, and backache. It consists of lighting a swab of cotton held on a fork, then placing the swab in an inverted glass, thereby creating a vacuum in the glass, which is then placed on the back of the ill person. The skin on the back is drawn into the glass. This procedure is repeated 8 to 12 times. An alternative method, for particularly serious cases, is the *kofte*, "cut *vendousa*." Here, the same procedure is followed, except that a cut in the shape of a cross is made on the skin. When the glass is placed over this cut, blood is drawn into the glass. The therapeutic rationale for using *vendousas* surrounds its counterirritant effect; the technique increases and revitalizes the circulation, draws out poisons and "cold," and prevents coagulation of blood. Fourth-generation community members rarely use *vendousas*.

- The primary barriers to health care for Greek and Greek Cypriots in America and Britain include a reliance on self-care in the family context and a general distrust of bureaucracies.

- Self-medicating behaviors are common, with herbal remedies and over-the-counter medications used widely for specific symptoms. **Encourage full disclosure of over-the-counter drug use.**

- Mental illness is accompanied by social stigma, with negative consequences for the afflicted person as well as the family and relatives. Shame originates in the notion that mental illness is hereditary; afflicted people are viewed as having lifelong conditions that "pollute" the bloodline. The stigma is so wide-ranging that people labeled as mentally ill and their families may experience the loss of friends and social isolation. As a result, families place a wide variety of behaviors within the range of "normal" to delay receiving the stigmatized label.

- Individuals with mental illness often present with somatic complaints such as dizziness and paresthesias on initial visits to health-care practitioners. Recent immigrants tend to have higher rates of mental disorders, which perhaps result from the stress of culture change. **Do not disclose emotional or psychiatric disorders to people outside the immediate family.**

- A folk model for *nevra* is a socially acceptable and culturally condoned medium for the expression of otherwise unacceptable emotions. *Nevra* is experienced most commonly by those in positions of least power, such as women and people living in poverty. It encompasses a wide variety of symptoms and provides a metaphor for social disorders, such as conflict between close kin or intergenerational conflict. Ideally, *nevra* are treated through medications for the relief of symptoms instead of through talk therapy.

- Individuals with physical illnesses such as asthma, diabetes, and arthritis are most accepted, followed by people with disfiguring illnesses such as cerebral palsy. Individuals and families experiencing mental retardation, psychiatric illness, and acquired immunodeficiency syndrome are less accepted. People in the most stigmatized groups are those with social deviance, such as addictions or delinquency.

- *Ponos* (pain) is the cardinal symptom of ill health and an evil that needs eradication. The person in pain is not expected to suffer quietly or stoically in the presence of family. The family is relied on to find resources to relieve the pain or, failing that, to share in the experience of suffering. In the presence of outsiders, the lack of restraint in pain expression suggests lack of self-control, and therefore it is considered *endropi*. **Provide adequate pain relief to help the patient maintain control.**
- The key aspect of the sick role is for the sick to fully rely on the family for sustenance. When an individual is ill, it is particularly important that he or she not be left alone.
- When hospitalization occurs, family members expect to stay with the individual, even during examinations and therapeutic procedures. Families are expected to ensure that sick family members are not harmed and are receiving the best care possible. Protection even includes shielding the sick from a serious diagnosis, such as cancer, until the family feels the individual is ready to learn about the diagnosis. **Make arrangements to accommodate multiple visitors. Determine the spokesperson for the family and obtain his/her assistance in visitor control. Seek assistance from the family spokesperson or next of kin before informing the patient of a grave diagnosis.**
- On the basis of the Christian Orthodox belief in the physical resurrection of the body, some Greeks and Greek Cypriots may reject the concept of autopsy and do not readily accept organ donation. However, the Greek Orthodox church is strongly pro-life and more recently has been encouraging organ donation as an act of love.
- Blood transfusions are wholly acceptable and are common for people with thalassemia.

HEALTH-CARE PRACTITIONERS

- A woman who cures, particularly one who cures the evil eye, is known as a *magissa*, which is usually translated as "witch" but means "magician"; she may also be called doctor. In the United States and Britain, "wise women" from one's own family conduct most lay healing. Occasionally, for particularly difficult cases of *matiasma*, a woman with particular gifts in diagnosis and healing may be called. The priest may also be called on for advice, blessings, exorcisms, and direct healing. **Assist patients and family in obtaining a priest or magissa.**

- Many Greeks and Greek Cypriots display a general distrust of all professionals. Considerable shopping around for physicians and other professionals to obtain additional opinions is relatively common even in Britain where health care is provided free to all citizens. This is particularly true if the sick person does not receive the diagnosis or the amount of sympathy judged appropriate by the family. Inconsistencies in opinions or recommendations result in further concern. The use of several physicians simultaneously may result in untoward drug interactions from conflicting interventions or overdoses. **Encourage clients to disclose the use of all health-care providers seen and treatments used.**

- Hospitals are a particular source of mistrust both for Greeks and Greek Cypriots. When hospitalizations occur, the family may be perceived by staff as demanding or "interfering" as they enact their protective advocacy roles. Mothers may demand to sleep with their children and fear that the children may not receive appropriate care. There is also a fear that the sick person may be used as a subject for experimentation. **Encourage family members to participate in hospital procedures.**

References

Beratis, S. (1990). Factors associated with adolescent suicidal attempts in Greece. *Psychopathology, 23,* 161–168.

Greek Herbs (2002). Retrieved December 22, 2003, from www.e-greekherbs.com

Marjoribanks, K. (1994). Cross-cultural comparisons of family environments of Anglo, Greek, and Italian Australians. *Psychological Reports, 74,* 49–50.

Papadopoulos, I. & Lees, S. (2002). *Cancer and culture: Investigating meanings and experiences of cancer of men from different ethnic groups. A pilot study.* London: Research Centre for Transcultural Studies in Health, Middlesex University.

Purnell, L., & Papadopoulos, I. (2003). People of Greek heritage. In L Purnell and B. Paulanka (Eds.), *Transcultural health care: A culturally competent approach,* (2nd ed., chapter on CD). Philadelphia: F.A. Davis Company.

Time Almanac. (2001). Boston: Time Inc.

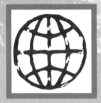

People of Haitian Heritage

Overview and Heritage

Haiti, located on the island of Hispaniola between Cuba and Puerto Rico in the Caribbean, shares the island with the Dominican Republic. With a population of 7 million and an area of 10,714 square miles, it is about the size of the state of Maryland. The capital and largest city, Port-au-Prince, has a population of more than 800,000. The per capita annual income is $248, with a daily wage rate of $3. The infant mortality rate is high, with 95.23 deaths per 1,000 live births; life expectancy is low at only 49.38 years, and only 13 percent of the people have access to potable water (*World Factbook,* 2003). Haiti defines itself as a black nation. Therefore, all Haitians are members of the black race. In Haiti, the concept of color differs from the concept of race. The Haitian system has been described as one in which there are no tight racial categories but in which skin color and other phenotypic demarcations are significant variables.

The Haitian population in the United States is not well documented because many are undocumented immigrants. According to the 2000 U.S. census, 500,000 Haitians live in the United States; others believe the number is closer to 1.5 million. Like other ethnic groups, Haitians are very diverse according to the primary and secondary characteristics of culture as described in Chapter 1.

Before 1920, Haitians traveled to North America only for educational purposes. After 1920, peasants were forced to go to Cuba and the Dominican Republic to cut sugarcane. Haitian land was taken and used for apple and banana plantations, and many acres of land throughout Haiti were controlled by the United States. The atrocities that accompanied the American occupation resulted in a small group of Haitians leaving Haiti and settling in the Harlem section of New York City, where they assimilated into American society.

When Duvalier was elected president-for-life in 1964, many Haitians covertly immigrated to the United States in small sailboats, resulting in their being labeled "boat people," a term that is associated with extreme poverty. Even though Haitians value education, only 15 percent are privileged enough to attain a formal education. The illiteracy rate of 80% continues to be a major concern in Haiti. Among Haitian immigrants in the United States, women often work in hotels, hospitals, and other service industries where they assume domestic and nursing assistant roles. Men work as laborers and factory helpers.

COMMUNICATIONS

- There are two official languages in Haiti, French and Creole. French is the dominant language of the educated and the elite, whereas Creole is the language of those who are suppressed: the lower classes. Creole, a rich, expressive language, is spoken by 100 percent of the population. Health-care providers should **develop video programs, audiocassettes, and picture brochures in Creole for providing health education.**
- Most individuals are very expressive with their emotions, including loud, animated speech. Pain and sorrow are very obvious in facial expressions.
- Most Haitians are affectionate, polite, and shy. The uneducated generally hide their lack of knowledge by

keeping to themselves, avoiding conflict, and sometimes projecting a timid air or attitude. They smile frequently and often respond in this manner when they do not understand what is being said.

- Many individuals pretend to understand by nodding; this sign of approval is given to hide their limitations. Because Haitians are very private, especially in health matters, it is inappropriate to share information with friends. Many clients may prefer to use professional interpreters, who will give an accurate interpretation of their concerns. Most important, the interpreter should be someone with whom they have no relationship and will likely never see again. Use simple and clear instructions. Ask family members to assist with interpretation only if an interpreter is not available.

- Voice intonations convey emotions, and some people speak loudly even in casual conversation. When the conversation is really animated, the conversants speak in close proximity and ignore territorial space. Sometimes the conversation is at such a high pitch and speed that, to an outsider, the conversation may appear disorganized or angry. Do not interpret loud conversations as anger.

- Traditionally, Haitians generally do not maintain eye contact when speaking with those in a position of authority. Maintaining direct eye contact can be considered rude and insolent, especially when speaking with superiors. Do not interpret lack of eye contact as not listening or not caring.

- Haitians touch frequently when speaking with friends. They may touch you to make you aware that they are speaking to you. Do not take offense from a casual touch on the arm or shoulder.

- Haitians greet each other by kissing and embracing in informal situations. In formal encounters, they shake hands and appear composed and stern. Men usually do not kiss women unless they are old friends or relatives. Children greet everyone by kissing them on the cheek. Children refer to adult friends as uncle or auntie.

- Temporal orientation is a balance among the past,

Haitian

present, and future. The past is important because it lays the historical foundation from which one must learn. The present is cherished and savored. The future is predetermined, and God is the only supreme being who can redirect it. The future is left up to God, who is trusted to do the right thing.

- Haitians have a fatalistic but serene view of life. Some believe that destiny or spiritual forces are in control of life events such as health and death. **To achieve acceptance, build trust, and ensure compliance, be clear, honest, and open when assessing individuals' perceptions and how they perceive the forces that have an influence over life, health, and illness.**
- Most do not respect clock time; flexibility with time is the norm, and punctuality is not valued. Most Haitians hold to a relativistic view of time, and although they try, some find it difficult to respond to predetermined appointments. It is not considered impolite to arrive late for appointments, even medical appointments. **Make reminder calls for appointments, and encourage the client about the importance of timeliness.**
- Most Haitians have a first, middle, and last name; sometimes the first two names are hyphenated as in Marie-Maude. The family name is very important in middle- and upper-class society, promoting and communicating tradition and prestige. Families usually have an affectionate name or nickname for individuals.
- When a woman marries, she takes her husband's full name. She loses her name except on paper. Most names are of French origin, although many Arabic names are also heard. Most are formal and respectful. **Address clients by their title: Mr., Mrs., Miss, Ms., Doctor, or other title.**

FAMILY ROLES AND ORGANIZATION

- Traditionally, the head of the household has been the man, but today most families are matriarchal. The man is generally considered the primary income provider for the family, and daily decision-making is considered his province. Women are expected to be faithful, honest, and respectable.

- Children are valued among Haitians because they are key to the family's progeny, cultural beliefs, and values. Children are expected to be high achievers. Children are expected to be obedient and respectful to parents and older people. They are not allowed to express anger to older people.

- Physical punishment, often used as a way of disciplining children, is sometimes considered child abuse by U.S. standards. Fear of having their children taken away from them because of their methods of discipline can cause parents to withdraw or not follow through on health-care appointments if such abuse is evident (e.g., bruises or belt marks). Educate parents about American methods of discipline and laws so they can learn new ways of disciplining their children without compromising their beliefs or violating American laws.

- In the summer, parents engage their children in health promotion activities such as giving them *lok* (a laxative), a mixture of bitter tea leaves, juice, sugarcane syrup, and oil. Children are also given *lavman* (enemas) to ensure cleanliness. This rids the bowel of impurities and refreshes it, prevents acne, and rejuvenates the body.

- Boys are given more freedom than girls and are even expected to receive outside initiation in social and sexual life. Girls are educated toward marriage and respectability. Even when they are 16 or 17 years of age, girls cannot go out alone because any mishap can be a threat to the future of the girl and bring shame to her family. Assist children and family members to work through these cultural differences related to proper age for dating while conveying respect for family and cultural beliefs.

- The expression "blood is thicker than water" reflects family connectedness. An important unit for decision-making is the family council, which is composed of influential members of the family, including grandparents. The family structure is authoritarian and includes linear roles and responsibilities. Any action

Haitian

taken by one family member has repercussions for the entire family; consequently, all share prestige and shame. Health-care providers should **suggest the family seek counsel for family health-care decision-making.**

- The family system includes the nuclear, consanguine, and affinal relatives, some or all of whom may live under the same roof. **Include family members in the care of loved ones to achieve more trusting relationships and greater compliance with treatment regimens.**

- When family members are ill and in the hospital, there is an obligation to be there for them; all family members try to visit. **Suggest alternate locations for family members to gather, and ask a family member to help regulate the number of visitors at any one time.**

- When grandparents are no longer able to function independently, they move in with their children. Older people are highly respected and are often addressed by an affectionate title such as aunt, uncle, grandma, or grandpa, even if they are not related. Their children are expected to care for and provide for them when self-care becomes a concern. The elderly are family advisers, babysitters, historians, and consultants.

- Most Haitians are reluctant to place their elderly family members in nursing homes.

- Homosexuality is taboo; gay and lesbian individuals usually remain closeted. If a family member discloses homosexuality, everyone keeps it quiet; there is total denial. Gay and lesbian relationships are not talked about; they remain buried. **Do not disclose lesbian and gay relationships to family members.**

- Although divorce is common, family members, friends, the church, and elders try to counsel the couple before the divorce becomes final. **Approach divorce carefully, and establish a trusting relationship before discussing it.**

- Single parenting, widespread in Haiti, is well accepted and closely tied to the issue of concubinage. In Haitian society it is a well-accepted practice for men to have both a wife and a mistress. Both women bear children. The mistress raises her children alone and with minimal support from the father. Haitian women in general know that their husbands are involved in extramarital relationships but pretend not to know. **Approach health education, birth control, and safe-sex issues with sensitivity and acceptance within cultural boundaries.**

BIOCULTURAL ECOLOGY

- Different assessment techniques are required when assessing dark-skinned people for anemia and jaundice. Examine the sclera, oral mucosa, conjunctiva, lips, nail beds, palms of the hands, and soles of the feet when assessing for cyanosis and low blood hemoglobin levels. To assess for jaundice, examine the conjunctiva and oral mucosa for patches of bilirubin pigment because dark skin has natural underlying tones of red and yellow.
- Prevalent diseases in Haiti include cholera, parasitosis, and malaria. Haiti has no mosquito control. Assess newer immigrants for signs of malaria such as chills, fever, fatigue, and an enlarged spleen.
- Other diseases of increased incidence among immigrants are hepatitis, tuberculosis, HIV/AIDS, venereal diseases, and parasitosis from inadequate potable water sources in their homeland. Haitians living in Haiti were routinely vaccinated with bacille Calmette-Guérin, thus making all subsequent skin tests positive.
- High rates of diabetes, cancer, hypertension, and cardio-vascular disease are a reflection of genetics and diet, which is high in fat, cholesterol, and salt. **Encourage a low-fat, low-salt diet while recommending culturally preferred food choices.**

HIGH-RISK HEALTH BEHAVIORS

- Behaviors that may be considered high-risk in American society are generally viewed as recreational or unimportant among Haitians.
- Alcohol plays an important part in society and is culturally approved for men. Women drink socially and in moderation. Cigarette smoking is practiced by men,

Haitian

whereas Haitian women have a very low rate of tobacco use.

- Other high-risk behaviors include non-use of seat belts and helmets when driving or using a motorcycle or bicycle because Haitians are not accustomed to these safety measures in Haiti. **Educate clients about traffic laws, seat belt use, car seats for youngsters, and the need for helmets. Use graphic videos or skits when instructing clients about these safety practices. Use Haitian radio stations for educational programs when they are available. Promote behavioral changes using church and community group activities.**

NUTRITION

- For many, food means survival; however, food is also relished as a cultural treasure, and most Haitians retain their food habits and practices after emigrating. They prefer eating at home, take pride in promoting their culture through their food choices to their children, and discourage fast food. When hospitalized, many individuals would rather fast than eat non-Haitian food. They do not eat yogurt, cottage cheese, or "runny" egg yolks. They drink a lot of water, homemade fruit juices, and cold fruity sodas. **Encourage family members to bring food from home for the hospitalized patient.**
- The typical breakfast consists of bread, butter, bananas, and coffee. Children are allowed to drink coffee, which is not as strong as that consumed by adults.
- The largest meal is eaten at lunch, which includes rice and beans, boiled plantains, a salad made of watercress and tomatoes, and stewed vegetables and beef or corn-meal cooked as polenta.
- "Hot and cold," "acid and non-acid, " and "heavy and light" are the major categories of contrast when discussing food. Illness is caused when the body is exposed to an imbalance of *fret* (cold) or *cho* (hot) factors. For example, soursop, a large green prickly fruit with a white pulp that is used in juice and ice cream, is

considered a cold food and is avoided when a woman is menstruating; eating white beans after childbirth is believed to induce hemorrhage.

- Foods that are considered heavy, such as plantain, cornmeal mush, rice, and meat, are to be eaten during the day because they provide energy. Light foods, such as hot chocolate milk, bread, and soup, are eaten for dinner because they are more easily digested.

- To treat a person in the hot-and-cold system, a potent drink or herbal medicine of the class opposite to the disease is administered. For example, cough medicines are considered to be in the hot category, and laxatives are in the cold category.

- Teenagers are advised to avoid drinking citrus fruit juices such as lemonade to prevent the development of acne.

- After performing strenuous activities or any activity that causes the body to become hot, one should not eat cold food because that will create an imbalance, causing a condition called *chofret*. A woman who has just straightened her hair by using a hot comb and then opens a refrigerator may become a victim of *chofret*. This means she may catch a cold and/or possibly develop pneumonia.

- When ill, pumpkin soup, bouillon, or a special soup made with green vegetables, meat, plantains, dumplings, and yams is consumed.

- Eating right entails eating sufficient food to feel full and maintain a constant body weight, which is often higher than weight standards medically recommended in the United States. Men like to see "plump" women. **Negotiate a desirable weight with clients.**

- Weight loss is considered one of the most important signs of illness. In addition, a healthy diet includes tonics to stimulate the appetite and the use of high-calorie supplements such as *Akasan*, which is prepared either plain or made as a special drink with cream of cornmeal, evaporated milk, cinnamon, vanilla extract, sugar, and a pinch of salt.

- **Ask clients about food rituals when designing individu-**

Haitian

alized dietary plans to facilitate compliance with dietary
regimens that promote a healthier lifestyle.
- Many women and children who come from rural areas
  have significant protein deficiencies. A cultural factor
  that contributes to this problem is the uneven distribution of protein among family members. The problem
  is not one of net protein deficiency in the community
  but rather the unwise distribution of the available
  protein among family members. Whenever meat is
  served, the major portion goes to the men on the
  assumption that they must be well fed to provide for
  the household. Being aware that men receive the largest
  protein servings enables health-care practitioners to
  prepare nutritional plans that meet clients' dietary
  needs.

PREGNANCY AND CHILDBEARING PRACTICES

- Pregnancy and fertility practices are not readily used.
  Most Haitians are Catholic and are unwilling to overtly
  engage in conversation about birth control or abortion.
- Abortion is viewed as a woman's issue and is left to her
  and her significant other to decide. Be cautious in
  assessing and gathering information related to fertility
  control.
- Pregnancy is not considered a health problem; rather, it
  is a time of joy for the entire family. Because pregnancy
  is not a disease, many women do not seek prenatal care.
  Pregnancy does not relieve a woman from her work.
- Pregnant women are restricted from eating spices that
  may irritate the fetus. They eat vegetables and red fruits
  because these are believed to improve the fetus's blood.
  They are encouraged to eat large quantities of food
  because they are eating for two.
- Pregnant women who experience increased salivation
  may rid themselves of the excess at places that may
  seem inappropriate. They may even carry a "spit" cup
  in order to rid themselves of the excess saliva. They are
  not embarrassed by this behavior because they feel it is
  perfectly normal.

- During labor, the woman may walk, squat, pace, sit, or rub her belly. Generally, women practice natural childbirth and do not ask for analgesia. Some may scream or cry and become hysterical, whereas others are stoic, only moaning and grunting. **Women in labor need support and reassurance. Applying a cold compress on the woman's forehead demonstrates caring and sensitivity of the practitioner.**
- Cesarean birth is feared because it is abdominal surgery.
- Fathers do not generally participate in labor and delivery, believing that this is a private event that is best handled by women. The woman is not coached; female members of the family give assistance as needed.
- Postpartum, the woman takes an active role in her own care. She dresses warmly after birth as a way to become healthy and clean.
- Many believe that the bones are "open" after birth and that a woman should stay in bed during the first 2 to 3 days postpartum to allow the bones to close. Wearing an abdominal binder is another way to facilitate closing the bones.
- The postpartum woman also engages in a practice called "the three baths." For the first 3 days, the mother bathes in hot water boiled with special leaves that are either bought or picked from the field. She also drinks tea boiled from these leaves. For the next 3 days, the mother bathes in water prepared with leaves that are warmed by the sun. At this point, the mother takes only water or tea warmed by the sun. Another important practice is for the mother to take a vapor bath with boiled orange leaves to enhance cleanliness and tighten the internal muscles. At the end of the 3rd to 4th week, the new mother takes the third bath, which is the cold bath. A cathartic may be administered to cleanse her intestinal tract. When the process is completed, she may drink cold water again and resume her normal activities.
- In the postpartum period, women avoid white foods such as lima beans, okra, mushrooms, and tomatoes because they are believed to increase vaginal discharge. Strength foods include porridge, rice and red beans,

Haitian

plantains boiled or grated with the skins and prepared as porridge (the skin is high in iron), carrot juice, and carrot juice mixed with red beet juice.

- Breast-feeding is encouraged for up to 9 months postpartum. Breast milk can become detrimental to both mother and child if it becomes too thick or too thin. If it is too thin, it is believed that the milk has "turned," and it may cause diarrhea and headaches in the child and, possibly, postpartum depression in the mother. If milk is too "thick," it is believed to cause *bouton* (impetigo).
- Breast-feeding and bottle feeding are accepted practices. If the child develops diarrhea, breast-feeding is immediately discontinued. Encourage and support practices that do not put the mother or the child at risk.
- *Lok*, similar to the one administered to the older children in the summer, is given to infants to hasten the expulsion of meconium. Stress the risks associated with *lok* and the need to prevent dehydration.

DEATH RITUALS

- Generally, Haitians prefer to die at home rather than in the hospital.
- When death is imminent, the family may pray and cry uncontrollably, sometimes even hysterically. Try to meet the person's spiritual needs by encouraging family members to bring religious medallions, pictures of saints, or fetishes.
- When the person dies, all family members try to be at the bedside and have a prayer service. If possible and if it is not too disturbing to other clients, encourage a family member to assist with postmortem care.
- Generally, a male kinsman of the deceased makes the arrangements. This person may also be more fluent in English and more accustomed to dealing with the bureaucracy. The kinsman is responsible for notifying all family members, wherever they might be in the world, an important activity because family members' travel plans influence funeral arrangements.

Additionally, he is responsible for ordering the coffin, making arrangements for prayer services before the funeral, and coordinating plans for the funeral service.

- The preburial activity is called *veye*, a gathering of family and friends who come to the house of the deceased to cry, tell stories about the deceased's life, and laugh. Food, tea, coffee, and rum are in abundant supply. The intent is to show support and to join the family in sharing this painful loss.

- Another religious ritual is the *dernie priye,* a special prayer service consisting of 7 consecutive days of prayer, which facilitates the passage of the soul from this world to the next. It usually takes place in the home.

- On the seventh day, there is a mass called *prise de deuil,* which officially begins the mourning process. After each of these prayers, there is a reception/celebration in memory of the deceased.

- Most Haitians are very cautious about autopsies. If foul play is suspected, they may request an autopsy to ensure the patient is really dead. This alleviates their fear that their loved one is being zombified. According to the belief, this can occur when the person appears to have died of natural causes but is still alive. About 18 hours after the burial, the person is stolen from his or her coffin; the lack of oxygen causes some of the brain cells to die, so the mental facilities cease to exist while the body remains alive. The zombie then responds to commands, having no "free will," and is domesticated as a slave.

SPIRITUALITY

- Catholicism is the primary religion of Haitians but a number are Protestant.
- Although most Haitians are deeply religious, their religious beliefs are combined with voodooism, a complex religion with its roots in Africa. Voodooism involves communication by trance between the believer and ancestors, saints, or animistic deities. Participants

Haitian

gather to worship the *loa*, deities or spirits, who are
believed to have received their powers from God, and
who are capable of expressing themselves through
possession of a chosen believer.

- Believers in voodooism attribute their ailments or
  medical problems to the doings of evil spirits. In such
  cases, they prefer to confirm their suspicions through
  the *loa* before accepting natural causes as the problem,
  which would lead to seeking Western medical care.
  Belief in the power of the supernatural can have a great
  influence on the psychological and medical concerns of
  clients.
- The extended family is a primary source of strength to
  most.
- Recognizing and accepting clients' beliefs alleviates
  barriers and may make clients feel more at ease to
  discuss their beliefs and needs.

HEALTH-CARE PRACTICES

- Good health is seen as the ability to achieve internal
  equilibrium between *cho* and *fret*. To become balanced,
  one must eat well, give attention to personal hygiene,
  pray, and have good spiritual habits. To promote good
  health, one must be strong, have good color, be plump,
  and be free of pain. To maintain this state, one must eat
  right, sleep right, keep warm, exercise, and keep clean.
- Illness is perceived as punishment, considered an assault
  on the body, and may have two different causes: natural
  illnesses, known as *maladi Bondye* (disease of the Lord),
  and supernatural illnesses.
- Natural illnesses may occur frequently, are of short
  duration, and are caused by environmental factors such
  as food, air, cold, heat, and gas. Other causes are
  movement of blood within the body, disequilibrium
  between hot and cold, and bone displacement.
- Supernatural illnesses are caused by angry spirits. To
  placate these spirits, clients must offer feasts called
  manger morts. If individuals do not partake in these
  rituals, misfortunes are likely to befall them. Illnesses of

supernatural origin are fundamentally a breach in rapport between the individual and his or her protector. The breach in rapport is a response from the spirit and is a way of showing disapproval of the protégé's behavior. Health can be recovered if the client takes the first step in determining the nature of the illness. This can be accomplished by eliciting the help of a voodoo priest and following the advice given by the spirit itself. **To accurately prescribe treatment options, differentiate between natural and supernatural causes of illness and disease.**

- Most individuals believe that gas may provoke pain and anemia. Gas can occur in the head, where it enters through the ears; in the stomach, where it enters through the mouth; and in the shoulders, back, legs, or appendix, where it travels from the stomach. When gas is in the stomach, the client is said to suffer *kolik* (stomach pain). Gas in the head is called *van nan tet* or *van nan zorey,* which literally means "gas in one's ears," and is believed to be a cause of headaches.

- Gas moving from one part of the body to another produces pain. Thus, the movement of gas from the stomach to the legs produces rheumatism, to the back causes back pain, and to the shoulder causes shoulder pain. **Ask clients what they think is causing their pain.**

- Foods that help dispel gas include tea made from garlic, cloves, and mint; plantain; and corn. To deter the entry of gas into the body, one must be careful about eating leftovers, especially beans. After childbirth, women are particularly susceptible to gas; to prevent entry of gas into the body, they tighten their waist with a belt or a piece of linen.

- Most Haitians engage in self-treatment and consider these activities as a way of preventing disease or promoting health, trying home remedies as a first resort for treating illness. If they know someone who had a particular illness, they may take the prescribed medicine from that person.

- Haitians tend to keep numerous topical and oral medicines on hand. In Haiti, many medications can be purchased without a prescription, a potentially dangerous practice. Admonishing clients may cause them to withdraw and not listen to instructions. Be very discreet in assessing, teaching, and guiding the client toward safer health practices. Inquire if the patient has been taking medication that was prescribed for someone else.

- Many Haitians in America ask friends or relatives to send medications from Haiti. Such medications may consist of roots, leaves, and European manufactured products that are more familiar to them. Ascertain what the client is taking at home to avoid serious complications.

- Constipation is treated with laxatives, herbal tea, or *lavman* (enemas).

- A primary respiratory ailment is *oppression*, a term used to describe asthma. However, the term really describes a state of anxiety and hyperventilation rather than the condition. Oppression is considered a "cold" state, as are many respiratory conditions. A home remedy for oppression is to take a dry coconut and cut it open, fill it half with sugarcane syrup and half honey, grate one full nutmeg and add it to the syrup mix, reseal the coconut, and then bury it in the ground for a month. The coconut is reopened, the content is stirred and mixed, and one tablespoon is administered twice a day until it is finished. By the end of this treatment, the child is supposed to be cured of the respiratory problem.

- Many Haitians have low-paying jobs that do not provide health insurance, and they cannot afford to purchase it themselves. Thus, economics acts as a barrier to health promotion. Additionally, those who do not speak English well have difficulty accessing the health-care system, explaining their needs fully, or understanding prescriptions and treatments. Obtain an interpreter when necessary.

- The root-work system is a folk medicine that provides a framework for identifying and curing folk illnesses. When illness occurs or when a person is not feeling well or is "disturbed," root medicine distinguishes whether the symptoms and illness have a natural or unnatural origin. An imbalance in harmony between the physical and spiritual world, such as dietary or lifestyle excesses, can cause a natural illness.

- Diabetes is considered a natural illness; however, most do not seek immediate medical assistance when they detect the symptoms of polyuria, excessive thirst, and weight loss. Instead, they attempt symptom management by making dietary changes on their own by drinking potions or herbal remedies. When the person finally seeks medical attention, he or she may be very sick. Use a culturally specific approach when explaining the medical regimen, diet, and medications for diabetes.

- Pain is commonly referred to as *doule*. Many Haitians have a very low pain threshold. Their demeanor changes, they are verbal about the cause of their pain, and they sometimes moan. They are vague about the location of the pain because they believe that it is not important; they believe that the whole body is affected because disease travels, making it very difficult to assess pain accurately. Injections are the preferred method for medication administration, followed by elixirs, tablets, and capsules.

- Chest pain is *doule nan ke mwen*, abdominal pain is *doule nan vent*, and stomach pain is *doule nan ke mwen* or *doule nan lestomak mwen*.

- Nausea is expressed as *lestomak/mwen ap roule, M santi m anwi vomi, lestomak/mwen chaje,* or *ke mwen tounin*. Because of modesty, they may discard vomitus immediately so as not to upset others. Specific instructions should be given regarding keeping the specimen until the practitioner has had a chance to see it.

- Oxygen should be offered only when absolutely necessary because the use of oxygen is perceived as an indicator of the seriousness of the illness.

- Fatigue, physical weakness known as *febles*, is interpreted as a sign of anemia or insufficient blood. Symptoms are generally attributed to poor diet. Clients may suggest that they need special care; that is, to eat well, take vitamin injections, and to rest. To counteract *febles* the diet includes liver, pigeon meat, watercress,

Haitian

bouillon made of green leafy vegetables, cow's feet, and red meat.

- Another condition is *sezisman* (fright). Various external and internal environmental factors are believed to cause *sezisman*, thereby disrupting the normal blood flow. *Sezisman* may occur when someone receives bad news, is involved in a frightful situation, or suffers from indignation after being treated unjustly. When this condition occurs, blood is said to move to the head, causing partial loss of vision, headache, increased blood pressure, or a stroke. To counteract this problem, the client may sit quietly, put a cold compress on the forehead, drink bitter herbal tea, take sips of water, or drink rum mixed with black unsweetened coffee.

- The stigma attached to mental illness is strong, and most individuals do not readily admit to being depressed. A major factor to remember is the strong prevalence of *voudun*, which attributes depression to possession by malevolent spirits or punishment for not honoring good, protective spirits. Depression can be viewed as a hex placed by a jealous or envious individual. Ask clients what they think is causing their depression. Negotiate treatment accordingly.

- In the case of an unnatural illness, the person's poor health is attributed to magical causes such as a hex, a curse, or a spell, which has been cast by someone as a result of family or interpersonal disagreement. The curse takes place when the intended victim eats food that contains ingredients such as snake, frog, or spider egg powder, which cause symptoms of burning skin, rashes, pruritus, nausea, vomiting, and headaches. These symptoms often coincide with psychological problems manifested by violent attacks, hallucinations, delusions, or "magical possession."

- Most individuals are extremely afraid of diseases associated with blood irregularities. Blood is the central dynamic of body functions and pathologic processes; therefore, any condition that places the body in a "blood need" state is believed to be extremely dangerous. Clients and their families become emotional about blood transfusions. Thus, they are received with much apprehension. Additionally, blood transfusions are feared because of the potential for HIV transmission. Factually explain the need for a blood transfusion, and carefully explain the procedure along with the involved risks. Involve clients and their families in the care as much as possible. Explain precautionary measures that have been taken to prevent blood contamination.

- The body must remain intact for burial. Thus, organ donation and transplantation are not generally discussed or practiced. A prime concern is transference, the belief that through the organ donor the donor's personality will "shift" to the recipient and change his or her being. Assess clients' beliefs about organ donation, and involve a religious leader to provide support and help facilitate a decision regarding organ donation or transplantation.

HEALTH-CARE PRACTITIONERS

- Most Haitians resort to symptom management with self-care first and then spiritual care. They commonly use traditional and Western practitioners simultaneously.
- Physicians and nurses are well respected. Physicians are men, and nurses are women. Nurses are referred to as "Miss." Haitians who have had limited contact with American health-care systems may have limited understanding of biomedical concepts. Explain and re-explain relevant points to compensate for clients' knowledge deficit or language limitations.

Haitian

References

Colin, J., & Paperwalla, G. (2003). People of Haitian heritage. In L. Purnell and B. Paulanka (Eds.), *Transcultural health care: A culturally competent approach* (2nd ed., chapter on CD). Philadelphia: F.A. Davis Company.

The World Factbook. (2003). *Haiti*. Retrieved August 23, 2003, from www.odci.gov/cia

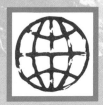

People of Hindu Heritage

Overview and Heritage

More than a billion people inhabit India. Eighty percent of the population are Hindus, followers of Hinduism. Asian Indians living in America represent a segment that includes Sikhs, Punjabis (people of the state of Punjab), Moslems, and Christians. Although different religious sectors share many common cultural beliefs and practices, they differ according to the primary and secondary characteristics of culture as presented in Chapter 1. India is divided into north and south, based primarily on Dravidian and Aryan cultural variations. These two heartlands mark two distinctive variants of the basic Indian culture. Physical characteristics influencing the history and civilization of India are the size of the country and the comparative isolation provided by the Himalayas.

Immigrants to the United States come predominantly from urban areas, including all major Indian states. Earlier immigrants represented a small and transitory community of students, Indian government officials, and businessmen. Asian Indians represent a diverse linguistic, religious, regional, and caste population. Immigration to America has come in two waves. The first wave began in the early 20th century and continued to the mid-1920s. Conditions such as racial discrimination and lack of access to economic advancement made it difficult for the first wave of Asian Indians to sustain themselves or their culture in America. The second wave of immigration began after 1965 and still continues. Most individuals from this wave are highly educated. More than 1,600,000 Asian Indians are living in the United States, with 33 percent living in the Northeast, 17.5 percent in the Midwest, 26.3 percent in the South, and 23.3 percent in the West. Most come to the United States to attain a higher standard of living, better working conditions, and job opportunities. Secondary reasons include opportunities for additional education as well as Indian perceptions of America as a country of opportunity and freedom. Immigrants include parents, who come for the sake of children, and those who come on student visas and later change to permanent resident status.

COMMUNICATIONS

- Many Indian state borders are reorganized in accordance with language limitations. Languages fall into two main groups: Indo-Aryan in the north and Dravidian in the south. Regional variations in the languages are distinct. Hindi, with 1,652 dialectical variations, is the national language, along with English and one of many Indo-Aryan languages. Although Hindi is the predominant language spoken in the north, English is the language among the educated. Because of regional dialects in the main language, be simple and direct in communication and clear in enunciation. With parents and grandparents, who may not speak English, have a bilingual interpreter available.
- Women often speak in a soft voice, making it difficult to understand or decipher what they say. Men may become intense and loud when they converse with other family members. To an onlooker, it might seem disruptive but, in general, this form of communication

Hindu

can be construed as meaningful when it is conducted with close friends.

- Women are expected to strictly follow deference customs; that is, direct eye contact is avoided with men, although men can have direct eye contact with each other. Direct eye contact with older people and authority figures may be considered a sign of disrespect.

- Touching and embracing are not acceptable for displaying affection. Even between spouses, a public display of affection such as hugging or kissing is frowned upon, being considered strictly a private matter.

- Temporality is past-, present-, and future-oriented. Time is conceived in cycles of four ages, which start with the "age of perfection" and end with the "age of degeneration."

- Punctuality in keeping scheduled appointments may not be considered important. Do not misconstrue being late for appointments as a sign of irresponsibility or not valuing health.

- The woman refers to the man in plural *Avar and Aap,* meaning "you" (with respect), whereas the man can use singular "you" like *Ne, Aval,* or *Thum. Aap* means "thou" and is used for elderly family members and for strangers.

- Older family members are usually not addressed by name but as elder brother, sister, aunt, or uncle. A woman never addresses a man by name because the woman is not considered an equal or superior.

- Strangers are greeted with folded hands and a head bow that respects their personal territory.

FAMILY ROLES AND ORGANIZATION

- No institution in India is more important than the family. The hierarchical structure of authority is the patriarchal joint family, based on the principle of superiority of men over women. Thus, families of the men join together, and when men get married the women go with the man's family. Most women remain subservient to their closest male relatives.

- The male head of the family is legitimized and considered sacred by caste and religion, which delineate relationships. Central relationships in this system are based on continuation and expansion of the male lineage through inheritance and ancestor worship, related to the father-son and brother-brother relationships.
- A matrilineal system exists in a few areas in the southwestern and northeastern regions of the country; however, power rests with the men in the woman's family.
- A submissive and acquiescent role is expected of women in the first few years of married life, with little or no participation in decision-making. Strict norms govern contact and communication with the men of the family, including a woman's husband. The nuclear family system continues to retain the hierarchical structure of authority and power significant in the patriarchal family.
- Parents want their children to be successful and strongly encourage and emphasize scholastic achievement in fields that promise good employment and a high social status. Parents in America want their children to maintain ties with their families and the Indian community.
- The desire for a male rather than a female child is prevalent.
- Although many parents expect and accept the Westernization of their children, the question of marriage is still a concern for parents who have opinions about how their children should be married, whether "arranged" or partly arranged. Hindu parents or Indians from all religious traditions want their children to marry other Indians.
- Arranged marriages at a young age are considered most desirable for women. This practice is related to the importance of virginity and restrictions placed on marriage within the same clan. The practice of an arranged marriage continues in the United States in order to minimize the stress associated with differences in castes, lifestyles, and expectations between the male and female hierarchy.

Hindu

- The two major types of transfer of material wealth accompanying marriage are bride price and a dowry. Bride price is payment in cash and other materials to the bride's father in exchange for authority over the woman, which passes from her kin group to the bridegroom's kin group.
- In the joint family structure, Hindu women are considered "outsiders" and are socialized and incorporated in such a way that "jointness" and residence are not broken up. This means that a close relationship between the husband and wife is disapproved because it induces favoring the nuclear family and dissolving the joint family. The marital union is a matter for the husband and wife, society, guardians, and supernatural powers that symbolize spirituality. Therefore, a marriage is regarded as indissoluble.
- Family elders are held in reverence and cared for by their children when they are no longer able to care for themselves. Families believe that knowledge is transmitted through an oral tradition that is derived from experience and that the elderly are repositories of such knowledge.
- Understand the various types of families (joint, extended, or nuclear), and determine which individual has control within the hierarchy.
- Single-parent, blended, and communal families are not well accepted by Hindus.
- Homosexuality may cause a social stigma. Refer lesbian, gay, or bisexual Hindu Americans to national support groups such as TriKone, a nonprofit group for lesbian, gay, and bisexual South Asians located in the San Francisco Bay area, the National AIDS hotline, or Asians Together in Washington, DC. Do not disclose same-gender relationships to other family members.

BIOCULTURAL ECOLOGY

- Asian Indian Hindus evidence a diversity of physical types and can be divided into three general groups according to the color of their skin: white in the north and northwest, yellow in areas bordering Tibet and Assam, and black in the south.

- *Indids* (whites) have a light-brown skin color, wavy black hair, dark- or light-brown eyes, are tall or of medium height, and are either dolichocephalic (long-headed) or brachycephalic (short-headed). The physical type of the *Indid* varies according to regions, ranging from a lighter to a darker brown skin color.
- Black-skinned people, *Melanids*, are often referred to as the Dravidians, the population of southern India. The *Melanids* have dark skin ranging from light brown to black, elongated heads, broad noses, thick lips, and black, wavy hair; and they are usually shorter than 5 feet 6 inches tall. The most characteristic *Melanids* are the Tamils, a major linguistic and cultural group in South India.
- Pallor in brown-skinned patients presents as a yellowish brown tinge to the skin. Pallor in dark-skinned individuals is characterized by the absence of the underlying red tones in the skin. Jaundice may be observed in the sclera. The oral mucosa of dark-skinned individuals may have a normal freckling or pigmentation. Inspection of the nail beds, lips, palpebral conjunctiva, and palms of the hands and soles of the feet shows evidence of cyanosis.
- People migrating from the tropical regions may present with symptoms of malaria. Filariasis may be present in people coming from the Malabar and Coromandel coasts. Tuberculosis and pneumonia are widely prevalent in immigrants. When performing health assessments, health screening, and physical examinations, be alert to possible signs and symptoms and risk factors associated with diseases linked to migration from different regions of India.
- Heart disease tends to develop at a very early age in Asian Indians. Diabetes mellitus, hypertension, central obesity, rheumatic heart disease, sickle cell disease, and dental caries and periodontal disease are prevalent. Breast cancer is one of the leading causes of morbidity and premature death among women.
- Many individuals require lower doses of lithium,

antidepressants, and neuroleptics, and they may experience side effects even with the lower doses. They are also more sensitive to the adverse effects of alcohol, resulting in marked facial flushing, palpitations, and tachycardia. Question therapeutic regimens that do not consider racial or ethnic differences.

HIGH-RISK HEALTH BEHAVIORS

* Alcoholism and cigarette smoking among Hindu Americans, especially among men, cause significant health problems. Refer to "stop smoking" clinics, and encourage low alcohol consumption.
* Beriberi is found in people coming from rice-growing areas, pellagra in maize-millet areas, and lathyrism in khesari-growing areas of Central India. Thiamine deficiency is common among people who are mostly dependent on rice. Thorough milling of rice, washing rice before cooking, and allowing the cooked rice to remain overnight before consumption the following day results in the loss of thiamine.
* Lathyrism is a crippling disease causing paralysis of leg muscles; it occurs mostly in adults who consume large quantities of seeds of the pulse khesari, *lathyrus sativus*, over a long period.
* Lactose intolerance affects up to 1 percent of infants and more than 10 percent of adults.
* Goiters are common along the sub-Himalayan tracts, resulting from an iodine deficiency in food and water.
* Osteomalacia is prevalent in northwest India, where diets are deficient in calcium and vitamin D.
* Endemic dropsy is prevalent in west Bengal as a result of the use of mustard oil for cooking.
* The high incidence of stomach cancer in the south may be due to the excessive intake of fried fatty foods, chilies, and rapid food consumption.
* Cancers of the mouth and lip are common because of chewing *pan* and tobacco.
* Fluorosis occurs in parts of Punjab, Haryana, Andhra Pradesh, and Karnataka, resulting from drinking water with large amounts of fluoride.

NUTRITION

- Dietary habits are complex and regionally varied. Most believe that food was created by the Supreme Being for the benefit of man. The influence of religion is pervasive in food selection, customs, and preparation methods.
- Classification of regional food habits can be two-fold, based on the types of cereals and fresh foods consumed. In the first category are rice and bread eaters; in the second category are vegetarians and nonvegetarians. Vegetarianism is firmly rooted in culture; the term *nonvegetarian* is used to describe anyone who eats meat, eggs, poultry, fish, and sometimes cheese. Many Brahmins in North India consider eating meat to be religiously sanctioned. In some parts of India, eating fish is acceptable to Brahmins, whereas in other parts eating meat is sacrilegious. Assess cultural food choices upon admission to the health-care facility.
- Dietary staples include rice, wheat, jowar, bajra, jute, oilseeds, peanuts, millet, maize, peas, sugarcane, coconut, and mustard. Cereals supply 70 to 90 percent of the total caloric requirements. A variety of pulses or lentils, cooked vegetables, meat, fish, eggs, and dairy products are also consumed. Heavily spiced (curry) dishes with vegetables, meat, fish, or eggs are favored, and hot pickles and condiments are common. Spice choices include garlic, ginger, turmeric, tamarind, cumin, coriander, and mustard seed. Vegetable choices include onions, tomatoes, potatoes, green leaves, okra, green beans, and root vegetables.
- Milk is used in coffee and tea and in preparing yogurt and buttermilk. Water is the beverage of choice with meals and is preferred as a thirst quencher. Coffee is popular in South India, whereas tea is the beverage of choice in the rest of the country.
- In North India wheat is the staple food. Other cereals are *jowar*, *bajra*, and *ragi*, consumed in porridges, gruels, and *rotis* (baked pancakes).
- *Bajra*, a staple food in Maratha families, is not considered favorably in Uttar Pradesh. People from Punjab do not favor fish, and people from the south

generally dislike the idea of meat of any kind. In Saurashtra in the south, fish, fowl, flesh, and eggs are taboo practically everywhere.

- Women generally serve the food but may eat separately from men. Women are not allowed to cook during their menstrual periods or have contact with other members of the family. **Assess food rituals practiced by Hindus in relation to meal times and food selections before attempting dietary counseling.**

- Foremost among the perceptions of Hindus is the belief that certain foods are "hot" and others are "cold" and therefore should only be eaten during certain seasons and not in combination. The geographic differences in the hot and cold perceptions are dramatic; many foods considered hot in the north are considered cold in the south. Such perceptions and distinctions are based on how specific foods are thought to affect body functions. The belief is that failure to observe rules related to the hot and cold theory of diseases results in illness. A more detailed description of the hot and cold theory of diseases is provided under Health-Care Practices. **Given the diversity of Hindus in America, individually assess dietary practices and nutritional deficiencies of clients according to their ethnic origins and area of residence.**

PREGNANCY AND CHILDBEARING PRACTICES

- Birth control methods include intrauterine devices, condoms, and rhythm and withdrawal methods. **Women may desire education in family planning from a same-sex health-care provider as well as assistance with delivery from female physicians, midwives, or female nurse practitioners.**

- Grandmothers, mothers, and mothers-in-law are considered to have expert knowledge in the use of home remedies during pregnancy and the postpartum period. Many older women frequently travel to the United States to assist new mothers in antenatal and postnatal care that is consistent with traditional customs.

- The birth of a son is a blessing because the son carries the family name and takes care of the parents in their old age. The birth of a daughter is cause for worry and concern because of the traditions associated with dowry, a ritual that can impoverish the lives of those who are less affluent.
- Box 17–1 describes various cultural practices related to pregnancy.

BOX 17–1 • Practices During Pregnancy

- Based on the hot and cold theory of disease, certain "hot" foods like eggs, jaggery, coconut, groundnut, maize, mango, papaya, fruit, and meat are avoided during pregnancy because of a fear of abortion caused by heating the body or inducing uterine hemorrhage.
- Pregnancy is a time of increased body heat; hence "cold" foods such as milk, yogurt, and fruits are considered good. Buttermilk and green leafy vegetables are avoided because of the belief that these foods cause joint pain, body aches, and flatulence. Minor swelling of the hands and feet is thought to result from increased heat and is not of much concern.
- Morning sickness is caused by an increase in body heat. Burning sensations during urination, scanty urine, or a white vaginal discharge are considered serious signs of significant overheating.
- Overeating and consumption of high-protein foods, including milk, are avoided because such foods result in an exaggerated growth of the baby that may lead to a difficult delivery.
- Anemia caused by iron deficiency is one of the nutritional disorders affecting women of childbearing age. This condition may be aggravated because of the practice of reducing the consumption of leafy vegetables to avoid producing a dark-skinned baby.

Hindu

- There is no taboo against the father being in the delivery room, but men are usually not present during birthing. Instead, they tend to wait outside the delivery room and allow female relatives to support the pregnant mother during labor and delivery. Report labor progress to fathers who prefer to stay in the waiting room.
- Because self-control is valued, women suppress their feelings and emotions during labor and delivery. Closely observe nonverbal communication, such as a change in body posture, restlessness, and facial expressions, during labor, and provide assistance as necessary.
- Beliefs and practices used during the postpartum period are discussed in Box 17–2.

BOX 17–2 • Postpartum Beliefs and Practices

- During the postpartum period, the mother remains in a warm room and often keeps the windows closed to protect her against cold drafts. Exposure to air conditioners and fans, even in warm weather, may be considered dangerous. **Provide warm clothing and additional blankets for the mother and baby to keep them warm.**
- After the birth, both the mother and the baby undergo purification rites on the 11th day. The postpartum mother is considered to be impure and is confined to a room. The pollution lasts for 10 days. This period of necessitated and mandatory confinement assists in bonding between the mother and the newborn and provides the mother with adequate rest and time to tend to the baby's needs. The baby is officially named on the 11th day during the "cradle ceremony," and several rituals are performed to protect the baby from evil spirits and to ensure longevity.
- A sponge bath for the newborn is recommended until the umbilical cord falls off.
- Soft massage to the extremities is recommended before bathing the infant.

- Washing the infant's hair daily is believed to improve the quality of the hair.
- During the postpartum period, hot foods such as brinjals, drumsticks, dried fish, dhal, and greens are good for lactation. Cold foods are thought to produce diarrhea and indigestion in the infant. Cold foods such as buttermilk and curds, gourds, squashes, tomatoes, and potatoes are restricted because they produce gas. Such abstentions are primarily practiced for the baby's health because harmful influences might be transmitted through the mother's breast milk.
- Some believe that colostrum is unsuited for infants. Most women think that the milk does not "descend to the breast" until their ritual bath on the third day and, as a result, newborns are fed sugar water or milk expressed from a lactating woman.
- Breast milk is commonly supplemented with cow's milk and diluted with sugar water. A child's stomach is considered weak as a result of diarrhea; therefore, the child is given diluted milk.
- Sources of protein such as eggs, curds, and meat are avoided because they might adversely affect the baby.
- The mother's diet the first few days is restricted to liquids, rice, gruel, and bread.
- Boiled rice, eggplant, curry, and tamarind juice are added to the diet between 6 months and a year after the birth of the baby.
- **Obtain dietary preferences and practices from the family before planning nutritional counseling.**

DEATH RITUALS

- A tenet of Hinduism is that the soul survives the death; death is a rebirth. Therefore, by performing a ritual bath, sprinkling holy river water over the body, covering the body with new clothes, daubing parts of the body with ghee, and chanting Vedic utterances, the deceased

Hindu

is considered purified and strengthened for the post-mortem journey.

- Hindus prefer to die at home. The eldest son is responsible for the funeral rites.
- The death rite is called *antyesti*, or last rites. The priest pours water into the mouth of the deceased and blesses the body by tying a thread around the neck or wrist. The priest may anoint with water from the holy Ganges River or put the sacred leaf from the *Tulsi* plant in the mouth. The eldest son completes prayers for ancestral souls, but all male descendants perform the rites; each offers balls of rice on behalf of the deceased ancestor.
- The body is usually cremated rather than interred. The ashes are immersed or sprinkled in the holy rivers. Such immersions are of great benefit to the souls of the dead. Hindus may save their family's ashes to later scatter them in holy rivers when they return to their homeland.
- Women may respond to the death of a loved one with loud wailing, moaning, and beating their chests in front of the corpse, attesting their inability to bear the thought of being left behind to handle situations by themselves. Offer support and understanding with respect for death and grief behaviors.

SPIRITUALITY

- Of Hinduism, Christianity, Islam, and Zoroastrianism, Hinduism is the largest religion and the oldest tradition practiced in India. Hinduism represents a set of beliefs and a definite social organization. Hinduism denotes belief in the authority of Vedas and other sacred writings of the ancient sages, immortality of the soul and a future life, existence of a Supreme God, the theory of karma and rebirth, worship of ancestors, social organization represented by the four castes, theory of the four stages of life, and the theory of four *Purusarthas*, or ends of human endeavor.
- Orthodox Hindus view society as divinely ordained on the basis of the four castes: (1) *Brahmin*, the highest

caste, priests and scholars, emerged from the head of God; (2) *Kshtriya*, warriors, from the arms; (3) *Vaisya*, merchants, from the waist; and (4) *Sudra*, menials, from the feet of God. The four-fold caste system is a theoretical division of society to which tribes, clans, and family groups are affiliated. Although religion does not bestow the caste system with a religious sanction, the great Hindu legal codes are based on the caste system. **Identify Hindu religious beliefs and practices, and incorporate these beliefs into clients' care.**

- Worship includes praying, singing hymns, reciting scripture, and repeating the names of deities. Temples are important for Hindus who do not live close to them. Various kinds of worship are performed in the temples at the request of the sponsoring Hindus who live far away, and the blessing of the offering to God is mailed back to these worshipers. **Assess the extent to which religion is a part of the individual's life, how religious beliefs are related to the individual's perception of health and illness, and the individual's daily religious practices. Assessing spiritual life is essential for identifying resources and solutions for therapy.**
- Women often fast one day a week or for a lunar month to fulfill a vow made to a deity in supplication for a particular blessing. Wives frequently fast to secure the continued health of their husbands and families.
- Shrines may be set up in the living room or the dining room but are most often located in a back room or in a closet. The shrine typically contains representations or symbols of one or more deities.

HEALTH-CARE PRACTICES

- Physical examinations are especially traumatic to women who may not have experienced or heard about Pap tests and mammography examinations.
- Most individuals believe that illnesses attack an individual through the mind, body, and soul. The body is the objective manifestation of a subjective mind and consciousness.

- The actions of supernatural forces and certain human excesses can be identified as a source of illness. Some believe that excessive consumption of sweets may cause roundworms and that too much sexual activity and worry are associated with tuberculosis. Others believe that diarrhea and cholera are caused by a variety of improper eating habits. **Explain factual information about parasitic and infectious diseases.**

- Suffering of any kind produces hope, which is essential to life. To maintain harmony between self and the supernatural world, the belief that one can do little to restore health by oneself provides a basis for ceremonies and rituals.

- Worshiping goddesses, pilgrimages to holy places, and pouring water at the roots of sacred trees are believed to have medicinal effects in healing the sick person and in appeasing the planets to help prevent illnesses and misfortunes.

- Medical beliefs are a blend of modern and traditional theories and practices. In *Ayurveda,* the traditional system of medicine in India, the primary emphasis is on the prevention of illnesses. Individuals have to be aware of their own health needs. One of the principles of Ayurveda includes the art of living and proper health care, advocating that one's health is a personal responsibility. The key to health is an orderly daily life in which personal hygiene, diet, work, and sleep and rest patterns are regulated. A daily routine has to be established and changed according to the season.

- A common health problem is self-medication. Those migrating to America are accustomed to self-medicating and may bring medications with them or obtain medications through relatives and friends. **Specifically ask clients about folk practices, use of over-the-counter medicines, and medicines brought from India.**

- The traditional healers, *nattuvaidhyars*, use Ayurvedic, Siddha, and Unani medical systems. These systems are all based on the Tridosha theory. The Ayurvedic system uses herbs and roots; the Siddha system, practiced mainly in the southern part of India, uses medicines;

and the Unani system, similar to the Siddha, is practiced by Muslims.

- According to the Tridosha theory, the body is made up of modifications of the five elements: air, space, fire, water, and earth. These modifications are formed from food and must be maintained within proper proportions for health. A balance among three elements, or humors—phlegm or mucus, bile or gall, and wind—corresponds to three different types of food required by the body. Box 17–3 shows the three types of foods and the allopathic equivalents of diseases associated with them.

BOX 17–3 • Bodily Manifestations of Various Foods

- Heat-producing foods: *brinjals*, dried fish, green chilies, raw rice, and eggs. *Pittham* foods include cluster beans, cowgram, groundnuts (peanuts), almonds, millet, oil, and runner beans. Allopathic equivalents of *sudu* diseases include diarrhea, dysentery, abdominal pain, and scabies. Allopathic equivalents of *pittham* diseases include vomiting, jaundice, and anemia.
- Cooling foods: tomatoes, pumpkin, kul, gourds, greens, oranges, sweet limes, carrots, radishes, barley, and buttermilk. Cold, headache, chill, fever, malaria, and typhoid are allopathic equivalents of cool diseases.
- Gas-producing foods: root vegetables such as potato, sweet potato, and elephant yam; plantain; and drumstick. Joint pains, paralysis, stroke, and polio are disorders related to gas-producing foods.
- Heating and cooling effects are produced in the body and hence are not related to the temperature or spiciness of foods. An imbalance leads to disease. If too much heat is in the body from consuming heat-producing foods, then cold foods need to be eaten to restore balance.

Hindu

- Cultural patterns in India are regionally specific. Be aware of practices related to the hot and cold theory of disease causation and treatment.
- Because of their religious beliefs of karma, Hindus may attempt to be stoic and may not exhibit symptoms of pain. Pain is attributed to God's will, the wrath of God, or a punishment from God and is to be borne with courage. Because of stoicism, rely more on nonverbal manifestations when assessing for pain.
- Families tend to be protective of ill members. They may not want to disclose the gravity of an illness to the patient or discuss impending disability or death for fear of the patient's vulnerability and loss of hope, resulting in death. The conflict between medical ethics and patients' values may pose a problem for health-care professionals, who need to be cognizant of the importance of the family members' wishes and values regarding the care of their loved ones.
- The sick role is assumed without any feeling of guilt or ineptness in doing one's tasks. The individual is cared for and relieved of responsibilities for that time.
- Psychological distress may be demonstrated through somatization, which is common, especially in women. The symptoms may be expressed as headaches, a burning sensation in the soles of the feet or in the forehead, and tingling pain in the lower extremities. Because of the stigma attached to seeking professional psychiatric help, many do not access the health-care system for mental health problems. Mental illness is considered to be God's will.
- No Hindu policy exists that prevents receiving blood or blood products. Donating and receiving organs are acceptable.

HEALTH-CARE PRACTITIONERS

- Although Hindus in general have a favorable attitude toward American physicians and the quality of medical care received in the United States, relatives and friends are usually consulted before health-care professionals.

- Physicians are considered omnipotent because God grants cures through physicians. Clients tend to be subservient and may not openly question physicians' behavior or treatment. If they are not pleased with the treatment, they just change physicians. However, they tend to be appreciative of the information that physicians provide about their illness. **Provide factual information about diseases and illnesses.**

- The physician is also viewed like an older person in the family; a protective, authoritative, and responsible relationship; a parent-child relationship; and a *guru-chela* (teacher-disciple) relationship. **Clients expect physicians to teach them about the disease and how to get cured in a friend-to-friend relationship.**

- Physicians are considered the leaders of health-care teams, and other medical personnel take on a lower status. The acceptance of traditional and folk practitioners is highly variable among Western health-care providers and may depend on their previous experiences with complementary care providers.

- In mental health, traditional healers, such as *Vaids*, practice an empirical system of indigenous medicine; *mantarwadis* cure through astrology and charms; and *patris* act as mediums for spirits and demons. **Specifically ask clients if they are using folk practitioners and what treatments have been prescribed.**

- Women are especially modest, generally seeking female health-care providers for gynecologic examinations. **Respect modesty by providing adequate privacy and assigning same-gender caregivers whenever possible.**

- **Explain the procedures, provide privacy, and assign a female health-care provider to decrease the stress and discomfort associated with a pelvic examination.**

References

Ferro-Luzzi, G. E. (1974). Food avoidances during the puerperium and lactation in Tamilnad. *Ecology of Food and Nutrition, 3,* 7–15.

Hindu

Jambunathan, J. (2003). People of Hindu heritage. In L. Purnell and B. Paulanka (Eds.), *Transcultural healthcare: A culturally competent approach* (2nd ed., chapter on CD). Philadelphia: F.A. Davis Company.

Kilara, A., & Iya, K. K. (1992). Food and dietary habits of the Hindu. *Food Technology, 46,* 94.

Levy, R. A. (1993). Ethnic and racial differences in response to medicines: Preserving individualized therapy in managed pharmaceutical programmes. *Pharmaceutical Medicine, 7,* 139–165.

Noble, A. G., & Dutt, A. K. (1982). *India: Cultural patterns and processes.* Boulder, CO: Westview Press.

U.S. Census Bureau. (2001). *Statistical abstract of the United States.* Washington, DC: U.S. Government Printing Office.

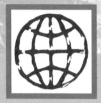

People of Iranian Heritage

Overview and Heritage

From 400,000 to more than 1 million Iranians live in the United States. Nearly half live in California. Despite the focus in this book on commonalities, Iranians vary enormously, from highly traditional to highly acculturated, in their reasons for leaving Iran as well as in the primary and secondary characteristics of culture (see Chapter 1). Most of Iran's 70 million people live in the North and Northwest. The capital, Tehran, has nearly 12 million residents, and a large proportion of the population lives in the cities. The terms *Persian* and *Iranian* are used interchangeably in this chapter because some people call themselves Persian for historical and political reasons. In 1935, the country's name was changed from Persia to Iran to present an image of progress and in an attempt to unify into one nation the enormous diversity of urban dwellers and rural tribes, ethnic groups, and social classes.

Reza Shah Pahlavi and his son instituted powerful social and economic reforms from the mid-1930s to the 1979 revolution, including national public health and education programs and a more secular society with decreased power for tribal chiefs, clergy, and landed aristocracy. During this period, women were allowed to go unveiled, gained access to university education, and were fully enfranchised in 1963. However, despite these economic and social changes, Mohammed Reza Shah reinstituted the secret police and had no tolerance for political opposition.

After conservative Moslem protests that led to the 1978 violence, martial law was declared, and a military government was appointed to deal with striking oil workers. Early in 1979, the Shah fled Iran to the United States. The "reform" instituted by the new Islamic government was deeply colored by the traditional religious ideology. Since then, Iran has once again come to externally resemble the more conservative Muslim countries.

Immigrants have faced considerable ethnic bias because of events in Iran and the September 11, 2001, disaster in the United States. Of the three waves of Iranian immigration to the United States, the first (1950 to 1970) consisted mostly of students from the social and professional elite class, many of whom remained after completing their education. The second wave (1970 to 1978) comprised immigrants who were more varied in social class background but who were predominantly urban and affluent. They came mainly to pursue higher education, professional or economic opportunities, or to join family members. The third wave, 1975 to 1980, included a higher proportion of minorities, such as Baha'is and Jews escaping religious persecution as well as more women and elderly. The third wave began with the Islamic revolution and included a large number of political exiles and forced migrants, who came mainly for personal or economic security.

Iranians are among the most highly educated immigrant group in the United States. Education is greatly valued, and advanced degrees are highly respected. Children are expected to do well in school and to attend college. Many middle-aged physicians, engineers, professors, army generals, and government officials who were unable to find comparable work in the United States have gone into business for themselves. Jobs that require manual labor are not respected, and some cannot accept that they have to take such menial jobs because of their limited skills in English.

COMMUNICATIONS

- Farsi (Persian) is the national language of Iran. Nearly half the population speaks different languages: Turkish, Kurdish, Armenian, Baluchi, or other Iranian dialects. Well-educated and well-traveled immigrants may speak three or more languages, often using French as a cultural language or English in business settings.
- Many foreign invasions and strict control by each ensuing government have influenced Iranians' interaction with outsiders, making them suspicious of foreigners. The disclosure of personal thoughts to strangers is generally perceived to have detrimental consequences. Not verbalizing one's thoughts is considered a customary and useful defense; overt expressions of emotions to strangers may be culturally stigmatized.
- Among women, patterns of speech may appear restrained or refined to avoid too much self-disclosure or to prevent loss of face. Most women give considerable detail rather than use blunt and succinct messages.
- Most Iranians are very concerned with respectability, a good appearance of the home, and a good reputation. They are embarrassed by financial troubles and even conceal such problems from relatives. *Zerangi* (cleverness) is valued but only among non-intimates; it means knowing how to manipulate bureaucratic structures and is used because government organizations were not trusted to function for the good of the people in Iran.
- The influence of intimate versus public spheres and hierarchical social relationships is seen clearly in the practice of *ta'arof* (ritual expressed courtesy), which is not practiced with intimates. *Ta'arof* expresses the public face, with its respectful forms of speech and behavior, and is used when dealing with individuals whose status is unequal to one's own.
- Communication is structured by social hierarchy and varies according to *baten* and *zaher*. *Baten* (inner self) is the true vulnerable self, a collection of freely expressed personal feelings. In contrast, *zaher* is proper and

Iranian

controlled behavior, a public face to protect and buffer the vulnerable world of the *baten* within. Silence is used to guard confidential matters and to manage impressions.

- Privacy is important; family matters remain within the family and are not for others' ears.

- Most Iranians refrain from showing anger or other strong emotions to outsiders because self-control is valued; showing anger can produce embarrassment, shame the family, or damage someone's reputation. To avoid embarrassment and to save face, they may agree or say that they understand an outsider, whether they do or not. Because politeness and saving face prevail, do not assume that a positive response means a definite "yes."

- At the beginning of any health-care encounter, the provider should take time to "warm up" with social conversation before "getting down to business." Any kind of bad news must be handled carefully by revealing it gently and gradually, in several meetings if possible, or only to the family spokesperson. A person should never be given bad news alone; for example, being informed of a death or serious diagnosis.

- Among the more traditional, men and women do not hold hands or show affection toward each other in public. However, women often show affection for women and men for men by walking hand in hand or greeting each other with a kiss on each cheek.

- Strangers and health-care providers are greeted with both arms held at the sides or with a handshake. A slight bow or nod while shaking hands shows respect. It is appropriate to offer something, e.g., a prescription, with both hands, which shows respect.

- Slouching in a chair or stretching one's legs toward another person is considered offensive. It is considered rude to show the sole of one's foot. Beckoning is done by waving the fingers with the palm down. Do not beckon clients; call them formally by name.

- Tilting the head up quickly means "no." Tilting the head to the side means "what?", and tilting it down means "yes." Extending the thumb (as in "thumbs up") is considered a vulgar sign. **Refrain from using nonverbal behaviors that may be offensive.**

- Personal distance is generally closer than that of Americans or northern Europeans. Respect for a health-care provider's role and education might be demonstrated by keeping a wide distance.
- Most individuals maintain intense eye contact between intimates and equals of the same gender, but the traditional tend to avoid eye contact. Younger people and those of lower status do not sustain eye contact with those they perceive as being older or of higher status. When speaking, smiling and using the arms and hands help to convey the message and to increase the expressiveness.
- Temporal relationships are a combination of present and future orientation. The future orientation enhances the effectiveness of health education. At the same time, a fatalistic theme in many Iranians' beliefs may hinder their understanding of teaching about risk reduction and health promotion.
- Iranians are not clock-watchers; rather, they are mood- and feeling-oriented. While social time is flexible, Iranians meet the social expectations for timeliness in work and appointments.
- In highly traditional families, privacy demands that husbands do not mention their wife's first name to other men.
- Close friends and children may be called by their first name by family members, but others should not do so. Shaking hands with a child shows respect to the parents, but **a man should wait for a woman to extend her hand first. One is expected to greet every member of the family with a handshake. Health-care providers should heed nonverbal cues and greet Iranians in culturally congruent ways.**

FAMILY ROLES AND ORGANIZATION

- Iranian culture is patriarchal and hierarchical. The father rules the family and expects obedience and submission from family members. In the father's absence, the oldest son has authority.

- Families were traditionally large in Iran, with male children being highly desirable. In more traditional families, older male siblings have the authority to make decisions about younger siblings, even in the father's presence. **Never underestimate the power of this hierarchy or of the family in general in decision-making. Individuals usually cannot or will not make decisions.**
- Men see their role as protecting and providing for the family, managing the finances, and dealing with matters outside the home. Women maintain the home; even working women may place their priorities on the family and home and do the cooking, cleaning, and laundry.
- In traditional families, both daughters and sons stay at home until married, and in rural areas marriages are often arranged. In the United States, young people are free to select their own marriage partners, but families usually want to approve because of the importance of marriage alliances between families.
- Parents pay much attention to their children and are willing to sacrifice for their welfare, especially for their higher education.
- Children are expected to be loyal to their families and behave respectfully toward their elders. Manners are considered important even outside the home, where children are expected to be clean and well behaved and to refrain from rowdiness.
- Girls are expected to behave and dress more modestly than boys, especially as they approach adolescence. Children and teens are usually included in adult gatherings. Young children are rarely left with babysitters.
- Taboo behaviors for teens include smoking, drugs, alcohol, and sex, in that order.
- Young women are expected to remain virgins until they marry, but sexual activity by men outside marriage is tolerated.
- Dating is not allowed in the most traditional families,

but this varies depending on ethnic group and amount of time in the United States.

- Family members often live close to each other so they can visit whenever possible. Most maintain strong intergenerational involvement with grandmothers, mothers, and children in the domestic sphere and with male family members, who are often employed in the family business.
- Iranians often remove their shoes at the door and wear slippers. Outside the home, they tend to dress conservatively, but more traditional or religious women in the United States avoid bright colors, cover their arms and legs, and conceal their heads with head covers or scarves (*hijab*). In Iran, these coverings are mandatory, not a matter of choice. However, there is great variety in dress, depending on age and tradition.
- Age is a sign of experience, worldliness, and knowledge. Regardless of kinship or relationship, an elder is treated with respect. When grandparents reach an age when they can no longer care for themselves, they live with and are cared for by the family. Caring for the elderly is an obligation. Respect for age is shown not only to grandparents but also to aunts, uncles, older siblings, and neighbors.
- Older and more traditional Iranians may be uncomfortable with unrelated members of the opposite sex. Most strongly disapprove of the American practice of living together before marriage. Although divorce is viewed negatively, its rate has been increasing among Iranians in the United States, partly as a result of the increase in intercultural marriages. Cultural mores also advocate ignoring or denying minor marital discord and acceptance of suffering for the sake of maintaining family stability.
- In Iran, out-of-wedlock teen pregnancy is neither talked about nor prevalent, although it can have a devastating outcome. If it happens in the United States, it may be taken care of quietly to preserve the face of the family.
- Homosexuality is highly stigmatized and not discussed; gays and lesbians remain "in the closet." Since 1979,

when the legal and religious systems became synonymous, homosexuality, which is considered unnatural
and sacrilegious, has been a capital offense punishable
by death. Take caution, and do not expose lesbian and
gay relationships to family members.

BIOCULTURAL ECOLOGY

- As white Indo-Europeans, skin tones and facial features
  resemble those of other Mediterranean and Southern
  European groups. Coloring ranges from blue or green
  eyes, light-brown hair, and fair skin to nearly black
  eyes, black hair, and brown skin. Because of the
  variations in skin color, health-care professionals may
  need to assess jaundice and anemia in Iranians by
  examining the sclera and oral mucosa rather than by
  relying solely on skin assessments.
- Malaria is widespread in Baluchistan (Southeast), with
  serologic test results sometimes showing more than
  one strain in a single client. In rural areas that lack
  standardized sanitary systems, viral and bacterial
  meningitis, hookworm, and gastrointestinal dysenteries
  caused by parasites are prevalent. Screen newer
  immigrants for cholera, malaria, and parasitic disease.
- Hypertension is widespread, with 2 million cases (one-
  sixth of the population) reported in Tehran. Ischemic
  heart disease is rising, and the rise is generally perceived
  as being related to the stress of living with daily
  uncertainties.
- Birth defects associated with marriages between cousins
  include epilepsy, blindness, several forms of anemia, and
  hemophilia.
- Other illnesses and diseases common with immigrants
  include diabetes, thalassemias, vitamin B_{12} or folic
  acid deficiencies linked to an enzyme deficiency, and
  Mediterranean glucose-6-phosphate dehydrogenase
  (G-6-PD) deficiency. G-6-PD deficiency can precipitate
  a hemolytic crisis when fava beans are eaten; it affects
  drug metabolism, such as increasing sensitivity to
  primaquine.

HIGH-RISK HEALTH BEHAVIORS

- Smoking is more prevalent in Iran than in the United States among both men and women. **Encourage decreasing or stopping smoking.**
- Some alcohol and street-drug abuse occurs in the immigrant population, but the rate is no higher than that of the population at large.
- Alcohol is prohibited by the Qur'an (Holy Book), although many are not religious and drink socially; a few to excess. In some people, years of opium use in Iran can create both psychological and physical addiction. Family responses to drug use range from complete support of the family member to disownment.
- Children and young adults are more physically active than their elders and exercise as frequently as their peers in nonimmigrant groups.
- Most individuals comply with seat-belt and child-restraint laws, valuing the safety of their children.

NUTRITION

- Food is a symbol of hospitality for Iranians. Iranian food is flavorful and takes hours to prepare. Presentation is important.
- Food is classified into two categories, *garm* (hot) and *sard* (cold), which sometimes correspond to high-calorie and low-calorie foods. The key is balance. At any given table, there is usually a pleasing mixture of foods of different colors and ingredients, composed of a balance of *garm* and *sard*.
- Too much of one category can cause symptoms of being "overheated" or "chilled." Such symptoms are treated by eating food from the opposite group. Becoming overheated, sweating, itching, and rashes may result from eating too many hot foods, such as walnuts, onions, garlic, spices, honey, or candy. The stomach may become chilled, causing dizziness, weakness, and vomiting, after eating too many cold foods, such as grapes, rhubarb, plums, cucumbers, or yogurt or from drinking beer.

- Tea and fruit are served for dessert after each meal. Iranians prefer to use only the freshest foods, although in some cases cost is a factor in their using some dried herbs. Canned, frozen, and fast foods are perceived to have less nutritional value and contain preservatives that can affect health.
- Hot tea is the most popular drink among Iranians. The most common starchy foods are rice and wheat bread. Long-grained, fluffy, and white rice is preferred. Bread is usually baked flat like lavash or pita. Corn and potatoes are used but less favored. Beans and legumes, for example, lentils, pinto, mung, kidney, lima and green beans, and split and black-eyed peas make up a fairly high proportion of the dietary intake and are commonly used in rice mixtures.
- Dairy products are dietary staples, particularly eggs, milk, yogurt, and feta cheese as well as dairy by-products, such as *doog* (yogurt soda) and *kashk* (milk by-product).
- Favorite meats are beef, chicken, fish, and lamb. Shellfish is sometimes eaten. Fresh fruit is always found in Iranian houses.
- Green leafy vegetables are used in cooking, and herbs such as parsley, cilantro (coriander), dill, fenugreek, tarragon, mint, savory, and green onions are served fresh at a meal.
- Islam has a strict set of dietary prescriptions *(halal)* and proscriptions *(haram)*. Slaughter of poultry, beef, and lamb must be done ritually to make the meat *halal*. Strict Muslims avoid pork and alcoholic beverages; a few avoid shellfish.
- Food is eaten with the right hand, and foods or objects are passed with the right hand alone or with both hands. Make adjustments to accommodate traditional food practices; make provisions for the family to bring food from home if the client prefers.
- Women are believed to be more susceptible to *sardie* than *garmie*, a digestive problem resulting from having eaten too much hot food. Incorporate Iranian foods

and dietary practices into health teaching to improve compliance with special dietary restrictions.

PREGNANCY AND CHILDBEARING PRACTICES

- Menstrual blood is believed to be ritually unclean and physically polluting to the body. Menstruating women are not allowed to touch holy objects or to have intercourse. Menstruation is also considered a time of great fragility when a woman should not exercise or shower excessively, because these activities might cause a hemorrhage. At the end of the menses, the woman must wash and purify herself thoroughly before partaking in any religious rituals.
- Birth control methods used by Iranians include the pill, intrauterine devices, and natural methods. Vasectomies are just beginning to gain acceptance.
- Pregnancy after marriage is desirable because women believe that their bodies are in a less healthy state and are polluted with excess menstrual blood until they have given birth.
- A woman's prestige is at its height when she delivers her first child, particularly if the child is a boy. Delivering the first child relieves anxiety and gives the young wife a more respected and cherished position with her in-laws. Providing factual information regarding family planning is one area in which health-care professionals can improve family care.
- Food cravings must be satisfied lest a miscarriage occur from not meeting the fetus's needs.
- Pregnant women avoid fried foods and foods that cause gas; fruits and vegetables are recommended, with special attention to the balance of hot and cold foods.
- Heavy work is thought to cause a miscarriage.
- Sexual intercourse is allowed until the last month.
- The pregnant woman receives considerable support from female kin, including relieving the pregnant and postpartum woman of household tasks. This assistance begins in the 6th month and continues until after the birth.

- In more traditional families, the father is usually not present at the birth.
- The postpartum period is 30 to 40 days. Because of the belief in the polluting nature of blood, postpartum women are required to take a ritual bath after they stop bleeding so they can resume normal religious activities.
- To strengthen the postpartum woman, a *ghorse kamar* (a brown, flat disk of dried herbs) is mixed with eggs and placed on her lower back a few hours before bathing.
- New mothers avoid cold water for bathing, ablutions, or cleaning, although they now bathe sooner than the traditional first 30 days.
- Baby boys are considered "hotter" than baby girls, and mothers of sons are considered to have hotter bodies, hotter milk, and hotter temperaments than mothers of girls.
- Mothers of girls are given a mixture of honey and other nutrients, an herbal extract called *taranjebin*, to raise their bodily heat to ensure that the next child is a boy.
- Some families keep an infant home for the first 40 days; at which time the baby is strong enough to fight off environmental pathogens.
- The baby is given a ritual bath between the 10th and 40th days. **Ask the childbearing family about prescriptive, restrictive, and taboo cultural practices that they customarily follow, and incorporate these practices in care.**

DEATH RITUALS

- Some families may demand that strenuous efforts be made to prolong life. **Assess each family individually about life-prolonging medical treatments.**
- To discuss termination of life support with a practicing Muslim, begin the conversation by noting God's will for human beings and His power over our destiny, followed by a dialogue about life and death as necessary steps toward immortal life in heaven. Muslims may need only a gentle reminder that death is not a termination of life but rather the beginning of a new and better life.

- Some individuals may oppose stopping life support, viewing it as "playing God," even though they may have no objection to beginning life support, viewing it as the "gift" of medical technology.
- Among religious Muslims, the deathbed should be turned to face Mecca so family members can read prayers from the Qur'an to ensure that the dying person hears this at the time of death. Determine the direction of Mecca, and rearrange furniture as necessary so that the dying person can face Mecca.
- After death, another Muslim should wash the body in a ritual manner, using soap and water and proceeding from head to toe and front to back. All body orifices must be closed and slightly packed with cotton to prevent leakage of bodily fluids (considered unclean). The final rinse is performed with water. The body is then wrapped in a special white cotton shroud. Prayers and verses from the Qur'an are read during the procedure. A non-Muslim health-care provider should wear gloves when touching the body.
- No specific religious rules exist against autopsy. However, the body of the dead is to be respected; the reason for the autopsy must be made clear, and some may still refuse.
- Iranians may express their grief over the death of a loved one by crying, wailing loudly, or even striking themselves or an object.
- After a Muslim's death, relatives, friends, and acquaintances gather on the 3rd, 7th, and 40th days after the death. Clergy, family, relatives, and friends read prayers. Special foods are served, and grieving may be expressed loudly. All wear black, and women relatives wear little or no makeup. On the anniversary of the death, the family gathers again to pay respect to the deceased.

SPIRITUALITY

- Specific Muslim practices include prayers, read in the name of one of the 12 imams, to provide peace of mind or to plead for a miracle.
- Devout Muslims pray five times daily and need privacy

and water for ritual washing. **Make arrangements for praying.**

- Most Muslims fast from sunrise to sundown during Ramadan, although pregnant women and the ill are exempt from fasting. **Arrange meals and medications to accommodate Ramadan.**
- Family relationships and friendships are sources of strength and meaning in life for many individuals. **Adjust visiting policies in health-care settings to accommodate family and friends.**
- *Tagdir*, God's will and power over one's fate in life and death, is a common belief, fostering a sense of passivity and dependence on a superior force.
- Death is not a finalization; rather, it is a graduation to a higher level of being.

HEALTH-CARE PRACTICES

- Traditional health beliefs and therapeutic processes are a combination of three traditions of medicine: Galenic (humoral), Islamic (sacred), and modern biomedicine. In classic humoral theory, illness arises from an imbalance (excess or deficiency) in the basic qualities of, for example, hot and cold or wet and dry. The purpose of treatment is to restore balance.
- In Galenic-Islamic thought, every individual has a distinctive balance of four humors, resulting in a unique temperament. Physical and emotional illnesses are caused by an imbalance in humors of the body and mind that may coexist; thus, an emotional upset can cause physical illness and vice versa.
- Sacred medicine is from the Qur'an and *hadith*, and holy men are considered able to heal. The sacred tradition includes beliefs in the "evil eye" and *jinns* as disease agents as well as healing by means of manipulating impurity.
- A balanced intake of hot and cold foods to maintain health is a daily consideration, although it may be practiced subconsciously and not articulated.
- *Narahati* is a general term used to express a wide range

of undifferentiated, unpleasant emotional or physical feelings, such as feeling depressed, uneasy, nervous, disappointed, or not fully well. *Narahati* is often expressed by silence, sullenness, crying, or avoidance of food. Many individuals somatize in a subconscious effort to communicate *narahati* or distress that cannot be otherwise expressed verbally. By somatizing, they construct an illness that is culturally sanctioned and socially understood. The source can be personal, social, spiritual, or psychological.

- Somatization also allows individuals to distance themselves from the actual problem while putting the responsibility and focus on the metaphoric body. Because Iranians generally shy away from overt expressions of "personal self," the "somatic self" becomes a focal point in the health-care encounter. When *narahati* is caused by fright, the evil eye, or *jinns*, it may be treated with religious cures. If it is considered caused by problems of blood, nerves, or humoral imbalance, it is treated with herbs or biomedicine.

- *Ghalbam gerefteh (narahatiye qalb*, or distress of the heart) may be expressed as a feeling that the heart is being squeezed and can range in severity from mild excitation of the heart or palpitations to fainting and heart attack.

- Fright or being startled by bad news negatively affects health. Symptoms caused by fright include extreme fatigue with chills and fever as well as more severe symptoms. A client might be given salt or a mixture of hard sugar candy and water, taken to a physician, or be given herbal medicines or a religious cure.

- A sudden ailment or symptom of puzzling origin may be attributed to the evil eye, or *cheshm-i-bad*, which is the belief that the eyes of another person can cause illness. *Cheshm-i-bad* can be unintentional (enthusiastically complimenting someone without saying "In the name of God") or intentional (cast out due to jealousy or enmity).

- Most individuals expect immediate relief or cures from the health-care system and may shop around until they find a provider they like. At the same time, they may seek advice from those who can suggest herbal remedies.

- Herbal remedies are used primarily to relieve symptoms. Mint tea and cilantro seeds are used to promote relaxation and sleep.
- Iranians also protect their health by getting enough rest and exercise, by taking vitamins, and by keeping warm or dressing adequately.
- Most Iranians practice self-medication and use prescription and over-the-counter medications as well as home-made herbal remedies. Antibiotics, codeine-based analgesics, mood-altering drugs in the benzodiazepine family, and intramuscular vitamins are available over-the-counter in Iran, and immigrants often bring these medications with them to the United States. Many Iranians believe that complementary treatments are more effective than a single treatment. Ask clients in a non-judgmental manner about full disclosure of prescription and nonprescription medicines and herbal treatments.
- Self-adjusting dosage of prescribed medications is common.
- When ill, most individuals are inclined to be passive and cared for by health-care providers and family members.
- When an individual is hospitalized, family members are expected to visit frequently or to be present continuously until the client is discharged from the hospital or is fully functioning again. Self-care should be implemented by encouraging family members to assist with care of the sick person.
- Common herbal remedies include dried flowers, seeds, leaves, and berries, steeped in hot or cold water and drunk for a variety of purposes, such as digestive problems, "cleaning the blood or kidneys," coughs, aches and pains, fevers, nerves, or fear. Some common herbal medications include *gol-i-gov zabon* (dried foxglove flowers) for an imbalance in the digestive system or nervous upsets, which is sometimes taken with *nabat*, a concentrated sugar. *Khakshir* (flat, brown rocket seed) is used for stomach problems and "dirty

blood"; *razianeh* is used for halitosis; quince seeds are sucked for sore throats; and *sedr* prevents and treats dandruff. *Neshasteh* (wheat starch) is combined with boiling water and drunk for sore throats or coughs and is also used to stop diarrhea. Mint extracts are used to relieve excess stomach gas. *Shatareh* is thought to cure fever.

- Most Iranians are expressive about their pain. Some justify suffering in light of later rewards.
- Mental illness is highly stigmatized and is thought to be genetic. If a family member has a mental illness, it is likely to be called a "neurological disorder" to avoid stigmatizing the family. Psychotherapeutic help may be avoided either because of stigma or because it is perceived as irrelevant.
- Before 1979, the disabled were hidden at home because they brought stigma on the family and because few treatment options were available. Today, rehabilitation, such as physical therapy and music therapy, is embraced as the way to bring the disabled into the mainstream.
- Blood transfusions, organ donations, and organ transplants are widely practiced. In Iran, donation of organs is often a business transaction—if a kidney is needed, it is purchased.

HEALTH-CARE PRACTITIONERS

- A frequent source of difficulties, even for immigrants with good English skills, is differing expectations regarding the proper roles of health-care providers and clients and the differences in diagnostic styles between Iranian and American physicians. Immigrants think that Iranian doctors make more authoritative and quicker diagnoses, using minimal technology, even if they may be uncertain or wrong. American physicians who are tentative, ask the client to describe the problem, or order too many tests may be viewed as incompetent.
- Most Iranians prefer to be cared for by health-care providers of the same sex. Iranian women are modest in front of men. Some very traditional families may

consider taking a woman client elsewhere or avoid care until the situation is acute, if only male health providers are available. **If possible, male health-care providers should not ask women to undress fully for an examination or procedure.**

- The most respected health-care provider is an experienced, middle-aged to elderly male physician, with several degrees, and preferably with a high position in the hospital or university. He is considered the authority and is expected to act like one, making diagnoses quickly and prescribing remedies that cure the client.
- The least respected health-care providers are students; immigrant families sometimes refuse student caregivers. Nurses are accorded little respect compared with physicians. Male nurses or women who have gray hair and positions of authority are accorded more respect than young, single, female nurses. Nurses who encourage self-care may be perceived as uncaring or even incompetent.

References

Hafizi, H., & Lipson, J. (2003). People of Iranian heritage. In L. Purnell and B. Paulanka (Eds.), *Transcultural health care: A culturally competent approach* (2nd ed., pp. 177–194). Philadelphia: F.A. Davis Company.

Klessig, J. (1992). The effect of values and culture on life-support decisions. *Western Journal of Medicine, 157*(3), 316–322.

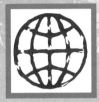

People of Irish Heritage

Overview and Heritage

The Republic of Ireland, whose capital city is Dublin with 1 million people, is also known as Eire and the Emerald Isle and covers most of the island bearing its name. The remainder of the island, Northern Ireland, is part of Great Britain. With a population of 3.8 million, the Republic of Ireland has a landmass of 32,500 square miles, slightly larger than the state of West Virginia. The Irish Sea and St. George's Channel separate Ireland from Great Britain. Ireland had a population of 8.5 million until the great potato famine of 1846 to 1848, when the population decreased to 3.4 million; since then it has remained relatively stable. During the potato famine, thousands of Irish died from malnutrition, typhus, dysentery, and scurvy, and millions immigrated to America. Ireland is the land of practical joking, red-haired leprechauns with pots of gold at the end of the rainbow, fairy tales, queens of the underworld, banshees, and superstitions.

More people of Irish descent (38.8 million) live in the United States than in Ireland. Irish is the second largest ancestry in the United States. As a result of Irish influence, the

265

United States celebrates a day in honor of St. Patrick, the patron saint of Ireland, on March 17. The Irish in America are a diverse group and vary in their beliefs according to the primary and secondary characteristics of culture as described in Chapter 1. The Irish immigrated to America in large numbers for almost three centuries beginning in the 1600s. The earliest settlements of Irish Catholics in America were in the colonies of Virginia and Maryland. The Irish ship, *St. Patrick*, arrived in Boston harbor in 1636. By 1699, Irish Catholic immigration was restricted in Virginia, Maryland, and South Carolina. For most of the 18th century, immigration from Ireland was dominated by Presbyterians. In the 19th and 20th centuries, most of the Irish immigrants were Catholic. From initial experiences of bigotry and prejudice, the Irish in America brought their values of education, a strong work ethic, and the importance of children. Religious persecution and deplorable economic conditions were primary reasons for early immigration to America. Most of the experiences of the Irish in America were similar to those of other immigrant groups, except for three features. First, the period of immigration lasted for well over a century. Many first-generation Irish in America saved money so other family members could come to America. Second, Irish women immigrated as single women rather than as part of a family group. This was in contrast to other immigrant groups and was without parallel in the history of European immigration. Third, the established Catholic churches fulfilled a cultural and religious role for the Irish in America, became the center of their lives, and a symbol of identity. The Catholic parish was the cornerstone of the Irish community in America.

Most Irish immigrants settled in industrial areas in the northeastern United States along the Atlantic coast. The cities of Philadelphia, New York, and Boston have the largest Irish settlements, followed by the commercial centers in Ohio, Illinois, and Michigan. Early Irish towns have been described as models for latter-day ghettos occupied by other groups whose race, religion, and nationality set them apart. In the early 20th century, first-generation Irish lived in urban areas. However, second- and third-generation Irish families began leaving these areas around that time and moving to the suburbs. Suburban Irish became known as lace-curtain Irish, and those left in the city became known as shanty Irish.

The Irish attained success in America because they spoke the same language, had the same physical appearance as other European Americans, and mastered the political system. They may have assimilated less than other ethnic groups because it was easier for them to blend with the rest of society. Many Irish children in America went to work at a young age, often at the expense of their education, because they were needed to help provide for the family and to send money to Ireland for other family members. Early Irish male immigrants contributed to the growth of America by helping build the Erie Canal, the transcontinental railroad, and skyscrapers. They served their new country by fighting in major military conflicts. They have made significant contributions to their new homeland in politics, the labor movement, the Catholic Church, the arts, and service to their country. One-third of U.S. presidents trace their lineage to Irish descent. Three early presidents, Andrew Jackson, James Buchanan, and Chester Arthur were sons of Irish immigrants. The priesthood was the leading career choice for second-generation Irish men in the early 1900s.

COMMUNICATIONS

- The major languages spoken in Ireland are English and Irish (Gaelic); the latter is the official language and is spoken primarily in West Ireland. Modern-day Irish priests, politicians, and others share the love of using many words and playing with language not only for communication but also for enjoyment and entertainment. The Irish enjoy puns, riddles, limericks, and storytelling.
- This Irish accent has a nasal quality and is spoken with a strong inflection on the first syllable of a word, resulting in a loss of weak syllables. Words ending in a vowel weaken the consonants following them. When one becomes accustomed to hearing the Irish-accented English used by the newer immigrants, there is little difficulty in understanding the speaker. Irish is

Irish

low-context English, using many words to express a thought. This low contextual use of the English language has its roots in the Celtic folk tradition of storytelling.

- Some common Gaelic words and their meanings are: *shamrock* for "emblem," *limer* for "folklore character," *colleen* or *lassie* for "girl," *sonsie* or *sonsy* for "handsome," *cess* for "luck," *brogue* for "shoe," *dudeen* for "pipe tobacco," and *paddy* for "Irishman."

- Even though most Irish delight in telling long stories, when discussing personal matters they are much less expressive unless they are talking with close friends and family. Even then, many are still reluctant to express their innermost thoughts and feelings.

- Humility and emotional reserve are considered virtues. Displays of emotion and affection in public are avoided and are often difficult in private. Family members are expected to know that they are loved without being told. To many, caring actions are more important than verbal expressions.

- The Irish use direct eye contact when speaking with each other. Not maintaining eye contact may be interpreted as a sign of disrespect, guilt, or evidence that the other person cannot be trusted.

- Personal space is important to the Irish, who may require greater distance in spatial relationships than other ethnocultural groups. When speaking, they stand farther apart than other European Americans.

- Although the Irish may be less physically expressive with hand and body gesturing, facial expressions are readily displayed, with frequent smiling even during times of adversity.

- The Irish in America, with their strong sense of tradition, are typically past-oriented. They have an allegiance to the past, their ancestors, and their history. The past is often the focus of Irish stories. However, many are past-, present-, and future-oriented. While respecting the past, they balance "being" with "doing," and they plan for the future by investing in education

and saving money. Many Irish see time as being elastic
and flexible. Therefore, Irish Americans may have to be
encouraged to arrive early for appointments.
- *Mac* before a family name means "son of," whereas the
  letter O in front of a name means "descended from."
  Gaelic names such as Brian, Maureen, Sheila, Sean, and
  Moira have become popular first names for American
  children. Otherwise, names are written with the
  surname, and the person is called by his or her first
  name in informal situations.

FAMILY ROLES AND ORGANIZATION

- The traditional Irish family is nuclear, with parents
  and children living in the same household. The Irish
  have a strong sense of family obligation, and this
  pattern continued when they immigrated to America.
  The roles of Irish American families are changing from
  traditional gender-divided roles with a move toward
  more egalitarian relationships in which men assist with
  household duties and child care.
- Children are cherished, and primary socialization is
  aimed at making them productive members of society,
  providing necessary educational experiences, and
  conferring status on the family.
- Kinship and sibling loyalty are important to the Irish.
  Families emphasize independence and self-reliance in
  children. Boys are allowed and expected to be more
  aggressive than girls, who are raised to be respectable,
  responsible, and resilient. Children are expected to have
  self-restraint and self-discipline and to be respectful and
  obedient to their parents, elders, and church and
  community figures.
- Adolescent years are a time for experiencing emotional
  autonomy, independence, and attachment outside the
  family while remaining loyal to the family and
  maintaining the traditional Irish belief in the importance
  of family. Peer-group pressures at school may have a
  significant influence and are often incongruent with the
  belief systems of Irish Americans. While parents see this

Irish

rebellion negatively, it can provide a functional benefit for teenagers by helping them to become autonomous, successful individuals of whom the family can be proud. Family relationships with teenagers contain mixed motivations of love and hatred. Because it is difficult for many Irish Americans to express their feelings, encourage openness between parents and teenagers.

- The extended family is important to the Irish. Although sentimental emotions are not expressed freely, and many Irish families have infrequent contact with extended family members, these members are available to assist when needed. Provisions are made in Irish homes for care of elderly family members, a task that becomes increasingly difficult when both parents work outside the home. Irish respect the experience of elderly people and seek their counsel for decision-making. Include elders into decision-making regarding health-care activities.

- The Irish value physical strength, endurance, work, the ability to perform work, children, and the ability to provide their children with the needed education to attain respectable socioeconomic status and professional accomplishments.

- Members of the clergy in all religions are respected.

- Additional status can be gained by remaining in traditional ethnic Irish neighborhoods. Middle-aged and older family members voice pride in their ethnic neighborhoods.

- Although no data could be found on divorce and single parenting among the Irish, one could expect that for some, a minor stigma continues for these groups.

- No information on alternative lifestyles specific to Irish in America was found in the health-care literature. A net search revealed the Irish Lesbian and Gay Organization, with links to other resources (www.ilgo2000.com). However, it has been reported that cases of AIDS related to homosexuality are low among the Irish. This may be related to the Catholic church's teaching against homosexuality and the value placed on chastity among the Irish. Same-sex relationships continue to carry a stigma for some.

Do not disclose same-sex relationships to family members or others.

BIOCULTURAL ECOLOGY

- Most Irish have dark hair and fair skin or red hair, ruddy cheeks, and fair skin; however, other variations exist in hair and skin color. The fair complexion of the Irish places them at risk for skin cancer. The Irish are taller and broader in stature than average European Americans, Asians, or Pacific Islanders. Explain the harmful effects of the sun, and encourage the use of sun block and other types of protection from the sun.
- Because mining is an important economic activity in Ireland, miners are at increased risk for respiratory diseases. In addition, the cool maritime climate of Ireland increases susceptibility to respiratory diseases. Assess newer immigrants who worked in mining industries for respiratory illnesses.
- Irish Americans have high mortality rates from coronary heart disease. Provide education and counseling regarding lifestyle and dietary changes to reduce risks associated with cardiovascular diseases.
- Osteoporosis is a significant health problem affecting older Irish women. Screen for osteoporosis in women in their late 60s or even younger if assessment data indicate it.
- The major cause of infant mortality in Ireland is congenital abnormalities. Other conditions with a high incidence among Irish newborns are phenylketonuria (PKU), neural tube defects, and fetal alcohol syndrome. Most states require screening of all newborns for PKU. Encourage women who give birth at home to seek PKU screening for their infants. Discourage alcohol intake during pregnancy.

HIGH-RISK HEALTH BEHAVIORS

- Smoking has been identified as the major risk factor causing premature mortality from cancer in Ireland and among the Irish in America. Encourage clients to stop

Irish

smoking, and assist them in finding smoking cessation programs with group and one-to-one counseling.

- The use of alcohol and intravenous drugs are major health problems among Irish Americans. Alcohol problems in Ireland are among the highest internationally. Alcoholism researchers generally agree that Irish ancestry puts individuals at risk for developing drinking problems. Irish pubs are popular establishments that have become synonymous with alcohol intake, lively music, and a vivacious time. This image of the Irish pub perpetuates the stereotype of Irish as heavy drinkers; do not ascribe this label to all Irish Americans. Because drinking may be a way of coping with problems, assist Irish clients in exploring more effective coping strategies, and caution them against the dangers of mixing alcohol with medications.
- The incidence of AIDS among the Irish is related primarily to the use of intravenous drugs. The incidence of AIDS associated with homosexual behavior is low. Direct health promotion at educating about high-risk behaviors for the prevention of AIDS.

NUTRITION

- Irish food is unpretentious and wholesome if eaten in recommended proportions. Food is an important part of health maintenance and celebrations. Eating balanced meals is considered important even if it means the individual is late for an appointment. Vitamins are commonly used as a dietary supplement.
- Traditional Catholic holidays celebrated with food include the Solemnity of Mary (Mother of God), January 1; Easter Sunday; Ascension Thursday, 40 days after Easter; the Feast of the Assumption, August 15; All Saints Day, November 1; the Feast of the Immaculate Conception, December 8; and Christmas, December 25. More devout Catholics fast and abstain from meat on Ash Wednesday, Good Friday, and all Fridays in Lent. Fasting is viewed as a discipline.
- Meat, potatoes, and vegetables are dietary staples.

Lamb, mutton, pork, and poultry are common meats. Seafood includes salmon, mussels, mackerel, oysters, and scallops. Popular Irish dishes include Irish stew made with lamb, potatoes, and onions.

- Potatoes are used in a variety of ways. *Colcannon* is made with hot potatoes, mashed with cabbage, butter, and milk, and seasoned with nutmeg. This dish may be served at Halloween. *Champ* is a popular dish made with mashed potatoes and scallions. The scallions are cut in small pieces, including the green tops, boiled in milk until tender, and then added to the mashed potatoes and served with butter. Potato cakes, made with mashed potatoes, flour, salt, and butter, are shaped into patties and fried in bacon grease. Potato cakes are served hot or cold with butter and sometimes molasses or maple syrup. Another popular dish is Dublin coddle, made with bacon, pork sausage, potatoes, and onions. Oatmeal is popular in Ireland. Soda bread, another popular food, is made with flour, baking soda, salt, sugar, cream of tartar, and sour milk.

- Mealtimes are important occasions for Irish families to socialize and discuss family concerns. Meals are eaten three times a day, with a large breakfast in rural areas, lunch around noon, and a late dinner. Some Irish Americans continue the afternoon tradition of "tea," a light sandwich or biscuit with hot tea. Because the Irish diet has the potential for being high in fats and cholesterol, assist clients with balanced food selections and preparation practices that reduce their risk of cardiovascular disease.

Irish

PREGNANCY AND CHILDBEARING PRACTICES

- Because fertility and sexuality practices for many Irish are influenced by Catholic religious beliefs, some Irish may have a tendency to view sexual relationships as a "duty." For Catholic Irish, the only acceptable methods of birth control are abstinence and the rhythm method. Women practice other means of birth control, but no statistics are available on their exact numbers.

- The birth of a baby is a joyous occasion for the Irish, with family and friends celebrating the birth with food and gifts. Consistent with many other cultural groups, a baby boy receives something blue; a baby girl receives something pink. If a gift is purchased before the birth and the sex of the baby was unknown, then the gift should be green or yellow.
- Prescriptive beliefs for a healthy pregnancy include eating a well-balanced diet. The Irish believe that not eating a well-balanced diet or not eating the right kinds of food may cause the baby to be deformed.
- The Irish share the belief, common to many other ethnic groups, that the mother should not reach over her head during pregnancy because the baby's cord may wrap around its neck. A taboo behavior in the past, which some women still respect, is that if the pregnant woman sees or experiences a tragedy during pregnancy, a congenital anomaly may occur.
- Eating a well-balanced diet after delivery continues to be a prescriptive practice for ensuring a healthy baby and maintaining the mother's health. Plenty of rest, fresh air, and sunshine are also important for maintaining the mother's health. Going to bed with wet hair or wet feet causes illness in the mother.

DEATH RITUALS

- The typical Irish reaction to death is a combination of the pagan past and current Christian faith. The Irish are fatalists and acknowledge the inevitability of death. The American emphasis on technology and dying in the hospital may be incongruent with the Irish American belief that family members should stay with the dying person. **Make arrangements for family to stay with family in the hospital and in long-term care facilities.**
- Whereas men are expected to be more stoical in their bereavement, women are more expressive. **Expect and accept a wide variety of grief expression among the Irish.**
- After a death, family and friends make every effort to be

present for the funeral. The wake continues as an important phenomenon in contemporary Irish families and is a time of melancholy, rejoicing, pain, and hopefulness. The occasion is a celebration of the person's life. The wake represents the Irish people's stubborn refusal to believe death is the end.

- Cremation is an individual choice, and there are no proscriptions against autopsy if required.

SPIRITUALITY

- The predominant religion of most Irish is Catholicism, and the church is a source of strength and solace. Other religions common among Irish in America include various Protestant denominations, such as the Church of Ireland, Presbyterian, Quaker, and Episcopalian.
- In times of illness, Irish Catholics receive the Sacrament of the Sick, which includes anointing, communion, and a blessing by the priest. The Eucharist, a small wafer made from flour and water, is given to the sick as the food of healing and health. Family members can participate if they wish. Inquire whether sick individuals want to see a member of the clergy, even if they have not been active in church.
- Attending mass daily is a common practice among many traditional and devout Irish Catholic families. Prayer is an individual and private matter. In times of illness, the clergy may offer prayers with the sick as well as with the family. Give clients privacy for prayer whether or not a clergy member is present.
- For Irish Catholics who practice their religion regularly, holy day worship begins at 4 PM the evening preceding the holy day; all Sundays are considered holy days. The obligation to fast and abstain from meat on specified days is relinquished during times of illness.
- Many Irish are fatalistic and view human beings as subjected to the harshness of nature. They gain meaning in their life through home, religion, the church, and the pub, which are centers of life in Irish communities.
- Some Irish may wear religious medals to maintain

Irish

health. Religious emblems provide solace and should not be removed.

HEALTH-CARE PRACTICES

- The Irish fatalistic outlook and external locus of control influences health-seeking behaviors. Many Irish use denial as a way of coping with physical and psychological problems. The Irish view of life is illustrated in the belief that life is black with long suffering, and the less said about it, the better. For some Irish, illness behavior does little to relieve suffering and perpetuates a self-fulfilling prophecy of fatalism.

- Many Irish ignore symptoms and delay seeking medical attention until symptoms interfere with the ability to carry out activities of daily living. Irish Americans limit and understate problems and handle problems by using denial. Because Irish people may not be very descriptive about their symptoms, treatment may be more difficult. Encourage early intervention and seeking health professionals for illnesses. Factually explain the importance of early intervention.

- Illness or injury may be linked to guilt and considered to be the result of having done something morally wrong. Restraint is a *modus operandi* in the Irish culture; temptation is ever-present and must be guarded against.

- Most Irish believe one is obligated to use ordinary means to preserve life. Therefore, extraordinary means may be withheld to allow the person to die a natural death. The sick person and family define extraordinary means; finances, quality of life, and effects on the family usually influence the decision. Arrange for a family conference to address issues and concerns in terminal care.

- Although some Irish attribute illness to sin and guilt, they readily excuse sick people from their obligations and become sources of support by assuming the normal roles of the sick until they are able to function again.

- In most Irish families, nuclear family members are

consulted first about health problems. Mothers and older women are usually sought for their knowledge of folk practices to alleviate common problems such as colds. The Irish believe that having a strong religious faith, keeping one's feet warm and dry, dressing warmly, eating a balanced diet, getting enough sleep, and exercising are important for staying healthy. **Optimize compliance for reducing health risks by emphasizing these important cultural values.**

- Irish folk practices include eating a balanced diet, getting a good night's sleep, exercising, dressing warmly, and not going out in the cold air with wet hair. Other folk practices include wearing religious medals to prevent illness, using cough syrup made from honey and whiskey, taking honey and lemon for a sore throat, drinking hot tea with whiskey for a cold, drinking hot tea for nausea, drinking tea and eating toast for a cold, and putting a damp cloth on the forehead for a headache. Some folk practices may be harmful, such as the use of senna to cleanse the bowels every 8 days, eating a lot of oily foods, and avoiding seeing a physician. **Encourage clients to reveal all traditional and home remedies being used to treat symptoms. Provide factual information about potentially harmful folk and traditional practices.**
- The behavioral response of the Irish to pain is stoic, usually ignoring or minimizing it.
- One explanation for high rates of mental illness may be associated with the Irish having difficulty describing emotions and expressing feelings. **Encourage the expression of emotions and feelings before symptoms become a problem.**
- In the past, the mentally and physically ill were taken care of in the home, not because of the stigma associated with mental illness and the family's desire to shield them, but rather because of the Irish family's preference for caring for each other whenever possible. **Assist families in finding resources for providing care at home.**
- Blood transfusions are acceptable to most Irish

Irish

Americans. Many participate in organ donation and indicate their willingness to do so on their driver's licenses. Obtain organ-donor status on an individual basis; be sensitive to client and family concerns; explain procedures involved with organ donation and procurement; answer questions factually; and explain the risks involved.

HEALTH-CARE PRACTITIONERS

- The Irish respect all health-care professionals.
- Although the Irish are not noted for being overly modest, some may prefer to receive intimate care from someone of the same gender. In general, men and women may care for each other in health-care settings as long as privacy and sensitivity are maintained.

References

Dezell, M. (2001). *Irish America: Coming into the clover: The evolution of a people and a culture.* New York: Doubleday.

Purnell, L., & Foster, J. (2003a). Cultural aspect of alcohol use: Part I. *The Drug and Alcohol Professional, (3)*3, 1723.

Purnell, L., & Foster, J. (2003b). Cultural aspect of alcohol use: Part II. The *Drug and Alcohol Professional (3)*2, 3–8.

Neill, K. (1993). Ethnic pain styles in acute myocardial infarction. *Western Journal of Nursing Research, 15*(5), 531–547.

Robins, J. (Ed.) (1997). *Reflections on health: Commemorating fifty years of the Department of Health 1947–1997.* Dublin, Ireland: Department of Health.

Time Almanac. (2002). Boston: Time Inc.

Wilson, S. (2003). People of Irish heritage. In L. Purnell & B. Paulanka (Eds.), *Transcultural health care: A culturally competent approach* (2nd ed., pp. 194–204). Philadelphia: F.A. Davis Company.

Zborowski, M. (1969). *People in pain.* San Francisco: Jossey-Bass.

Zola, I. K. (1983). *Socio-medical inquiries: Recollections, reflections, and reconsideration.* Philadelphia: Temple University Press.

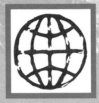

CHAPTER 20

People of Italian Heritage

Overview and Heritage

Italy, which includes Sicily and Sardinia, has a population of 57.6 million people. Italy is famous for the marvels of ancient Rome, such as the Coliseum, Pantheon, libraries, museums, and St. Peter's Square; the Leaning Tower of Pisa; the canals and Piazza San Marco in Venice; the Ravenna opera; the ruins of Pompeii; the Portofino lace-makers, wineries, and marble; and artists such as Michelangelo and Leonardo da Vinci. An Italian, Christopher Columbus, is credited with discovering North America, which is named after the Italian explorer, Amerigo Vespucci.

Italians in America are bound by the commonalities of language, home country, heredity, religion, and history. Italian American immigrant groups include (a) first-generation, mostly traditional, older Italians living primarily in enclaves; (b) second-generation, less traditional Italians living in suburban and urban neighborhoods with ethnic enclaves; (c) third-generation, usually more educated, Italians living primarily in the suburbs; and (d) a relatively small group of newer immigrants with strong ties to their homeland. Because of the

279

primary and secondary characteristics of culture as described in Chapter 1, Italians are not a homogeneous group. This chapter focuses on the beliefs and practices of the Italians from the mainland of Italy, although Italians with a heritage from Sicily and Sardinia may share some of these characteristics. Most of the 14.7 million Italians in the United States live in New York, New Jersey, Massachusetts, Pennsylvania, and California. Italian enclaves, or "Little Italies," can be found in major cities throughout the United States. Because of their general distaste for abstract values, ambivalent attitude toward formal schooling, and desire to remain close to family, a disproportionate number of second- and third-generation Italian Americans seek employment in blue-collar jobs. Even though many have made great strides in various occupations, only 20 percent have obtained professional status.

COMMUNICATIONS

- The official language of Italy is Italian; however, there are 19 dialects. Many second-generation Italian Americans do not speak Italian well or at all. When a dialect-specific interpreter is not available, the interpreter should select words that have pure meanings from Tuscan Italian.
- In many households, discussions can become quite passionate, with voice volume raised and many people speaking at once. High voice volume does not mean anger, rather passionate communication.
- Their willingness to share thoughts and feelings among family members is a major distinguishing characteristic. Positive and negative emotions and sentiments are permissible and encouraged with family members. Expressions of affection might erupt, and frequent kissing reaffirms the emotional bond among Italians.
- The "typical" kiss is a kiss on each cheek. Gestures convey a range of feelings, from poetic eloquence to intense anger, and are conveyed in an economical, subtle, flowing, and almost imperceptible manner. For example, a slowly raised chin means "I don't know."

Observe clients for nonverbal cues to obtain the full meaning of verbal communication.

- Touching and embracing family and friends are common. Touching between men and women, between men, and between women can be observed during verbal communication.
- Past orientation is evidenced by the pride they take in their home country's rich Roman heritage. Within the context of fatalism and their present orientation, they do not allow their imagination to stray too far, occupy themselves with concrete problems and situations, and accept things the way they are. Finally, they are future-oriented as evidenced by the importance given to planning ahead and saving for the future. First-generation and newer immigrants view time as an approximation rather than categorically imperative; second- and third-generation Italians adhere to clock time at least in the work situation and for appointments.
- The order of first and last names is frequently reversed in Italy. Pietropaolo Vincenzo is often used when Vincenzo is the person's first name and Pietropaolo is the last name. Nicknames are common and used among family and friends. A person is called by the first or given name in social situations and by a title such as Miss, Ms., Mr., Mrs., or Dr. and his or her last or family surname in the health-care environment. Ask recent immigrants the order of the name to assure an accurate health-care record.

FAMILY ROLES AND ORGANIZATION

- Traditional families recognize the father's authority as absolute; nothing is purchased, and decisions are not made without his approval. The father's decision may be accepted as law, even among his married children. To criticize one's father is considered a sacrilege. In old age and illness, the eldest son supersedes him, but even then, the father retains much of his prestige.
- Many husbands turn over their paychecks to their wives

Italian

to run the home, and thus women tend to have more power in economic decisions. Women also dominate decision-making on child-rearing issues and family social events. Even though traditional roles remain strong in second- and third-generation families, a trend toward more egalitarian relationships is evolving.

- The "typical" traditional father frequently demonstrates public and private affection for his children, but such demonstrations are less frequent in public for his wife.

- Children are taught to have good manners and respect for their elders. Boys and girls are encouraged to be independent and are expected to contribute to the family's support as soon as they are old enough to work. Adolescent girls are expected to remain virgins until they marry.

- While parents are alive, the home is most often the focus of family gatherings. Sons and daughters visit frequently during the week and after church on Sundays to share a large meal at the parents' house.

- To most older people, the ideal living situation is to maintain one's own home near one's children. Older people receive respect, gratitude, and love in return for their many sacrifices.

- Most Italian Americans have an actively functioning kinship and extended family system that is the primary focus of solidarity for the nuclear family. Because the extended family is close, and frequent visits are important, make special arrangements for visitation when clients are in acute or long-term care facilities.

- Social status for most families comes from family lineage. Titles are more important than names. Identify yourself with a title such as Mr., Mrs., Miss, Ms., or Dr. to increase compliance with health treatments and regimens.

- A weakened external restriction on premarital sex continues, but internal inhibitions remain strong. A strong sense of modesty and embarrassment may result in the avoidance of discussions related to sex and menstruation, hindering early diagnosis and primary prevention interventions.

- Most individuals do not reject another family member because of an infraction or alternative lifestyle such as divorce, living together before marriage, or being involved in a lesbian or gay relationship. The individual is accepted without consequences. When the need arises to make social support referrals for gays or lesbians, health-care practitioners can assist clients in contacting one of the gay and lesbian religious groups.

BIOCULTURAL ECOLOGY

- Italians as a group have varied physical characteristics. Those from a predominantly northern background have lighter skin, lighter hair, and blue eyes, whereas those from the south of Rome, particularly from Sicily, have dark, often curly hair, dark eyes, and olive-colored skin. In dark-skinned clients, the skin turns ashen instead of blue in the presence of cyanosis and decreased hemoglobin levels. Examine the sclera, conjunctiva, buccal mucosa, tongue, lips, nailbeds, and palms of the hands and soles of the feet. To assess for jaundice, look at the conjunctiva and in the buccal mucosa for patches of bilirubin pigment.
- People of Italian ancestry have some notable genetic diseases. Familial Mediterranean fever, recurrent polyserositis, is characterized by short attacks of fever, peritonitis, pleuritis, and arthritis, with death caused by amyloidosis if the disease progresses. No specific diagnostic test is available; treatment is symptomatic.
- Mediterranean-type G-6-phosphate dehydrogenase (G-6-PD) deficiency is an inherited, X-linked, recessive disorder most fully expressed in homozygous men, with a carrier state found in heterozygous women. Red blood cell damage begins after intense or prolonged administration of sulfonamides, antimalarial agents, salicylates, or naphthaquinolones; after ingestion of fava beans; or in the presence of hypoxemia or acidosis. Supportive therapy includes withdrawing the causative agent and administering blood transfusions and oral iron therapy, which usually results in spontaneous recovery.

Italian

- β-Thalassemia, of which there are two types, is caused by genetic defects in the synthesis of the hemoglobin A or B chain. Beta-chain production is depressed moderately in the heterozygous form, β-thalassemia minor, and severely depressed in the homozygous form, thalassemia major, which is also called Cooley's anemia. β-Thalassemia minor causes mild to moderate anemia, splenomegaly, bronze coloring of the skin, and hyperplasia of the bone marrow. Affected people are usually asymptomatic. Individuals with β-thalassemia major may experience severe anemia; death caused by cardiac failure can occur in early childhood if this condition is left untreated. No cure exists, but palliative therapy includes repeated transfusions of packed red blood cells. Mediterranean-type G-6-PD deficiency and β-thalassemias have a profound effect on drug metabolism. Because of conditions such as hypoxemia and acidosis, the ingestion of fava beans and the administration of sulfonamides, antimalarial agents, salicylates, and naphthaquinolones can exacerbate these conditions; take extra precaution when prescribing these drug therapies.
- There is a high incidence of hypertension and coronary artery diseases related to smoking and type A behavior.

HIGH-RISK HEALTH BEHAVIORS

- Many immigrants continue to smoke. Alcoholism also presents a risk in this group. Assess for illnesses related to smoking and alcohol use, especially among newer immigrants. Encourage clients to cease or decrease smoking. Promote responsible drinking.

NUTRITION

- Food is symbolic of a connection between a child and the parents; food represents the product of the father's labor, prepared with care by the mother. In a symbolic sense, meals are a communion of the family, and food is sacred because it is the tangible medium of that communion. A mother may demonstrate her affection by feeding her family and anyone else she likes. To the average "mom," love is a four-letter word: food.

- The diet, rich in vegetables, pasta, fruit, fish, and cheese, varies according to the region of Italy from which the individual originated. Northern Italian foods are rich in cream and cheese, resulting in a potential high intake of fat. Southern Italian foods are prepared in red sauces, spices, and added salt. **Because of regional variations in food selections and preparation practices, specifically inquire about the diet, preferably during intake assessments.**

- Dietary staples are spaghetti, lasagna, ravioli, pasta with pesto, and manicotti. Vegetables, fresh fruit, and beans are common. Other popular Italian foods include lentils, sausage, eggplant parmigiana, salami, olive oil, espresso and cappuccino coffee, wine, ice cream (gelato), pastries such as cannoli and biscotti, and cheeses such as provolone, ricotta, romano, and parmigiana. Other common dishes include escarole, Caesar salad, calzone, and pizza. Table 20–1 lists the Italian names of popular foods with their descriptions and ingredients. Wine is taken at almost every meal, and red wine, mixed with water, is given to children with meals to maintain healthy blood.

- A common practice for health promotion is eating a clove of garlic every night before going to bed to prevent upper respiratory infections. Garlic may also be worn around the neck when there is an epidemic of influenza or other upper respiratory ailments to prevent the wearer from getting the infection. Eating a fresh raw egg every morning keeps the person strong. Fresh dandelions are used to make a salad or are boiled to make soup to give the person strength.

PREGNANCY AND CHILDBEARING PRACTICES

- Many third-generation Italian Americans use birth control from the beginning of marriage; sex is commonly discussed in the family.

TABLE 20 – 1

Italian Foods

Common Name	Description	Ingredients
Calamari	Squid, fried or on pasta	Floured squid fried in olive oil or in red sauce
Frittata	Italian omelet	Eggs, peppers, and onions cooked in olive oil
Minestrone	Soup with greens	Escarole and beans with garlic and other herbs
Parmigiana di melanzana	Eggplant parmesan	Eggplant, tomato sauce, bread crumbs, Parmesan cheese, and mozzarella cheese
Pasta con pesto	Sauce served over linguine	Sauce of basil, nuts, olive oil, and garlic
Pasta e fagioli	Macaroni and beans	Shell-shaped pasta, kidney beans, and tomato sauce
Pasta marinara	Pasta in tomato sauce	Tomato sauce
Pizza fritta	Fried dough with sugar and cinnamon	Bread dough fried in oil and sprinkled with sugar and cinnamon
Prosciutto	Thinly sliced ham	Delicate thin ham served with melon
Spaghetti aglio olio	Spaghetti with olive oil	Spaghetti, olive oil, garlic, and red pepper
Tortellini	Little rounds of pasta in white or red sauce	Pasta dough stuffed with meat and cheese
Veal scaloppine	Medallions of veal	Veal sautéed with wine, butter, and lemon

- The belief that a mother does not conceive while nursing continues to be held by many Italian women. Sprinkling salt under and around the bed of a newly married couple is believed to make them fertile.
- Common beliefs and customs about pregnancy are shown in Box 20–1.
- Although many women still prefer having their children delivered at home by a family physician or a midwife, many women deliver their babies in hospitals. If labor does not progress rapidly enough, a neighbor has to spit out the window. This ritualistic spitting has the power to break any magic spell that might have brought the ill fortune of slow labor.
- A traditional postpartum woman is not allowed to wash her hair, take a shower, or resume her domestic chores for at least 2 or 3 weeks after birth so she can rest. The woman's mother and other female family members tend to the chores and assist with the care of the new baby.
- New mothers are expected to breast-feed to restore the health of the reproductive organs and keep the mother

BOX 20-1 • Beliefs About Pregnancy

Traditional beliefs related to pregnancy include the following:

- Coffee spills may result in the baby being born with a birthmark where the coffee was spilled.
- Women must abstain from sexual relationships while pregnant.
- If the expectant mother's cravings for a particular food are not satisfied, a congenital anomaly may occur, or the baby will be marked.
- If a pregnant woman is not given the food she smells, the fetus moves, and a miscarriage results.
- She should not reach over her head because harm may come to the baby.

Italian

and baby free of infections. Many believe that bigger babies are healthier. The size of the baby is perceived as an index of the successful maintenance of maternal and wifely responsibilities. Explain that a fat baby is not necessarily a healthy baby.

DEATH RITUALS

- Death is a great social loss and brings an immediate response from the community. It means sending food and flowers (chrysanthemums), giving money, and congregating at the home of the deceased. Friends and distant relatives bring food. The funeral procession to the cemetery is a symbol of family status, which is determined by the number of cars in the procession.
- Grief over the deceased is eased if a biomedical explanation for the cause of death is given and if it is explained that the death was inevitable. Within the context of fatalism in Catholicism, many Italians view death as "God's will"; thus, a fatal diagnosis may not be discussed with the ill family member.
- Emotional outpourings can be profuse. Women may mourn dramatically, even histrionically, for the whole family. They do not merely weep; they may rage against death for the harm it has done to the family. Family members may moan and scream for the deceased throughout the church service. Screaming is an effort to ensure that Jesus, Mary, and the saints hear what the bereaved are thinking and feeling.
- Family members get up constantly to touch and talk to the deceased loved one.
- Children are taught to let the female kin express their feelings for them.
- The real time of sorrow comes at the end of the ceremony when the priest and nonfamily congregation say good-bye to the deceased. At this time, the family is left on its own for a time with the loved one. Older women may throw themselves onto the casket, trying to prevent it from leaving the church.
- Then the priest intones the farewell: "May the angels

take you into paradise, may the martyrs welcome you on your way." While men mourn, they do so in the fashion of *pazienza* (patience). Their constant, silent, and expressionless presence may be their only act of public mourning. When the loss is a child or spouse, expressions of grief continue for years. **Be open to emotive and alternative expressions of grief.**

- More traditional families hold anniversary masses for the deceased and wear black for months or years.

SPIRITUALITY

- The predominant religion is traditional Roman Catholicism, the center of which is the celebration of Mass, the Eucharist, which is the commemoration of Christ's sacrificial death and of His Resurrection. Other sacraments are baptism, confirmation, confession, matrimony, ordination, and anointing of the sick.
- The workings of nature and the benefits and calamities caused by nature are attributed to (a) saints resembling pagan gods such as witches, ghosts, and demons; (b) the Christian God; (c) Satan; and (d) any and all possible combinations and alliances of these factors.
- When a loved one becomes ill, prayers are said at home and in church for the person's health. **Help clients obtain the basic rites of the Sacrament of the Sick, which includes anointing, communion and, if possible, a blessing by the priest.** Most pray to the Virgin Mary, the Madonna, and a number of saints.
- Even though Catholics are obligated to fast or abstain from meat and meat products on certain days of the year, the sick are not bound by this practice. **Despite the church's exception for the sick, many first-generation immigrants choose to fast.** Respect this wish.
- Most individuals view God as an all-understanding, compassionate, and forgiving being.
- Prayer and having faith in God and the saints help Italian Americans through illnesses. Italian men bypass praying to the Madonna because women are perceived to have a closer relationship with Her.

Italian

- Niceties of Catholic orthodoxy and enlightened learning are employed together with pagan practices such as beliefs in witches, ghosts, and demons. The lessons of common sense and science are freely mingled with those of magicoreligious beliefs. **Respect and acknowledge religious beliefs to gain the trust of clients.**
- Many traditional first-generation and newer Italian American families display shrines to the Blessed Virgin in their backyards.

HEALTH-CARE PRACTICES

- The beliefs of first-generation and newer immigrants about health and health care are similar to beliefs in their homeland. In traditional terms, illnesses are attributable to (1) wind currents that carry disease, (2) contamination, (3) heredity, (4) supernatural (God's will) or human causes, and (5) psychosomatic interactions.
- Leaving a body cavity, such as the abdomen, open too long during surgery exposes it to excess air and leads to a quicker death.
- Within the context of fatalism, diseases largely run their own course; thus, it is better to leave the investigation into health problems until a condition becomes so obvious that it cannot be neglected.
- Nervousness, hysteria, and many other mental illnesses are attributed to an evil spirit entering the body and remaining in the body until it is cast out by making its abiding place so unpleasant that it is forced to leave.
- The extended family may be the front-line resource for intensive advice on emotional problems. Mental health specialists are frequently perceived as inappropriate agents for meeting problems that are beyond the expertise of the family and local community. The mother assumes responsibility for the health of the children.
- *Il mal occhio* (the evil eye), which is also called *occhio cattivo* (bad eye), *occhio morto* (eye of death), and *occhio tristo* (wicked eye), has its roots in ancient

Greece. Individuals can protect themselves from the evil eye by using magical symbols and by learning the rituals of the *maghi* (witch). Amulets, miniature representations of natural or man-made weapons that fight off the evil eye include teeth, claws, and replicas of animal horns that are worn on necklaces or bracelets, held in a pocket, or sewn into clothing. *Cornicelli* (little red horns) can still be purchased in Italian neighborhoods as good-luck charms. Many believe in obtaining as much protection from the evil eye as possible. An array of pictures and statues of the Madonna and saints are liberally distributed throughout their homes and supplement these red horns, which are often hung over a door. **When clients bring amulets with them into health-care settings, do not remove them because they provide great solace to the clients.** The principal animals in folk prescriptions are the wolf, chicken, viper, lizard, frog, pig, dog, mouse, and sea horse. Body secretions such as saliva, urine, mother's milk, blood, and earwax are commonly used as folk medicines. Some Italian mothers use early morning saliva to bathe the eyes of children with conjunctivitis.

- Common plant derivatives used in folk healing are olive oil, lemon juice, wine, vinegar, garlic, onion, lettuce, and tobacco. A crown of lemon leaves is believed to cure a headache, as are wild fennel, deadly nightshade, and sorrel. The leaves and flowers of the wild mallow herb, *malva*, are used to make tea, providing cool energy and positive effects on the lungs and stomach. When suffering from a fever, a person is given hot rather than cold drinks. For indigestion, a mixture of coffee grounds and sugar is taken. Grain sprouts, especially those grown in the dark, in consecrated ground, in the churchyard, or in a crypt, are believed to protect against Satan and the forces of chaos.

- Baldness is treated with an application of warm cow's urine. Sulfur and lemon juice are mixed as an ointment for scabies, and potato or lemon slices are bound to the wrists to reduce fever.

- Many individuals do not use available resources because

Italian

they have little faith in medical practitioners. In addition, the high cost of institutional care may be a deterrent for many. **Provide a cultural broker for newer immigrants who have difficulty with the English language and who are unfamiliar with the health-care system.**

- Women are more likely to report pain experiences and express symptoms to the fullest extent; however, they expect immediate treatment. Most are expressive with chronic pain. **Be cautious to avoid an overdose of pain medication.**

- The sick role is not entered without personal feelings of guilt; thus, individuals may keep sickness a secret from their family and friends and are not inclined to describe the details because they blame themselves for the health problem. Suppressing emotions and stress from fear, guilt, and anxiety can cause illness. Most believe that people who have disabilities should be cared for at home by the family; very few individuals are placed in long-term care facilities.

- A person with a physical or mental disability is not stigmatized because the condition is believed to be God's will.

- Families may be ashamed to let neighbors know of an incident that may impair the social status of a family member. This applies especially to afflicted daughters and to a lesser extent to sons. A reputation of poor health unfavorably affects the value of a young woman's potential as a wife. When a family member is sick, other women in the family take over and assist until the sick person is well.

- Judicious use of medications and blood transfusions are permissible and morally acceptable as long as the benefits outweigh the risks to the individual; thus, there is little objection to accepting a blood transfusion. Organ donation is morally permissible when the benefits to the recipient are proportionate to the loss of the organ to the donor and when the organ does not deprive the donor of life or the functional integrity of the body. Otherwise, organ transplant is an individual decision.

HEALTH-CARE PRACTITIONERS

- Mystical powers are not limited to saints. For the traditional, certain humans are believed to have immediate and potent access to magical powers. These are the *maghi*, "male witch," and the *maghe*, "female witch," who are granted various amounts of black magic power at birth. A man or woman with more limited powers is often called *un'uomo di fuori* (a different or "outside" man). A powerful sorcerer is called *lupo mannaro* (werewolf). These extraordinary people are thought to possess or influence the evil eye. They have the power to cast spells, cause or cure ailments, and change events by using their own force— even their gaze is thought to be potent. These traditional beliefs may be practiced by first-generation and newer Italian immigrants but hold little value for second- and third-generation Italian Americans. Accept and incorporate folk practitioners' practices into treatment plans, along with providing written instructions for biomedical treatments.

- Success in persuading children to take medicine depends on the trust the mother has in the health-care provider. If the health-care provider is Italian or makes an effort to understand the Italian culture, the mother is more compliant. Assigning practitioners of the same culture, when possible, is advantageous.

References

Hillman, S. (2003). People of Italian heritage. In L. Purnell and B. Paulanka (Eds.), *Transcultural health care: A culturally competent approach* (2nd ed., pp. 205–218). Philadelphia: F.A. Davis Company.

Levy, R. (1993). Ethnic and racial differences in response to medicines: Preserving individualized therapy in managed pharmaceutical programmes. *Pharmaceutical Medicine, 7,* 139–165.

Mangione, J., & Morreale, B. (1993). *La storia: Five centuries of the Italian American experience.* New York: Harper Collins.

Italian

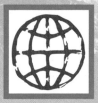

People of Japanese Heritage

Overview and Heritage

Nihon, or Nippon, as Japan is called in the Japanese language, is a 1,200-mile chain of islands in the northwestern Pacific Ocean. Japan borders Russia, Korea, and China, and its modern history has, until recently, been shaped by conflict with these countries. The population of more than 126 million resides mainly on the four largest islands. Japanese citizens residing in North America tend to locate in large commercial and educational centers. Over 500,000 million Japanese live in the United States.

Education is highly valued; the illiteracy rate in Japan is nearly zero. About 40 percent of all young people go on to higher education. The alumni network primarily provides job placements; the school one attends determines to a great extent where one is employed after graduation. Issei (first-generation Japanese immigrants) vary widely in their English-language ability. Nisei (second-generation immigrants) and sansei (third-generation immigrants) were educated under the American educational system to the extent that they were permitted; for example, educational access was limited or segregated during the World War II internment of American citizens of Japanese ancestry.

COMMUNICATIONS

- Japanese is the language of Japan, with the exception of the indigenous Ainu people.
- Because high school graduates in Japan complete 6 years of English, even newer Japanese immigrants and sojourners can speak, understand, read, and write the English language to some extent. **Whereas the language barrier may be an obstacle to verbal instructions or explanations in English-speaking health-care settings, Japanese clients are likely to use written materials effectively.**
- Their sensitivity to relative status and the need to constantly gauge one's behavior limits the circle of intimates with whom one can truly relax.
- Men tend to speak more coarsely and women with more gentility or refinement.
- Light social banter and gentle joking are a mainstay of group relations, serving to foster group cohesiveness.
- Polite discussion unrelated to business, often over *o-cha* (green tea), precedes business negotiations. Relationship-building and respect for personal privacy are important aspects of working relationships in all sectors.
- Open communication is discouraged, making it difficult to learn what people think. In particular, saying "no" is considered extremely impolite; rather, one should let the matter drop.
- A high value is placed on "face" and "saving face." Asking someone to do something he or she cannot do induces loss of face or shame. For people to be shown wrong is deeply humiliating. People feel shame for themselves and their group, but they are respected when they bear shame in stoic silence. Because of ethnic homogeneity, an ingrained sensitivity to the feelings of others and close contact with one's family, classmates, and work group, vague and intuitive communication is well understood by fellow group members.

- Traditional Japanese exhibit considerable control over body language. Anger or dismay may be quite difficult for Westerners to detect.
- Smiling and laughter are common shields for embarrassment or distress.
- Prolonged eye contact is not polite even within families.
- Social touching occurs among group members but not among people who are less closely acquainted. In general, body space is respected.
- Intimate behavior in the presence of others is taboo.
- When people greet one another, whether for the first time or for the first time on a given day, the traditional bow is performed. The depth of the bow, its duration, and the number of repetitions reflect the relative status of the parties involved and the formality of the occasion.
- An offer to shake hands by a Westerner is reciprocated graciously.
- Overall orientation is toward the future. Punctuality is highly valued.
- Family names are stated first, followed by given names. Seki Noriko would be the name of a woman, Noriko, of the Seki family. The family names of both men and women, married or single, are designated by the suffix -san, but one does not use that designation when referring to oneself.
- Women generally assume their husband's family name upon marriage. Schoolchildren may use given names when speaking to one another, also designated with the suffix -san. Work groups and business associates tend to use family names. Infants and young children are called by their first names, followed by -chan. Schoolboys, and increasingly schoolgirls, may be referred to by their first or last names, followed by -kun.
- Elders are referred to respectfully. The designation sensei (master) is a term of respect used with the names of physicians, teachers, bosses, or others in positions of authority. **Greet Japanese clients with a handshake, and call them formally by their last name.**

FAMILY ROLES AND ORGANIZATION

- The predominant family structure is nuclear. The role of wife and mother is dominant.
- Wives care for their husbands to a great extent. Japanese men are presumed not to be capable of managing day-to-day matters.
- The paramount family concern is for the children's education. It is the mother's responsibility to oversee the completion and quality of homework.
- Children are socialized to study hard, make their best effort, and be good group members. They are taught to take care of each other, and girls are taught to take care of boys. Self-expression is not valued.
- Be aware of differences in spousal relationships when assessing the quality of family dynamics and communication, sexual health, and sensitivity to risk for sexually transmitted diseases.
- The primary relationship within a family is the mother-child relationship, particularly that of mothers and sons. It is customary for a mother to sleep with the youngest child until that child is 10 years old or older, and when a new baby is born the older sibling may sleep with the father or a grandparent. Be aware of Japanese family sleeping practices and refrain from judgmental evaluation.
- Babies are not allowed to cry; they are picked up instantly. Women constantly hold their babies in carriers on their chests and sleep with them.
- Corporal punishment is acceptable in Japan. Explain U.S. child abuse laws to clients.
- Traditional teens and college students generally do not date. They typically join clubs, membership in which is taken seriously; most social activities, such as ski trips, are club activities. Japan has the lowest incidence of teen birth in the world. Do not assume that dating holds the amount of concern for Japanese young people that it does for American teens. Do not assume that Japanese youth are well informed about sexuality and sexual health risks.

Japanese

- Older people are respected and cared for by the family in the home, if at all possible, with the eldest son being the responsible family member. Be sensitive to Japanese clients' sense of obligation and commitment to older people. Help families network within the Japanese American community for both social support and for resources or good long-term care facilities.
- In Japan, a small segment of women have long lived outside the usual constraints for their gender. Women of "the floating world," or the entertainment industry, enjoy a fair amount of autonomy. The most traditional of these, the *geisha,* live in all-female communal arrangements. Geisha are not prostitutes, and they are now recognized as a cultural treasure. The women in the entertainment industry fulfill men's need to relax in a society that is highly constrained by social norms. At hostess bars, women sit with male customers, pour their drinks, and listen to them. In earlier eras concubines were accepted within families, and today infidelity is more tolerated in Japan than in North America. Geisha entertainment industries exist in North America.
- There is less tolerance for marriage of a Japanese person to a foreigner than in the United States.
- The existence of a gay and lesbian social network and of cross-dressing clubs is evident, although they are not generally talked about.

BIOCULTURAL ECOLOGY

- Racial features include the epicanthal skin folds that create the distinctive appearance of Asian eyes, a broad and flat nose, and "yellow" skin that varies markedly in tone. Hair is straight and naturally black, with differences in shade. Rely on color changes in the mucous membranes and sclerae to assess oxygenation and liver function.
- Negative blood types account for less than 1 percent of the population.
- The leading causes of death in Japan include, in descending order, cancers, heart disease, stroke,

pneumonia, accidents, motor vehicle accidents, suicide, renal disease, liver disease, diabetes, hypertension (related to the high sodium diet), and tuberculosis. Asthma, related to duct mites in the *tatami* (straw mats that cover floors in Japanese homes), is one of the few endemic diseases. These same conditions affect clients in the United States.

- Drug dosages may need to be adjusted for the physical stature of Japanese adults. Many Asians are poor metabolizers of mephenytoin and related medications, potentially leading to increased intensity and duration of the drugs' effects. Be aware that Asians tend to be more sensitive to the effects of some beta-blockers, many psychotropic drugs, and alcohol.
- They rapidly metabolize acetylate substances, which has an impact on metabolism of tranquilizers, tuberculosis drugs, caffeine, and some cardiovascular agents.
- Most individuals require lower doses of some benzodiazepines and neuroleptics.
- Opiates may be less effective analgesics, but gastrointestinal side effects may be greater than among whites. Take clients' body mass into consideration in dosing; even with that precaution, clients' responses to drugs need to be monitored carefully.

HIGH-RISK HEALTH BEHAVIORS

- Smoking rates are high among Japanese and Japanese Americans.
- Alcohol (rice wine) has ritual significance in the marriage ceremony, in offerings at Shinto shrines, and at the household ancestral shrine. Alcohol is part of many social rituals, such as picnics, to celebrate cherry blossoms, autumn leaves, or moon viewing. Adults commonly drink beer and sake in the home, and children may be seen purchasing alcohol. College students engage in beer drinking when they socialize.
- Once alcohol is consumed, one can relax and speak freely; they are forgiven for what they say because of the alcohol. Be aware of the prevalence of smoking and

heavy alcohol consumption, particularly among men. **Give individuals specific medical reasons why they must abstain, thus providing a socially acceptable excuse.**

- Mothers' time-honored strategy of rewarding academic diligence with candy and other treats contributes to the issue of the fitness of youth. **Encourage mothers to offer other rewards for academic excellence.**
- Public safety consciousness is high: readily using seatbelts and other safety measures such as seatbelts, child safety seats, and helmets.

NUTRITION

- All food groups are well represented in the Japanese diet. Staples include rice, beef, poultry, pork, seafood, root vegetables, cabbage, persimmons, apples, and tangerines.
- Rice is the mainstay of the traditional diet and is included in all three meals as well as snacks. A traditional breakfast includes fish; pickles; *nori* (various seaweeds used to flavor or garnish meals); a raw egg stirred into the hot rice; *miso* (soybean-based) soup; and tea. Some people prefer a Western breakfast of toast or cold cereal and coffee.
- Rice has a symbolic meaning related to the Shinto religion, analogous to the concept of the "bread of life" among Christians. A staple of schoolchildren's *o-bento* (lunch box) is a white bed of rice garnished with a red plum pickle, reminiscent of the Japanese flag. Meals combine elements of land and sea.
- Schoolchildren eat lunch on their *o-bento*, packed with rice, pickles, and meat or fish. A popular lunch among working people is a steaming bowl of ramen (noodles) in broth or cold noodles on a hot summer day. Instant broth, although high in sodium, is another popular quick lunch.
- A traditional dinner is a pot of boiled potatoes, carrots, and pork seasoned with sweet sake, garlic, and soy sauce or a stir-fried meat and vegetable dish.
- The daily intake of sweets can be high and often

includes European-style desserts, sweetbreads and cookies, sweet bean cakes, soft drinks, and heavily sweetened coffee, which may contribute to the high incidence of tooth decay.

- Increasingly, Westernized food tastes, resulting in higher fat and carbohydrate intake, have contributed to the rise in obesity and associated increases in diabetes, heart disease, and premature death.
- There is growing public awareness that the sodium content of the traditional soups and sauces contributes to the high rate of cerebrovascular accidents. General principles of nutrition are the same in America as in Japan, although the food preferences may differ. **Dietary assessment should be undertaken on admission. Incorporate traditional food practices and preparation practices in dietary counseling sessions.**
- Green tea, although high in caffeine, is a good source of vitamin C. Garlic and various herbs are used widely for their medicinal properties.
- Many individuals have difficulty digesting milk products due to lactose intolerance. **Encourage use of reduced-lactose milk and of tofu and unboned fish to meet calcium needs.**
- Iron deficiency anemia is a concern among young women and can be alleviated with dietary counseling or dietary supplements. *Nori* is a traditional food source for iron.

PREGNANCY AND CHILDBEARING PRACTICES

- Oral contraceptives became legal in Japan in 1999. Condoms remain the most common contraceptive method. Most women have several abortions during their married fertile lives.
- Pregnancy is highly valued within traditional culture as a woman's fulfillment of her destiny. Women may enjoy attention and pampering that they get at no other time. They may prepare themselves for the possibility of pregnancy when they become engaged and eliminate alcohol, caffeine, soft drinks, and tobacco.

- Women often return to their mother's home for the last 2 months of their pregnancy and through the first 2 months postpartum. **Explore a woman's expectations during pregnancy and the possibility that she might return to Japan. Finding another Japanese woman who has experienced childbearing in the United States and who can share her experiences would support the pregnant client.**
- Loud noises, such as a train or a sewing machine, are thought to be bad for the baby.
- Shinto shrines sell amulets for conception and easy delivery. Husbands do not commonly attend the births of their children.
- Vaginal deliveries are usually performed without medication. To give in to pain dishonors the husband's family, and mothers are said to appreciate their babies more if they suffer in childbirth. Japan enjoys the world's lowest infant mortality rate, at 3.2 per 1,000 live births.
- The postpartum period is taken seriously. Traditionally, postpartum women do not bathe, shower, or wash their hair for at least the first week.
- Breast-feeding is also taken seriously. Maternal rest and relaxation are deemed essential for success. If the mother is asleep, the grandmother feeds the baby formula. Women who give birth in the United States may resent the American expectation that they will resume self-care and child-care activities quickly. **Explain the expectations for postpartum care; exercise sensitivity and help plan for assistance upon discharge early in the pregnancy.**

DEATH RITUALS

- The taboo against open discussion of serious illness and death is evident. Hospice patients may not want to be told their diagnosis and prognosis in order to allow a peaceful death and to spare both the patient and the family the difficulty of having to discuss the situation. **Hospice workers may have to rely on implicit behaviors to admit clients for care.**

- When a person is dying, the family should be notified of impending death so they can be at the dying person's bedside. Traditionally, the eldest son has particular responsibility during this time.
- When death occurs, an altar is constructed in the home. Photographs of the deceased are displayed, and floral arrangements are placed within and outside the home. A bag of money is hung around the neck of the deceased to pay the toll to cross the river to the hereafter. Visitors bring gifts of money and food for the bereaved family.
- The mourning period is 49 days, the end of which is marked by a family prayer service and the serving of special rice dishes. At this time the departed has joined those already in the hereafter. Perpetual prayers may be donated through a gift to the temple. In addition, special prayer services can be conducted for the 1st, 3rd, 7th, and 13th annual anniversaries of the death.
- Beliefs are common that the dead need to be remembered and that failure to do so can lead the dead to rob the living of rest.

SPIRITUALITY

- Shinto, the indigenous religion, is the locus of joyful events such as marriage and birth.
- Many festivals are marked by offerings, parades, and a carnival on the grounds of the shrine.
- Buddhism has permeated artistic and intellectual life. Very few people regularly attend services, but most are registered temple members, if only to ensure a family burial plot.
- One percent of Japanese people is Catholic or Protestant. Most do not identify themselves solely with one religion or another, and even a baptized Christian might have a Shinto wedding and a Buddhist funeral.
- Many accept the Buddhist belief in reincarnation, and the eternal life of the soul is also recognized in the Shinto faith.
- *Kampo* (healers) often set up shop in the vicinity of the temple or shrine, and a person might be seen scooping incense smoke onto an ailing body part. Prayer boards

might bear requests for special healing. Newborns are taken to a shrine for a blessing. Additional blessings take place on November 15, when a child is 3, 5, or 7 years old. Visits to shrines and temples are social, recreational, and spiritual outings. Souvenirs and refreshments are usually available, and the hike into the prayer area provides exercise.

HEALTH-CARE PRACTICES

- There is greater tolerance of self-indulgence even during minor illnesses. Because Japanese people are less likely to express feelings verbally, this indulgence may be a way for people to affirm caring for one another nonverbally. Termination of pregnancy when the health of the fetus is in doubt is common, and most parents want medically compromised neonates to be treated aggressively when prognoses are not favorable. **Help clients with legal obligations who face value conflicts with termination of pregnancy and not treating medically compromised newborns.**

- The concept of *ki*, the life force or energy and how it flows through the body, is integral to traditional Chinese healing modalities, including acupuncture. Good health requires the unobstructed flow of *ki* throughout the body.

- The concepts of *yin* and *yang* are reflected in modern attitudes, as is the need to balance five energy sources: water, wood, fire, earth, and metal. Strategies that help to restore balance include use of herbal medicines, bed rest, bathing, and having a massage. One traditional form of massage, *shiatsu* (acupressure), involves redirection of energy along the Chinese meridians by application of light pressure to what we might recognize as acupuncture points.

- Whereas Chinese tradition calls for a restoration of balance when one is ill, Shinto calls for purging and purification. Preoccupation with germs and dirt is not likely to interfere with daily life. **Health-care providers who visit Japanese homes should note or** even ask whether the family removes their shoes upon entering.

- Many pharmacies stock traditional herbal *kampo* preparations.
- Most individuals make liberal use of both modern medical and traditional providers of health care. Residents in the United States have Internet and mail-order access to traditional medications, if they are not available locally. **A complete health assessment includes inquiry about home therapies.**
- *Morita* therapy is an indigenous strategy for addressing *shinkei shitsu*, excess sensitivity to the social and natural environment. Introspection is seen as harmful, and *Morita* therapy focuses on constructive physical activity to help clients accept reality as it is.
- *Naikan* therapy is one of reflection on how much goodness and love are received from others.
- *Shinryo Naika* focuses on bodily illnesses that are emotionally induced.
- **Be sensitive to family issues that may underlie illnesses among clients; if psychotherapy is indicated, the therapist must be someone familiar with the Japanese culture. Resources may be obtained through large academic medical centers or universities as well as through professional associations, Japanese churches, or other religious organizations where Japanese people gather.**
- Japanese high regard for the status of physicians decreases the likelihood of their asking questions or making suggestions about their care. The idea that clients should be given care options may be alien. **Provide ample opportunity for dialogue, and explain the choices that are offered. Use Japanese and Japanese American health-care providers to bridge gaps in understanding.**
- Some individuals may need assistance in seeking care. Their verbal English skills may be an impediment to making their needs known and to understanding the care they are offered, even though their ability to understand written information is very good.

- *Itami* (pain) may not be expressed, and bearing pain is considered a virtue and a matter of family honor. Addiction is a strong taboo in Japanese society, making clients reluctant to accept pain medication. **Use a schedule of analgesic administration rather than an as-requested or patient-controlled approach to ensure adequate pain management. Explain that physiological status and healing are actually enhanced by pain control.**
- Mental illness is taboo. Because emotional problems cannot be discussed freely, somatic manifestations are common and acceptable.
- Handicapped people may bring shame or heartache to the family, although they are treated kindly.
- Assumption of the sick role is highly tolerated by families and colleagues, and a long recuperation period is encouraged.
- Critical care and organ transplantation and donation issues need to be approached sensitively. People rely more heavily on the physician's opinion, and the family may have difficulty negotiating cessation of treatment. **The concept of advance directives is unknown to many. Carefully explain advance directives to clients. Be cautious in initiating extraordinary measures with family members.**

HEALTH CARE PRACTITIONERS

- Physicians, referred to as *sensei*, are highly esteemed.
- Self-care as a philosophy is not evident among most. Being told what to do by the physician or *kampo* practitioner is expected, and his (or, occasionally, her) authority is not questioned.
- Nurses and nursing are highly regarded, reflecting traditional taboos against illness and impurity as well as the status of women. Currently in Japan, nurses are well respected, even though women in general are not. In the past, nurses were not highly respected because "good women" did not touch people with an illness unless they were immediate family members. If she did touch

"sick bodies," the woman would become tainted and less pure.

- Home care and the orchestration of many community-based providers may be overwhelming for residents who expect long recuperations in the hospital. **Assist clients in understanding how the health-care delivery system works and the functions of the different health-care providers whom they encounter.**

Japanese

References

Immigration and Naturalization Service, U.S. Department of Justice (2000). *1998 Statistical yearbook of the Immigration and Naturalization Service.* Retrieved November, 6, 2003, from www.ins.usdoj.gov

Sharts-Hopko, N. (2003). People of Japanese heritage. In L. Purnell and B. Paulanka (Eds.), *Transcultural health care: A culturally competent approach* (2nd ed., pp. 218–234). Philadelphia: F.A. Davis Company.

Shinto Online Network Association (2000). Shinto. www.jinja.or.jp/english.

UNICEF (1996). *Progress of nations 1996. The industrial world.* Japan has lowest teen birth rate. Retrieved November 6, 2003, from www.unicef.org/pon96/inbirth.htm

United Nations, Department of Economic and Social Information and Policy Analysis/Statistical Division (1993). *Statistical yearbook 1990/1991* (38th ed.). New York: Author.

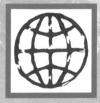

People of Jewish Heritage

Overview and Heritage

The term *Jewish* refers to both a people and a religion; it is not a race. The terms *Hebrew, Israelite*, and *Jew* are used interchangeably. In the Bible, Abraham's grandson, Jacob, was also called Israel. His 12 sons and their descendants became known as the children of Israel. The term *Jew* is derived from Judah, one of Jacob's sons. Judaism is both a religion and a culture. The religion is practiced along a wide continuum that ranges from liberal Reform to strict Orthodox. Instances occur within the ultra-Orthodox communities when individuals cannot make decisions without consulting their rabbis. The extent of religiosity is a major force in shaping the Jewish culture and the behaviors and beliefs of various groups. A child born to a Jewish mother is Jewish. A child born from the union of a Jewish father and a non-Jewish mother is recognized as Jewish by those in the Reform movement but not by those in the Orthodox movement.

There are 5.84 million Jews throughout the United States, with half living in the Northeast. Migration of Jews from

Europe began to increase in the mid-1800s because of the fear of religious persecution. The greatest influx occurred between 1880 and 1920. Many came from Russia and Eastern Europe after a wave of *pogroms* (religious persecutions). Most families in America today are descendants of these eastern European and Russian immigrants and are referred to as Ashkenazi Jews. Many Jews of Ashkenazi descent have stories of how some members of their families escaped to America, while others had relatives who were part of the six million Jews killed in the pogroms and the Holocaust. Sephardic Jews, on the other hand, are from Spain, Portugal, the Mediterranean, North Africa, and South and Central America. They represent a more diverse group. A *Sabra* is a Jew who was born in Israel. The *Falasha* are black Jews from Ethiopia.

Throughout their history, Jews have placed a major emphasis on education and social justice through social action. In general, this population is well educated. A high percentage has succeeded in science, medicine, law, and dentistry. Thirty-nine percent of Jewish men and more than 36 percent of Jewish women list their occupation as professional, compared with only 15 percent of the American white population.

COMMUNICATIONS

- English is the primary language of Jewish Americans. Although Hebrew is the official language of Israel and is used for prayers, it is generally not used for conversation. Many elderly Ashkenazi Jews who immigrated early in the 20th century or who are first-generation Americans speak Yiddish, a Judeo-German dialect.
- Many Yiddish terms have worked their way into English, including the following: *kvetch* (someone who complains a lot); *chutzpah* (clever audacity); *bagel* (a circular roll of bread with a hole in the middle); *challah* (braided white bread); *knish* (dumpling with filling); *nosh* (snack); *zaftig* (plump); *tush, tushie,* or *tuchus* (buttocks); *ghetto* (a restricted area where certain groups live); *klutz* (a clumsy person); *mentsch, mensh* (a respected person with dignity); *shlep* (drag or carry);

Jewish

kosher (legal or okay); and *oy, oy vey* (oh my), and *veys mir* (woe is me).

- Common expressions include *l'chaim* (to life), which is said during a toast of wine; *shalom aleichem* (peace be with you) a traditional salutation; *mazel tov* (congratulations), and *shabbat shalom* (a good and peaceful Sabbath), which is said from Friday evening at sunset until Saturday at sunset.
- Hebrew is read from right to left, and books are opened from the opposite side compared with English books.
- No religious ban or ethnic characteristics prevent Jews from sharing their feelings. Communication practices are more related to their American upbringing than to their religious practices.
- People are judged by their actions, not by what they say and feel, because only the actions last beyond the lives of individuals.
- As a way to cope and a way to communicate with others, Jews frequently use humor. However, jokes are considered to be insensitive when they reinforce mainstream stereotypes about Jews, such as implying that Jews are cheap or pampered (e.g., Jewish American princess). Any jokes that refer to the Holocaust or concentration camps are also inappropriate. However, self-criticism through humor is acceptable.
- Modesty, which involves humility, is a primary value, especially among the Orthodox. It is seen in the Orthodox style of dress and in one's actions. Jews are encouraged not to "show off" or constantly try to impress others.
- Hasidic men are not permitted to touch a woman other than their wives. They often keep their hands in their pockets to avoid touch. **They do not shake hands with women, and their failure to do so when one's hand is extended should not be interpreted as a sign of rudeness.**
- Because women are considered seductive, Hasidic men may not engage in idle talk with them nor look directly at their faces. Non-Hasidic Jews may be much more informal and may use touch and short spatial distance

when communicating. Only touch Hasidic men when providing direct care. "Therapeutic touch" is not appropriate with these clients.

- While most Jews live for today and plan for and worry about tomorrow, they are raised with stories of their past, especially of the Holocaust. They are warned to "never forget," lest history be repeated. Therefore, their time orientation is simultaneously to the past, the present, and the future.

- The Jewish calendar is based on both a lunar and solar year, with each month beginning with the birth of the new moon. The festivals and holidays are based on the phases of the moon, whereas the seasons are based on the solar year. The lunar year is 11 days shorter than the solar year. Therefore, an extra month is periodically added.

- The Jewish format for names follows the Western tradition. The given name comes first and is followed by the family surname. Only the given name is used with friends and in informal situations. In more formal situations, the surname is preceded by the appropriate title of Mr., Miss, Ms., Mrs., or Dr.

- Babies may be named after someone who has died or after a living person to keep the person's name alive. The format chosen depends on whether the family is of Ashkenazi or Sephardic heritage. In ultra-Orthodox circles, children are not referred to by their names until after the *bris or brit milah* (circumcision). Infants are also given a Hebrew first name that is used when they are older and are called to read from the Torah. An example would be Efraim ben Reuven (Frank son of Robert).

FAMILY ROLES AND ORGANIZATION

- The family is the core of society, and the needs of all family members are respected. Whereas the man is considered the breadwinner for the household, the woman is recognized for running the home and being responsible for the children.

Jewish

- According to Jewish law, the father has the legal obligation to educate his children in Judaism, to teach them right from wrong, to teach them to swim, and to teach his sons a trade. He must provide his daughters with the means to make them marriageable. The mother's role is to keep a Jewish home and to raise the children.

- In most families, both parents share the responsibilities of supporting the home and raising the children. Husbands are required to provide their wives with food, clothing, medical care, and conjugal relations and are prohibited from beating their wives, forcing them to have sex, or restricting their free movement.

- Children are valued treasures, are considered blessings, are treated with respect, and are provided with love. Jewish children are to be afforded an education, not only in studies that help them progress in society but also in studies that transmit their Jewish heritage and the laws. Jewish school-age children typically attend Hebrew school at least two afternoons a week after public school throughout the school year.

- Children play an active role in most holiday celebrations and services. Respecting and honoring one's parents is one of the Ten Commandments. Children should be forever grateful to their parents for giving them the gift of life.

- In Judaism, the age of majority is 13 years for a boy and 12 for a girl, at which age children are deemed capable of differentiating right from wrong and capable of committing themselves to performing the commandments. Recognition of adulthood occurs during a religious ceremony called a *bar or bat mitzvah* (son or daughter of the commandment). This rite of passage is usually accompanied by a family celebration.

- The goal of the Orthodox family is to live their lives as prescribed by *halakhah* (Code of Jewish Law), which emphasizes maintaining health, promoting education, and helping others.

- Marriage is considered the ideal human state for adults. The two goals of this union are to propagate the race

and companionship. Sexuality is a right of both men and women.
- Sexual intercourse is viewed as a pure and holy act when performed mutually within the relationship of marriage. Premarital sex is not condoned.
- Among the ultra-observant, women must physically separate themselves from all men during their menstrual periods and for 7 days after. No man may touch a woman or sit where she sat until she has been to the *mikveh*, a ritual bath, after her period is over.
- Judaism supports the need for sex education. The Jewish community sees this as its responsibility. This belief has been reemphasized during the AIDS epidemic, in which the goal is to protect the next generation and provide them with accurate information so they can make informed choices.
- Older people receive respect, especially for the wisdom they have to share. Honoring one's parents is a lifelong endeavor and includes maintaining their dignity by feeding, clothing, and sheltering them, even if they suffer from senility.
- The Bible, as interpreted by the Orthodox, prohibits homosexual intercourse; it says nothing specifically about sex between lesbians. Some of the objections to gay and lesbian lifestyles include the inability of these unions to fulfill the commandment of procreation and the possibility that acting on the recognition of one's homosexuality could ruin a marriage. The liberal movement within Judaism, however, supports legal and social equality for lesbians and gays.

BIOCULTURAL ECOLOGY

- Skin coloring for Ashkenazi Jews ranges from fair skin and blonde hair to darker skin and brunette hair. Sephardic Jews have slightly darker skin tones and hair coloring, similar to those from the Mediterranean area. There are also Jewish groups throughout Africa who are black, most notably the Jews originally from Ethiopia, known as *Falasha*.

- Genetic risk factors vary based on whether the family immigrated from Ashkenazi or Sephardic areas. There is a greater incidence of some genetic disorders among Ashkenazi individuals. Most of these disorders are autosomal-recessive, meaning that both parents carry the affected gene. Although the best known is Tay-Sachs disease, Gaucher's disease is more prevalent. Others include Canavan's disease. familial dysautonomia, torsion dystonia, Niemann-Pick disease, Bloom syndrome, Fanconi's anemia, and mucolipidosis IV (National Foundation for Jewish Genetic Diseases 2001). Torsion dystonia; Niemann-Pick disease, type A; Bloom syndrome; and mucolipidosis IV are more frequent in Ashkenazi Jews. Orthodox rabbis usually do not support genetic testing because it might cause couples to refrain from marrying or having children, thus preventing them from fulfilling the mitzvah of procreation. The Reform movement supports a couple's right to make the decision whether to have the testing done.
- Other conditions that occur with increased incidence in the Jewish population include inflammatory bowel disease (ulcerative colitis and Crohn's disease), colorectal cancer, and breast and ovarian cancer.
- Ashkenazi Jews have a higher rate of side-effects with clozapine; 20% develop agranulocytosis. Institute testing for agranulocytosis when Jewish clients are prescribed clozapine.

HIGH-RISK HEALTH BEHAVIORS

- Any substance or act that harms the body is not allowed. This includes smoking, suicide, taking nonprescription or illegal medications, and permanent tattooing.
- Alcohol, especially wine, is an essential part of religious holidays and festive occasions and is a traditional symbol of joy. Wine is appropriate and acceptable as long as it is used in moderation.
- Most Jews are health-conscious and practice preventive health care, with routine physical, dental, and vision

screening. This is also a well-immunized population. Encourage these positive health-promotion and disease-prevention practices.

NUTRITION

- Beside satisfying hunger and sustaining life, eating also teaches discipline and reverence for life. For those who follow the dietary laws, much attention is given to the slaughter, preparation, and consumption of food.
- Dietary practices serve as a spiritually refining act of self-discipline and a unifying factor as an instrument of ethnic identity.
- Perhaps the food identified as "Jewish" that receives the most attention is chicken soup, which has frequently been referred to as "Jewish penicillin," and is often served with *knaidle* balls in it (dumplings made of *matzoh* meal). Although it has no intrinsic meaning or religious value, it is a staple in religious homes, especially on Friday evenings to usher in the Sabbath and during times of illness. It is frequently associated with a mother's warmth and love.
- Common foods include *gefilte* fish (ground freshwater fish molded into oblong balls and served cold with horseradish); *challah* (braided white bread); *kugel* (noodle pudding); blintzes (crepes filled with a sweet cottage cheese); chopped liver (served cold); *hamentashen* (a triangular pastry with different types of filling); and lox and bagel sandwiches. Lox is cold smoked salmon, served with cream cheese and salad vegetables, on a bagel.
- The laws regarding which foods are permissible under religious law are referred to as the laws of *kashrut*. The term *kosher* means "fit to eat"; it is not a brand or form of cooking. Foods are divided into those that are considered *kosher* (permitted or clean) and those considered *treyf* (forbidden or unclean). A permitted animal may be rendered *treyf* if it is not slaughtered, cooked, or served properly. Care must be taken that all blood is drained from the animal before eating it.

Jewish

- Milk and meat may not be mixed together in cooking, serving, or eating. To avoid mixing foods, utensils used to prepare foods and the plates used to serve them are separated. Religious Jews who following the dietary laws have two sets of dishes, pots, and utensils: one set for milk products and the other for meat. Because glass is not absorbent, it can be used for either meat or milk products, although religious households still usually have two sets. Therefore, cheeseburgers, lasagna made with meat, and grated cheese on meatballs and spaghetti is unacceptable. Milk cannot be used in coffee if served with a meat meal. Nondairy creamers can be used instead, as long as they do not contain sodium caseinate, which is derived from milk.
- Some foods are *parve* (neutral) and may be used with either dairy or meat dishes. These include fish, eggs, anything grown in the soil (vegetables, fruits, coffee, sugar, and spices), and chemically produced goods.
- Mammals are considered clean if they meet the other requirements for their slaughter and consumption and have split (cloven) hooves and chew their cud. These animals include buffalo, cattle, goats, deer, and sheep. The pig is an example of an animal that does not meet these criteria. Although liberal Jews decide for themselves which dietary laws they will follow, many still avoid pork and pork products out of a sense of tradition and symbolism. Serving pork products to a Jewish client, unless specifically requested, is insensitive. Poultry that is acceptable includes chicken, one of the most frequently consumed forms of protein, as well as turkey, goose, and duck. Fish can be eaten if it has both fins and scales. Nothing that crawls on its belly is allowed, including clams, lobsters and other shellfish, tortoises, and frogs.
- In religious homes, meat is prepared for cooking by soaking and salting it to drain all the blood from the flesh. Broiling is acceptable, especially for liver, because it drains the blood.
- A U with a circle around it (Ⓤ) is the seal of the Union of Orthodox Jewish Congregations of America and is

used on food products to indicate that they are kosher. A circled K (Ⓚ) and other symbols may also be found on packaging to indicate that a product is kosher. **Do not bring food into the house without knowing whether the client adheres to kosher standards. If the client keeps a kosher home, do not use any cooking items, dishes, or silverware without knowing which are used for meat and which are used for dairy products. Health-care providers must fully understand the dietary laws so they do not offend the client, can advocate for kosher meals if they are requested, and can plan medication times accordingly.**

- Care must be taken in serving cheese to ensure that no animal substances are served at the same time.
- Breads and cakes made with lard are *treyf*, and breads made with milk or milk by-products (for example, casein) cannot be served with meat meals.
- Eggs from non-kosher birds, milk from non-kosher animals, and oil from non-kosher fish are not permitted.
- Butter substitutes are used with meat meals. Honey is allowed because it is produced from the nectar of flowers.
- Kosher meals are available in most hospitals. They arrive on paper plates and with sealed plastic utensils. **Do not unwrap the utensils or change the foodstuffs to another serving dish. If health-care providers have difficulty locating a supplier of kosher foods, they should contact a local rabbi. Determining a client's dietary preferences and practices regarding dietary laws should be done during the admission assessment.**
- One must always wash one's hands before eating. Religious Jews wash their hands while reciting a prayer. **Make facilities for clients to wash their hands before eating.**
- During the week of Passover, no bread or product with yeast may be eaten. *Matzoh* (unleavened bread) is eaten instead. Any product that is fermented or that can cause fermentation (souring) may not be eaten. Rather than attend synagogue, the family conducts the service (seder) around the dinner table during the first two

Jewish

nights and incorporates dinner into a service that includes all participants and retells the story of Moses and the exodus from Egypt.

- The Jewish calendar has a number of fast days. The most observed is the holiest day of the year, *Yom Kippur* (Day of Atonement). Jews abstain from food and drink as they pray to God for forgiveness for the sins they have committed during the past year. They eat an early dinner on the evening the holiday begins and then fast until after sunset the following day.

- Ill people, the elderly, the young, pregnant and nursing women, and the physically incapacitated are absolved from fasting and may need to be reminded of this exception to Jewish law. **If concerns arise about fasting, a consultation with the client's rabbi may be necessary. Schedule appointments and treatment to avoid religious days.**

PREGNANCY AND CHILDBEARING PRACTICES

- Couples who are unable to conceive should try all possible means to have children, including infertility counseling and interventions, including egg and sperm donation. Orthodox opinion is virtually unanimous in prohibiting ... artificial insemination when the semen donor is a man other than the woman's husband. When all natural attempts have been made, adoption may be pursued.

- Unless pregnancy jeopardizes the life or health of the mother, contraception is not looked on favorably among the ultra-Orthodox. Liberal Judaism recognizes that children have the right to be wanted and that they should be born into homes where their needs can be met. Therefore, the use of temporary birth control may be acceptable. Condom use is supported, especially when unprotected sexual intercourse poses a medical risk to either spouse.

- Reform Judaism supports the access of minors to reproductive health services that are unrestricted by parental notification or permission, including dispensing contraceptives.

- To the Orthodox, coitus interruptus and masturbation are not acceptable because they result in the needless expenditure of semen, although most Jews consider the latter practice a normal, healthy activity. Barrier techniques are not acceptable because they interfere with the full mobility of the sperm in its natural course. The birth control pill does not result in any permanent sterilization, nor does it prevent semen from traveling its normal route. Therefore, use of this method is the least objectionable to most branches of Judaism. Sterilization implies permanence, and Orthodox Jews probably oppose this practice, unless the life of the mother is in danger. Reform Judaism leaves the choice of what to use and whether to use contraceptives to the parents.

- The fetus is not considered a living soul or person until it has been born. Birth is determined when the head or "greater part" is born. If the physical or mental health of a pregnant woman is endangered by the fetus, all branches of Judaism consider the fetus an aggressor and require an abortion. Random abortion is not permitted by the Orthodox branch because the fetus is part of the mother's body and one must not do harm to one's body. Jewish law does allow for a reduction of fetuses in the case of multiple gestations when the potential viability of one or more are threatened by the others. Reform Judaism believes that a woman maintains control over her own body and that it is up to her whether to abort a fetus. The decision is not to be made without serious deliberation.

- A Hasidic husband may not touch his wife during labor and may choose not to attend the delivery because he is not permitted to view his wife's genitals. These behaviors should never be interpreted as insensitivity on the part of the husband. During the delivery in an ultra-Orthodox family, initiate the following interventions. Give the mother a hospital gown that covers her in the front and back to the greatest extent possible. Provide a surgical cap so that her head remains covered (because the hair is considered a private part of her body). Give the father the opportunity to leave during procedures and during the birth or, if he chooses to stay, drape the

Jewish

mother so that the husband may sit by his wife without viewing her perineum, including by way of mirrors or other means. Because the husband is not permitted to touch his wife, he may offer only verbal support. The female nurse may need to provide all of the physical care.

- Pain medication during delivery is acceptable.
- For male infants, circumcision, which is both a medical procedure and a religious rite, is performed on the 8th day of life by a *mohel*, an individual trained in the circumcision procedure, asepsis, and the religious ceremony. Although a rabbi is not necessary, it is also possible to have the procedure completed by a physician with a rabbi present to say the blessings.
- Attending a *brit milah* is the only mitzvah for which religious Jews must violate the Sabbath so that the brit can be completed at the proper time. Provide a space for a family celebration if the circumcision is done in the hospital.

DEATH RITUALS

- Death is an expected part of the life cycle. Traditional Judaism believes in an afterlife where the soul continues to flourish, although many dispute this interpretation. A dying person is considered a living person in all respects. Provide pain control even if it decreases the person's level of consciousness.
- Active euthanasia is forbidden for religious Jews. Passive euthanasia may be allowed depending on its interpretation. Nothing may be used or initiated that prevents a person from dying naturally or that prolongs the dying process. However, anything that artificially prevents death (cardiopulmonary resuscitation, ventilators, and so forth) may possibly be withheld, depending on the wishes of the patient and his or her religious views.
- Taking one's own life is prohibited and is considered a criminal act and morally wrong. To the ultra-religious, suicide removes all possibility of repentance.
- The dying person should not be left alone.

- Any Jew may ask God's forgiveness for his or her sins; no confessor is needed. Some Jews feel solace in saying the *Sh'ma* in Hebrew or English. This prayer confirms one's belief in one God. At the time of death, the nearest relative can gently close the eyes and mouth, and the face is covered with a sheet.
- The body is treated with respect and revered for the function it once filled. **Ask the closest relative of the deceased specifically about the practices to follow after death.**
- For the ultra-Orthodox, after the body is wrapped, it is briefly placed on the floor with the feet pointing toward the door. A candle may be placed near the head. However, this does not occur on the Sabbath or holy days. The dead body is not left alone until the funeral so as not to leave the body defenseless.
- Autopsy is usually not permitted among religious Jews because it results in desecration of the body, and it is important that the body be interred whole. Allowing an autopsy might also delay the burial, something that is not recommended. On the other hand, autopsy is allowed if its results would save the life of another patient who is immediately at hand. Many branches of Judaism currently allow an autopsy if (1) it is required by law; (2) the deceased person has willed it; or (3) it saves the life of another, especially an offspring.
- Cremation is prohibited because it unnaturally speeds the disposal of the dead body. Embalming is prohibited because it preserves the dead. However, in circumstances when the funeral must be delayed, some embalming may be approved. Cosmetic restoration for the funeral is discouraged.
- Funerals and burials usually occur within 24 to 48 hours after the death. The funeral service is directed at honoring the departed by only speaking well of him or her. It is not customary to have flowers either at the funeral or at the cemetery. The casket should be made of wood with no ornamentation. The body may be wrapped only in a shroud to ensure that the body and casket decay at the same rate. There is no wake or

Jewish

viewing. The prayer said for the dead, *kaddish*, is usually not said alone.

- After the funeral, mourners are welcomed at the home of the closest relative. Outside the front door is water to wash one's hands before entering, which is symbolic of cleansing the impurities associated with contact with the dead. The water is not passed from person to person, just as it is hoped that the tragedy is not passed. At the home, a meal is served to all the guests. This "meal of condolence" or "meal of consolation" is traditionally provided by the neighbors and friends.

- *Shiva* (Hebrew for "seven") is the 7-day period that begins with the burial. *Shiva* helps the surviving individuals face the actuality of the death of the loved one. During this period when the mourners are "sitting *shiva*," they do not work. When health-care providers are the ones experiencing the loss, it is important for supervisors to understand the mourning customs. In some homes, mirrors are covered to decrease the focus on one's appearance; no activity is permitted to divert attention from thinking about the deceased; and evening and morning services may be conducted in the closest relative's home. Condolence calls and the giving of consolation are appropriate during this time.

- Mourning lasts 30 days for a relative and 1 year for a parent.

- Crying, anger, and talking about the deceased person's life are acceptable.

- A common sign of grief is the tearing of the garment that one is wearing before the funeral service.

- In liberal congregations, a black ribbon with a tear in it is a symbolic representation of mourning. During *shiva*, the mourner sets the tone and initiates the conversation. Because there are such discrete periods of mourning, Judaism tells the mourner that it is wrong to mourn more than 30 days for a relative and for more than 1 year for parents.

- Mourning is not required for a fetus that is miscarried or stillborn. This is also true of any premature infant who dies within 30 days of birth. However, parents are required to mourn for full-term infants who die at birth or shortly thereafter.

- Within Orthodoxy, when a limb is amputated before death, the amputated limb and blood-soaked clothing are buried in the person's future gravesite because the blood and limb were part of the person. No mourning rites are required. In the case of an amputation, assist with arrangement for burial of the body part as needed.

SPIRITUALITY

- Judaism is more than 3,000 years old. Its early history and laws are chronicled in the Old Testament. Jews consider only the Old Testament as their Bible.
- Judaism is a monotheistic faith that believes in one God as the creator of the universe. No physical qualities are attributed to God; making and praying to statues or graven images are forbidden.
- The spiritual leader is the rabbi (teacher). He (or she, in liberal branches) is the interpreter of Jewish law. All Jews pray directly to God. They do not need the rabbi to intercede, to hear confession, or to grant atonement.
- Some of the major principles that guide Judaic bioethics are shown in Box 22–1.
- The practice of Judaism spans a wide spectrum. Although there is only one religion, there are three main branches or denominations of Judaism. The Orthodox are the most traditional. They adhere most strictly to the *halakhah* of traditional Judaism and try to follow as many of the laws as possible while fitting into American society. They observe the Sabbath by attending the synagogue on Friday evening and Saturday morning and by abstaining from work, spending money, and driving on the Sabbath. Orthodox Jews observe the Jewish dietary laws; men wear a *yarmulke* or *kippah* (head coverings) at all times in reverence to God. Women wear long sleeves and modest dress. In many Orthodox synagogues, the services are primarily in Hebrew, and men and women sit separately.
- Orthodox Jews and some Conservative men and women

Jewish

BOX 22–1 • Principles of Judaic Bioethics

- Man's purpose on earth is to live according to certain God-given guidelines.
- Life possesses enormous intrinsic value, and its preservation is of great moral significance.
- All human lives are equal.
- Our lives are not our own exclusive private possessions.
- The first five books of the Bible, also known as the five books of Moses, are handwritten in Hebrew on parchment scrolls called *Torah*. These scrolls are kept in the "Holy Ark" within each synagogue under an "eternal light." The Torah directs Jews on how they should live their lives; it provides guidance on every aspect of human life. The rest of the Bible includes sacred writings and teachings of the prophets.
- The 613 commandments within the Torah and the oral law derived from the biblical statutes determine Jewish law. These commandments ask for a commitment in behavior and also address ethical concerns. The commandments reflect the will of God, and religious Jews feel it is their duty to carry them out to fulfill their covenant with God. This makes Judaism not only a religion but also a way of life.

use the *tefillin* (phylacteries) during morning prayer services. These are two small black boxes with parchment containing biblical passages that are connected to long leather straps. These are wrapped around the arms and forehead as reminders of the laws of the Torah. The *tallis* (or *tallit*) is a rectangular prayer shawl with fringes, also only used during prayer but frequently used by both Conservative and Orthodox Jews. Ultra-Orthodox men wear a special garment under their shirts year-round.

- A *mezuzah* is a small container with scripture inside. Jewish homes have a mezuzah on the doorpost of the house. Some Jews wear a mezuzah as a necklace. Other religious symbols include the Star of David, a six-pointed star that has been a symbol of the Jewish community since the 1350s, and the *menorah* (candelabrum).

- Whereas Conservative Jews observe most of the halakhah, they do make concessions to modern society. Many drive to the synagogue on the Sabbath, and men and women sit together. Many keep a kosher home, but they may or may not follow all of the dietary laws outside the home. Women are ordained as rabbis and are counted in a *minyan*, the minimum number of 10 that is required for prayer. While a yarmulke is required in the synagogue, it is optional outside of that environment.

- The liberal or progressive movement is called Reform. Reform Jews claim that post-biblical law was only for the people of that time and that only the moral laws of the Torah are binding. They practice fewer rituals, although they frequently have a mezuzah on the doorpost of their homes, celebrate the holidays, and have a strong ethnic identity. They may or may not follow the Jewish dietary laws, but they may have specific unacceptable foods (for example, pork), which they abstain from eating. Men and women share full equality, and they engage in many social action activities.

- Of the many small groups of ultra-Orthodox fundamentalists, the Hasidic (or Chasidic) Jews are perhaps the most recognizable. They usually live, work, and study within a segregated area. They are usually easy to identify by their full beards, uncut hair around the ears (*pais*), black hats or fur *streimels*, dark clothing, and no exposed extremities.

- Women, especially those who are married, also keep their extremities covered and may have shaved heads covered by a wig and often a hat as well.

- A relatively new denomination, Reconstructionism (1.3 percent of American Jews), is a mosaic of the three main branches. It views Judaism as an evolving religion of the

Jewish people and seeks to adapt Jewish beliefs and practices to the needs of the contemporary world. In addition to these groups, many do not indicate any affiliation.

- The Jewish house of prayer is called a synagogue, temple, or *shul*. Jews may pray alone or may pray as a group anywhere that 10 Jews, over the age of 13 who have had their bar/bat mitzvah, are gathered together for prayer. This group is called a minyan. Orthodox Jews pray three times a day: morning, late afternoon, and evening. They wash their hands and say a prayer on awakening in the morning and before meals. Religious clients in hospitals may want their prayer items (yarmulke or kippah, tallit, tzitzit, tefillin) and may request a minyan. Disregard hospital policies regarding the number of visitors in the sick person's room in such instances.

- Visiting the sick is one of the social obligations of Judaism and ensures that Jews look after the physical, emotional, psychological, and social well-being of others. Remind visitors not to stay too long or tire the patient.

- The Sabbath begins 18 minutes before sunset on Friday. During this time, religious Jews do no manner of work, including answering the telephone, operating any electrical appliance, driving, or operating a call bell from a hospital bed. If an Orthodox client's condition is not life-threatening, medical and surgical procedures should not be performed on the Sabbath or holy days. A gravely ill person and the work of those who need to save him or her are exempted from following the commandments regarding the Sabbath.

- *Rosh Hashanah* (Jewish New Year) and Yom Kippur are high holy days and are usually in September or early October. On Yom Kippur, one fasts for a day to cleanse and purify oneself. Fasting for Yom Kippur may be broken for reasons of critical illness, labor and delivery, or for children under the age of 12 years.

- Other holidays include Passover, the Feast of the Unleavened Bread, which lasts for 8 days and celebrates

	TABLE 22–1		
	Jewish Holidays: 2004–2008		
Holiday	2004–2005	2005–2006	2006–2007	2007–2008
---	---	---	---	---
Rosh Hashanah	9/16–17	10/4–5	9/23–24	9/13–14
Yom Kippur	9/25	10/13	10/2	9/22
Sukkot	9/30–10/1	10/18–19	10/7–8	9/27–28
Chanukah	12/9–15	12/26–1/2	12/16–23	12/5–12
Purim	3/25	3/14	3/4	3/21
Passover	4/24–5/1	4/13–20	4/3–10	4/20–27
Shavuot	6/13–14	6/2–3	5/23–24	6/9–10

the Jews' Exodus from Egypt and freedom from slavery; *Chanukah*, an 8-day holiday, and *Purim*, both of which celebrate religious freedom. Table 22–1 provides a list of Jewish holidays for the years from 2004 through 2008.

HEALTH-CARE PRACTICES

- All people have a duty to keep themselves in good health, which encompasses physical and mental well-being. All denominations recognize that religious requirements may be laid aside if a life is at stake or if an individual has a life-threatening illness. Once it is clear that an individual is dying and that medical treatment is no longer working, individuals may choose not to interfere with death. **Hospice care is fully consonant with Jewish beliefs.**
- In ultra-Orthodox denominations of Judaism, taking medication on the Sabbath that is not necessary to preserve life may be viewed as "work" and is unacceptable. This belief may result in some people with conditions such as asthma not recognizing the severity of their condition; they may also be unaware of the laws that allow them to take their necessary medications. **Teach patients about the potential life-threatening sequelae of their condition as well as the**

exceptions to Jewish law that permit them to take their medications.

- The verbalization of pain is acceptable and common. Individuals want to know the reason for the pain, which they consider just as important as obtaining relief from pain.
- The sick role for Jews is highly individualized and may vary among individuals according to the severity of symptoms.
- Judaism opposes discrimination against people with physical, mental, and developmental conditions. The maintenance of one's mental health is considered just as important as the maintenance of one's physical health. Mental incapacity has always been recognized as grounds for exemption from all obligations under Jewish law.
- Jewish law considers organ transplants from four perspectives: those of the recipient, the living donor, the cadaver donor, and the dying donor. Because life is sacred, if the recipient's life can be prolonged without considerable risk, then transplant is ordained. For a living donor to be approved, the risk to the life of the donor must be considered. One is not obligated to donate a bodily part unless the risk is small. Examples include kidney and bone marrow donations. Organ donation at the time of death is acceptable if it saves a person's life. The concern has always been that the patient will be killed for the purpose of getting the organs sooner. Conservative and Reform Judaism approve using the flat EEG as the determination of death so that organs, such as the heart, can be viable for transplant. Burial may be delayed if organ harvesting is the cause of the delay. **Assist clients to obtain a rabbi when making a decision regarding organ donation or transplant.** The use of a cadaver for transplant is usually approved if it is to save a life. No one may derive economic benefit from the corpse. Use of skin for burns is also acceptable, although no agreement has been reached on the use of cadaver corneas.

HEALTH-CARE PRACTITIONERS

- Physicians are held in high regard. Although physicians must do everything in their power to prolong life, they are prohibited from initiating measures that prolong the act of dying.
- Only supportive care is required while the patient is dying and includes such care as food and water, good nursing care, and maximal psychosocial support.
- The more traditional Orthodox prefer that care be delivered by a same-gender health-care provider.

References

Dorff, E. (1998). *Matters of life and death: A Jewish approach to modern medical ethics.* Philadelphia: The Jewish Publication Society.

Robinson, G. (2000). *Essential Judaism: A complete guide to beliefs, customs, and rituals.* New York: Pocket Books.

Selekman, J. (2003). People of Jewish heritage. In L. Purnell and B. Paulanka (Eds.), *Transcultural health care: A culturally competent approach* (2nd ed., pp. 234–249). Philadelphia: F.A. Davis Company.

Washofsky, M. (2000). *Jewish living: A guide to contemporary reform practice.* New York: Union of American Hebrew Congregations Press.

Jewish

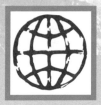

People of Korean Heritage

Overview and Heritage

Information in this chapter focuses on the commonalities among Koreans, with historical reference to the mother country, the Republic of South Korea. South Korea is a peninsula separated by North Korea to the north at the 38th parallel, by the former Soviet Union to the northeast, the Yellow Sea on the west, and the Sea of Japan to the east. South Korea has a landmass of 38,031 square miles, which is about the size of the state of Indiana, and has a population of 48 million people. The filming in Korea of the movie and television series, *M.A.S.H.,* has popularized this small nation, making it more familiar to people around the world. Korea, second only to China, is one of the two oldest continuous civilizations in the world.

The first major immigration from Korea occurred between 1903 and 1905, when more than 7,000 men arrived in Hawaii. Today, Koreans immigrate to America to increase socioeconomic opportunities and improve educational opportunities. More than 1.3 million Koreans live in the United States. They place a high value on education; South Korea has more citizens with PhDs per capita than any other country in the world. In the United States, many own their own businesses, which vary from "mom-and-pop" stores and gas stations, to grocery stores and real estate agencies, to retail shops. Their reputation for hard work, independence, and self-motivation has earned them the label of "model minority."

COMMUNICATIONS

- The dominant Korean language, *han'gul*, was the first phonetic alphabet in East Asia.
- Most Koreans in America can speak, read, write, and understand English to some extent. However, some Americans may have difficulty understanding their English, especially those who learned English from Koreans who spoke with their native intonations and pronunciations.
- A high value is placed on harmony and the maintenance of a peaceful environment. Most are comfortable with silence. Small talk may appear senseless and insincere. Most stand close when conversing.
- Touch in the realm of health care is readily accepted. Touching among friends and social equals is common and does not carry a sexual connotation, as it might in Western societies. Hugging and kissing are uncommon among parents and children as well as among children and older aunts or uncles.
- Age, gender, and social status determine the use of eye contact. Respect for those in senior positions is shown by not looking them directly in the eye.
- Feelings are infrequently communicated in facial expressions.
- More traditional Koreans are past-oriented. Much attention is paid to the ancestry of a family. Yearly, during the Harvest Moon in Korea, *chusok* (respect) is paid to ancestors by bringing fresh fruits from the autumn harvest, dry fish, and rice wine to gravesites.
- The younger and more educated generation is more futuristic and achievement-oriented.
- Punctuality is the norm for keeping important

Korean

appointments, making transportation connections, and reporting to work.

- The number of surnames in Korea is limited, with the most common ones being Kim, Lee, Park, Rhee or Yi, Choi or Choe, and Chung or Jung. Korean names contain two Chinese characters, one of which describes the generation and the other the person's given name.
- The surname comes first; however, because this may be confusing to many Americans, some Koreans in the United States follow the Western tradition of using the given name first, followed by the surname. Individuals should be addressed by their surname, with the title Mr., Mrs., Miss, Ms., Dr., or Minister, unless otherwise indicated. Determine Korean clients' language ability, comfort level with silence, use of eye contact, and spatial distancing practices when completing health assessments.

FAMILY ROLES AND ORGANIZATION

- Men are the primary financial providers. Women are expected to stay home and care for the children and domestic affairs unless they are professionals or it is necessary to work for economic purposes.
- Women have long been degraded in Korean society and seen as appendages of male family members. In earlier times, a woman's identity was determined by her role as someone's daughter, wife, or mother as well as by her responsibility for protecting the family with whom she was identified. While many still practice these gender relationships, more educated women and men no longer adhere to these Confucian values.
- Parenting in Korea is authoritative, although class differences play a more influential role in determining parenting styles and family roles.
- Children are expected to be well behaved because the whole family is disgraced if a child behaves in an embarrassing manner. Most children are not encouraged to state their opinions. Parents usually make the decisions.
- Discussing domestic violence violates Korean cultural norms. When family violence is suspected, the health-

care provider must approach the topic in an indirect manner.
- Dating is uncommon among high school students.
- Once young adults have entered a university, they receive their freedom and are permitted to make their own decisions about personal and study time. Group outings are common for meeting the opposite sex.
- With rapid acculturation, children often take on the values of the dominant society or culture, challenging parents who support traditional values and ideals. Assist parents in exploring alternative parenting practices.
- Education is a family priority.
- Parents expect their children to care for them in old age. *Hyo* (filial piety) is the obligation to respect and obey parents, care for them in old age, give them a good funeral, and worship them after death. The obligation to care for one's elderly parents is written into civil code in Korea.
- Elders are frequently consulted on important family matters as a sign of respect for their life experiences.
- Old age begins when one reaches the age of 60 years.
- Women who divorce may suffer social stigma. Living together before marriage is not customary in Korea. If pregnancy occurs outside marriage, it may be taken care of quietly and without family and friends being aware of the situation.
- Lesbian and gay relationships are frowned upon. Personal disclosure to friends and family jeopardizes the family name and may lead to ostracism. Assure that same-sex relationships are not disclosed to family members.

BIOCULTURAL ECOLOGY

- Common physical characteristics include dark hair and dark eyes, with variations in skin color and amount of hair darkness. Skin color ranges from fair to light brown, with those residing in the southern part of South Korea being darker.
- Epicanthal skin folds create the distinctive appearance of Asian eyes.

Korean

- Schistosomiasis and other parasitic diseases are endemic to certain regions of Korea.
- Korea continues to manufacture and use asbestos-containing products. There is a high rate of hypertension, renal failure, and stomach and liver cancer.
- Assess for stomach and liver cancer, tuberculosis, hepatitis, renal impairment, hypertension, parasites, and asbestos-related health problems.
- Be aware that many Koreans require lower dosages of psychotropic drugs.

HIGH-RISK HEALTH BEHAVIORS

- Smoking by women in public is taboo, but some women smoke at home.
- Men have a high incidence of alcohol consumption.
- Seat belts are worn infrequently in South Korea. Encourage moderate alcohol intake and smoking cessation. Explain the legal mandates of seat-belt and child restraint laws in the United States.

NUTRITION

- The traditional Korean diet includes steamed rice; hot soup; *kimchee*; and side dishes of fish, meat, or vegetables served in some variation for breakfast, lunch, and dinner. Breakfast is traditionally considered the most important meal.
- Rice is served with 5 to 20 small side dishes of mostly vegetables and some fish and meats.
- Food is flavorful and spicy. Cooking includes a variety of seasonings such as red and black pepper, garlic, green onion, ginger, soy sauce, and sesame seed oil.
- Most Korean Americans are at high risk for calcium deficiencies due to lactose intolerance. Determine individual cultural food choices that are high in calcium.
- A cultural treatment for the common cold is soup made from bean sprouts, anchovies, garlic, and other hot spices.

Common Korean American Dishes

- *Kimchee:* a spicy fermented cabbage made from a variety of vegetables but made primarily from a Chinese, or Napa, cabbage. Spices and herbs are added to the previously salted cabbage, which is allowed to ferment over time, and it is served with every meal in a variety of forms.
- *Beebimbap:* rice, finely chopped mixed vegetables, and a fried egg served in a hot pottery bowl. Hot pepper paste is usually added.
- *Bulgolgi:* thinly sliced pieces of beef marinated in soy sauce, sesame oil, green onions, garlic, and sugar and served after being barbecued.
- *Chopchae:* clear noodles mixed with lightly stir-fried vegetables and meats.
- **Adapt health teaching to Korean American food choices and practices.**

PREGNANCY AND CHILDBEARING PRACTICES

- Pregnancy is a highly protected time for women. Both pregnancy and the postpartum period are ritualized.
- Once a woman is pregnant, she starts practicing *Tae-Kyo*, which literally means "fetus education." The objective of *Tae-Kyo* is to promote the health and well-being of the fetus and mother by having the mother focus on art and beautiful objects.

DEATH RITUALS

- Death and dying are fairly well accepted in the Korean culture.
- Prolonging life may not be highly regarded in the face of modern technology. Families are expected to stay with family members and assist in feeding and personal care around the clock. **Include family in caring for their hospitalized family member.**

Korean

Pregnancy Beliefs

- Pregnant women who handle unclean objects or kill a living creature may experience a difficult birth.
- Women wear tight abdominal binders beginning at 20 weeks gestation or work physically hard toward the end of the pregnancy to increase the chance of having a small baby.
- Expectant mothers should avoid chicken, fish with scales, squid, or crab because eating these foods may affect the child's appearance. For example, eating duck may cause the baby to be born with webbed feet.
- Women attribute a variety of complaints to *naeng* (chill), a cold imbalance of the womb that brings on a heavy vaginal discharge and can cause women who experience it to become sterile.
- Eating blemished fruit causes a skin disease on the infant or an unpleasant face.
- Women commonly labor and deliver in the supine position. After the delivery, women are traditionally served seaweed soup, a rich source of iron, which is believed to facilitate lactation and to promote healing of the mother.
- Bed rest is encouraged after delivery for 7 to 90 days.
- Women are encouraged to keep warm by avoiding showers, baths, and cold fluids or foods in order to prevent chronic illnesses such as arthritis.
- The baby should be wrapped in warm blankets to prevent harm from cold winds.
- Postpartum women should care for their bodies by augmenting heat and avoiding cold, resting without working, eating well, protecting the body from harmful strains, and keeping clean. **To improve postpartum care, develop bilingual pamphlets that include medical terms used in the U.S. healthcare system.**

- Many believe that patients should not be told they have a terminal illness. Take cues from the patient and, if necessary, disclose terminal illnesses to the oldest son or designated family spokesperson, who will inform the patient when the family deems necessary.
- Crying and open displays of grief are common and signify the utmost respect for the dead.
- Relatives and friends come to pay respect by viewing photographs of the deceased instead of viewing the body.
- An ancestral burial ceremony follows death, with the body being placed in the ground facing south or north. Rice wine is sprinkled around the gravesite.
- The eldest son or male family member sits by the deceased, sometimes holds a cane, and makes a moaning noise to display his grief. The cane is a symbol of needing support. Provide a private room so family may grieve in culturally congruent ways.

SPIRITUALITY

- Organized religions include Christianity, Buddhism, and *Chondokyo*. The church is a powerful social support group for Korean immigrants.
- Christians believe the spirit goes to heaven; Buddhists believe the spirit starts a new life as a person or an animal. Each patient's spiritual practices need to be individually assessed.
- Family and education are central themes that give meaning to life.

HEALTH-CARE PRACTICES

- Many prescription drugs in the United States, such as antibiotics, anti-inflammatory and cardiac medications, and certain pain control medications, can be purchased over-the-counter in Korea.
- Herbal medicine may be used in conjunction with Western biomedicine. Herbal remedies include ginseng, seaweed soup, and *haigefen* (clamshell powder), which

Korean

has high levels of lead, causing abdominal colic, muscle pain, and fatigue. Ask about the use of traditional medicine, and include non-harmful practices into prescriptions.

- Complementary health practices include acupuncture, acumassage, acupressure, and moxibustion therapy.
- Some Korean Americans are stoic and are slow to express emotional distress from pain. Others are expressive and discuss their smallest discomforts. Monitor nonverbal cues and facial expressions for pain.
- Mental illness may be stigmatized. *Hwa-Byung*, a traditional Korean illness, occurs from the suppression of anger or other emotions. These emotions are expressed as physical complaints, ranging from headaches and poor appetite to insomnia and lack of energy.
- Organ donation and organ transplantation are rare, reflecting traditional attitudes toward integrity and purity.

HEALTH-CARE PRACTITIONERS

- More traditional individuals frequently prefer health-care providers who speak Korean and are older.
- Because of modesty, women prefer women for performing Pap smears, mammography, and breast examinations. Provide a same-gender health-care provider for intimate care whenever possible.

References

Purnell, L., & Kim, S. (2003). People of Korean heritage. In L. Purnell and B. Paulanka (Eds.), *Transcultural health care: A culturally competent approach* (2nd ed., pp. 249–264). Philadelphia: F.A. Davis Company.

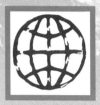

People of Mexican Heritage

Overview and Heritage

Great variations exist among people of Mexican ancestry, depending on their primary and secondary characteristics of culture as described in Chapter 1. However, a core of beliefs and practices are shared by those who self-identify as Mexican, Mexican American, Latino, Chicano, or Hispanic. Mexicans evolved from multiple races, all socioeconomic levels, various religions, and different educational and occupational backgrounds. Mexican Americans include newer immigrants and people who have been in the United States for six or seven generations. Some originate from high mountains and plateaus, some from low-lying swamp areas, and others from sea- and ocean-side communities. The topography of the region of origin in Mexico may be the key to accurate health assessments for illnesses and disease.

COMMUNICATIONS

- Great diversity exists in the Spanish language; 62 dialects are spoken in Mexico. Although most Mexicans use Spanish as their primary language, some speak only English, some speak both English and Spanish, and a few may only speak an indigenous Indian language.

- Significant importance is placed on verbal communication. Conversants may stand very close, even with people who are not well known to them. Loud voice volume in formal settings may connote anger.
- Whereas more traditional and older individuals do not maintain eye contact, acculturated and more educated people usually do maintain eye contact.
- Many Mexicans tend to be fatalistic and present-oriented. Many arrive late for appointments and delay seeking health care until the condition is more serious.
- Explaining the necessity of arriving on time for appointments is crucial.
- Touch is common between people of the same gender. However, men and women rarely touch in public. It is important to explain the necessity for touching private body areas during a physical.
- Formal names may be extensive and include a middle name and the mother and father's surnames. A married woman may take her husband's surname, thereby having three surnames. Greet adults formally with Señor, Señora, or Señorita unless told to do otherwise. Ask which name is preferred as well as which name is used for legal purposes.

FAMILY ROLES AND ORGANIZATION

- In traditional families, men are expected to provide financial support for the family.
- The stereotype of "machismo," in which men are the primary decision-makers in the household, is not accurate for all Mexicans and Mexican Americans.
- Women care for children and maintain the home. In most homes where the man and woman both work outside the home, they tend to share household chores and child-rearing responsibilities.
- Some households are patriarchal, some are matriarchal, and some are egalitarian. Regardless of who makes the

decision, the male traditionally is expected to be the spokesperson for the family. Specifically ask who makes which decisions for the family.

- Priorities for children are getting an education, having good manners, and respecting elders and people in high-status positions.
- Traditionally, adults expect children to live with their parents until marriage.
- Children born out of wedlock are loved regardless of the parents' marital status. Men usually remain involved with their children who are born out of wedlock.
- When possible, extended family members prefer living close to each other. The elderly frequently live with their children when self-care becomes a concern; in addition, the elderly are always respected for their wisdom. Extended family members can be a good resource for home care.
- Social status is gained through formal academic education, having a respected position, and having children and family members with good manners. The extensive name format represents status.
- Same-sex couples may be stigmatized. Do not disclose sexual orientation status to family members.

BIOCULTURAL ECOLOGY

- Most Mexicans have dark hair and dark eyes, but some may have blond hair and blue eyes. Many have a diverse gene pool that includes indigenous Indian groups, blacks, and whites. To assess for cyanosis and jaundice in those with dark skin, observe the sclera and conjunctiva, palms of the hands, soles of the feet, and buccal mucosa and tongue rather than relying on skin tone.
- Many adults suffer from lactose intolerance to some extent.
- High rates of diabetes are common. Diarrheal and parasitic diseases are common with newer immigrants. People emigrating from low-lying swampy areas need to be assessed for malaria and dengue fever symptoms such as lassitude, fever, weight loss, and failure to thrive,

Mexican

which are common in immigrants from these areas.
Assessments need to include exposure to pesticides,
parasitic diseases, and illnesses that are common in their
home country.

- Mexicans may require lower doses of antidepressants
  and experience more intense side-effects than non-
  Hispanic white populations. Many are also poor
  metabolizers of debrisoquine. Observe for side-effects
  of antidepressants.

HIGH-RISK HEALTH BEHAVIORS

- Smoking is more common among the more acculturated, but they smoke fewer cigarettes when they do
  smoke. Encourage smoking cessation.
- Some Mexicans use alcohol to make them emotionally
  and socially extroverted and are more likely to engage in
  binge drinking than other groups. When assessing alcohol consumption in this group, determine the amount of
  alcohol used both daily and during celebrations.
- Many newer immigrants may be reluctant to use seat
  belts and helmets because they are not used in their
  home countries. Explain the legal requirements of using
  seat belts and helmets as well as the safety issues
  involved to increase compliance.
- Men may object to condom use because it decreases
  sensitivity. Women may object to the use of condoms
  because of the suggestion that the woman is "dirty."
  Explain that condoms help prevent pregnancy and
  decrease the incidence of HIV/AIDS (SIDA) and other
  sexually transmitted diseases.

NUTRITION

- Food choices vary widely, depending on the region of
  Mexico from which the person comes. Rice, beans, and
  tortillas are food staples. Determine preparation
  practices because some people use coconut oil and
  animal fat for flavoring. Determine flavorings and
  ingredients as well as the major food choices because
  these can add significant calories to the diet. Encourage

use of corn tortillas instead of flour tortillas, leafy green vegetables, and soups and stews that use bones in them to increase calcium content in the diet and avoid lactose intolerance.

- Being overweight is seen as positive. Clients should be co-participants in deciding an acceptable weight.
- Sweetened fruit drinks are popular, and adding sugar to fresh fruit juice is common. Discouraging the use of sweetened fruit drinks and encouraging the use of natural juices without added sugar is one means of reducing calorie consumption, especially for diabetics.
- Mealtimes may not coincide with the dominant American schedule. For many, the noontime meal is the largest meal of the day, and the evening meal may be served very late in the evening. Determine the individual and family's meal times and adjust medication schedules accordingly.
- Many individuals balance food choices according to the "hot" and "cold" theory. Variations occur in the assignment of different foods for hot and cold properties. Herbal teas are commonly used to maintain health and treat illnesses. Individually determine the client's use of the hot and cold theory of food choices, which herbs and teas are used, how frequently they are used, and the amount used each time. Non-harmful practices should be incorporated into the plan of care.

PREGNANCY AND CHILDBEARING PRACTICES

- Fertility practices are primarily connected with religious beliefs usually associated with the Catholic Church. The church discourages the use of condoms, believing they promote promiscuity.
- The rhythm method or Norplant is usually deemed acceptable because they are more natural means of helping to prevent an unwanted pregnancy. Foams, creams, and intrauterine devices may not be acceptable because women are not supposed to touch their genitals except for purposes of bathing.
- Abortion is considered morally wrong. A few

individuals may see sterilization and other methods of birth control as acceptable. Determine on an individual basis acceptable methods of birth control, and counsel clients in a culturally congruent manner.

- Multiple births are more common among Mexicans. Pregnancy is considered a natural condition, with most advice for health care coming from family members; this may deter prenatal care. Stress that medical evaluation during pregnancy is necessary to help ensure the health of both the mother and baby. Encouraging female relatives to accompany the pregnant woman for prenatal check-ups may be helpful.
- For many, the delivery room is not a place for men, and many believe that allowing the father to see the woman or baby during the delivery may harm the mother or baby.
- Various cultural customs and beliefs are included in Box 24–1.

DEATH RITUALS

- Death is an extended family affair, and members are obligated to visit in the hospital or long-term care facility. Expect many visitors in the inpatient setting. Among more traditional Mexicans, a family member must remain with the dying person. Find a place where family members can be together, preferably in the unit with the dying person. In alternative settings, find another quiet place where the family can gather.
- Some families may want to have lighted candles in the room of the dying patient. Although in-patient facilities will not permit open candle flames because of fire safety, electric candles are acceptable to most.
- Death is considered part of life, and some, especially men, may approach death stoically. Just because someone does not openly display emotions about death does not mean the person does not care about the deceased.
- Some, especially women, may have an *ataque de nervios* on hearing about the death of a loved one. In this culture-bound syndrome, the person exhibits

hyperkinetic and seizure-like activity that releases strong emotions. This is a normal reaction, and treatment is usually not necessary except to remain with the person and provide emotional support. Use family members for assistance when possible.

BOX 24–1 • Common Cultural Beliefs and Customs

- Walking in the moonlight while pregnant may cause birth defects.
- Safety pins, metal keys, or other metal amulets are worn to prevent birth deformities.
- Raising one's arms over the head while pregnant will cause the cord to wrap around the infant's neck.
- Postpartum women are discouraged from taking baths, sitting in a bathtub, taking sitz baths, or washing their hair for 6 weeks.
- Bathing with a cloth, including the hair, is acceptable. Encourage use of warm compresses instead of sitz baths.
- Cutting the baby's hair or nails in the first 3 months is believed to cause blindness and deafness in the baby. **Ask permission before cutting an infant's nails or hair.**
- Placing a key, coin, or other metal object on the infant's umbilicus is believed to promote healing. **Teach how to clean the object to prevent infection.**
- Wearing an abdominal binder can prevent air from entering the uterus in postpartum women.
- Covering their ears, head, shoulders, and feet can prevent blindness, mastitis, frigidity, or sterility in women.
- **Recognize which practices are harmless, and respect the woman's beliefs as appropriate.**
- **Using videos and literature in Spanish and with pictures of Hispanics may help compliance with health interventions.**

Mexican

- Burial practices vary, but the more traditional do not practice cremation. Autopsy is not welcomed. Explaining the legalities of autopsy is conducive to having the family accept an autopsy.

SPIRITUALITY

- Although many other religions are practiced, the predominant religion is Roman Catholicism. However, do not assume that the practice of the Catholic religion is the same for all people. Each person's religious practices must be assessed on an individual basis. Many families have altars in their homes.
- The family is foremost. The individual's source of strength comes from being with family members. Priests and other religious leaders are major sources of emotional strength and support for most Mexicans. On admission to the health-care facility, inform the family of the availability of religious leaders.

HEALTH-CARE PRACTICES

- The family is considered the most credible source of health-care information among Mexicans. This practice can impede health-seeking behaviors. For many, good health means being free of pain and is largely due to the "will of God."
- Many migrant workers are not aware of the necessity of protecting themselves from pesticides and herbicide poisoning because they are not used in Mexico. Health teaching in this area should be a family affair.
- Almost all Mexicans use herbal medicines and teas. The specific herbs and teas vary among families. Most of these teas and herbs are beneficial or at least not harmful. A few can be harmful by themselves, whereas others may be harmful when included with prescription and over-the-counter medications. Ascertain if clients are using over-the-counter medicines and explain the hazards of excessive use of over-the-counter medications as well as using medicines that were originally intended for use by another family member. Assess for use of

herbs and teas. Two herbs commonly used by Mexican Americans are *azarcon* and *greta,* which are used for colic and stomach conditions in children. Both of these herbs contain lead and can be toxic, especially in children.

- Many Mexicans practice the hot and cold theory, according to which many diseases and illnesses are caused by a disruption in the hot and cold balance of the body. Thus, if too many cold forces in the body cause an illness, treatment is aimed at balancing the condition by introducing hot treatments and foods that are considered hot. *Hot and cold do not always coincide with temperature.*

- Hot conditions include infection, diarrhea, and sore throats and, therefore, are treated with such cold foods as fruits, vegetables, and dairy products. Cold conditions, such as cancer, malaria, and earaches, are treated with such hot foods as liquor, beef, port, and spicy foods. Tremendous variations exist between and among hot and cold conditions, depending on the family.

- The entire family must be included in health promotion and health teaching to increase compliance with health prescriptions and interaction.

- Frequently seen cultural illness or conditions are shown in Box 24–2.

- Perform an individual pain assessment; determine usual treatment modalities used for pain; ask what the patient thinks caused the pain; and determine what the patient usually does to relieve pain. Have pain scales in Spanish as well as visual scales for those who do not read Spanish. Explaining that pain medication will promote healing may encourage the patient to accept pain mediation.

- The sick role is easy to enter without personal feelings of inadequacy or blame. Family members readily take on the sick person's responsibilities. Family members usually care for the ill family member at home, if at all possible. Query the family to determine if they have the resources to care for a member at home. Not all Mexicans in the United States have the extended family to care for relatives at home. Because long-term care

Mexican

BOX 24–2 • Common Cultural Illnesses Among Mexicans

- *Empacho* (blocked intestines) may result from an incorrect balance of hot and cold foods causing a lump of food to stick in the gastrointestinal tract. Treatment includes massaging the stomach and back to dislodge the food bolus.
- *Mal de ojo* (evil eye) occurs when an older person looks at a younger person in an admiring fashion. Such eye contact can be voluntary or involuntary. Symptoms are numerous, including fever, anorexia and vomiting, or irritability. The spell can be broken if the person doing the admiring touches the person while admiring him or her. **Allopathic health-care providers are usually unable to cure *mal de ojo*. Making a referral to a folk practitioner is advisable.**
- *Caida de mollera* (fallen fontanel) has numerous causes, which may include removing a nursing infant too harshly from the nipple or handling an infant too roughly. Symptoms vary from failure to thrive to irritability. The usual treatment is to hold the infant upside down by the feet. **Assess for dehydration. A referral to a folk practitioner is also recommended.**
- *Susto* (magical fright or soul loss) is associated with epilepsy, tuberculosis, and other infectious diseases as well as an "overwhelming feelings of loss." Symptoms may be physical or psychological in nature and may also be consistent with depression. **Gear treatment to the underlying causes, and treat physical and psychological symptoms.**

facilities are either nonexistent or are of very poor quality in Mexico, family members may be very reluctant to place family members in such a facility. Suggesting a visit to one may be an option.

- Extraordinary means being used to preserve life are frequently frowned upon and are often determined by finances, education, and availability of services.
- Blood transfusions are acceptable, but some may be reluctant to accept transfusion or blood products for fear of HIV *(SIDA)*. The belief that the body must be buried whole deters organ donation. Organ transplantation may not be acceptable because of the belief that *mal aire,* bad air, will enter the body and increase one's risk for developing cancer. Dispel myths related to organ donation and organ transplantation. Eliciting the assistance of a priest may be helpful.

Mexican

HEALTH CARE PRACTITIONERS

- Many Mexicans use a number of folk practitioners who are usually well known to the client. See Box 24–3.

BOX 24–3 • Major Mexican Folk Practitioners

- ***Curanderos*** receive their gift from God or serve an apprenticeship. Some even prescribe over-the-counter medications. They usually treat traditional illnesses not caused by witchcraft.
- ***Espiritistas*** (spiritualists) treat conditions caused by witchcraft. Amulets and prayer are a large part of the treatment. Seeing an *espiritista* may carry a stigma among some Hispanics.
- ***Yerberos*** or ***Jerberos*** use herbs, teas, and roots to prevent or treat illnesses. Patients usually purchase the herbs from a *botanica,* a specialist herb shop that also sells religious figurines.
- ***Sobadores*** treat muscle and joint problems using massage and manipulation; usually they do not have formal training.
- **Ask patients if they are using folk practitioners and the reasons why they are using them, and have them fully disclose all treatments prescribed.**

- Health-care practitioners with the right qualities are well respected by Mexicans. Important qualities include addressing the client formally unless told to do otherwise, showing respect by asking questions, accepting the patient's ideas, taking an interest in the entire family, and being well groomed. Always ask permission, and explain the reason for the necessity of touching the client during a physical examination.

References

Zoucha, R., & Purnell, L. (2003). In L. Purnell and B. Paulanka (Eds.), *Transcultural health care: A culturally competent approach* (2nd ed., pp. 264–279). Philadelphia: F.A. Davis Company.

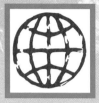

CHAPTER 25

Navajo Indians

Overview and Heritage

American Indians are the original inhabitants of North America. Although these groups are referred to as Native Americans and Alaskan Natives, many prefer to be called American Indians or names more specific to their cultural heritage. The amount of Indian blood necessary to be considered a tribal member or American Indian varies with each tribe. Navajo Indians claim the distinction of being the largest tribe: at least one-fourth Navajo blood is required to be considered a member of the tribe. Even among Native Americans, there is controversy concerning what constitutes an American Indian. This chapter describes primarily the cultural attributes, values, beliefs, and health-care practices of the Navajo.

The Bureau of Indian Affairs recognizes more than 500 different American Indian tribes, which extend throughout Alaska and Canada from Maine to Florida and from the east coast to the west coast. Although each of these American Indian cultures is unique, some share similar views regarding cosmology, medicine, and family organization. The Navajo Indians, the largest American Indian tribe, consist of approximately 200,000 people and have one of the largest reservations in the United States, covering portions of Arizona, Utah, and New Mexico. The Navajo Indians are nomadic and wander great distances, searching for adequate grazing grounds for their sheep. Because of severe economic conditions and high unemployment rates, significant migration occurs into and out of the reservations. Commercial activities on reservations are limited to businesses owned by Navajo Indians or partnerships in which a Navajo must own the controlling interest. Many Native Americans who leave their reservations experience culture shock resulting from a rapid and drastic change in environment. They usually return because of a lack of a social support system and loss of identity and self-esteem. Many Indians return to their reservation on a regular basis to refresh and renew themselves through Blessingway ceremonies.

Educational levels for American Indians are lower than those of similar populations, creating a barrier to employment. American Indians have consistently been identified as the most underrepresented of all minority groups in colleges and universities. Traditional educational values for most American Indians are reflected in learning the tribal culture that clarifies their roles in the clan and the community. Competitiveness is generally discouraged among American Indian populations, viewing group activities as more important than individual accomplishments. The health-care field severely lacks Navajo professionals. Nursing is perceived as an undesirable profession because Navajos believe it inadvisable to be around sick people. Navajos who choose to work in a hospital must sometimes have a special cleansing ceremony to protect themselves. Many American Indian students choose careers such as social worker, construction labor, arts, and weaving. Art is an important occupation and takes such forms as weaving rugs or baskets, making pottery, and beadwork. Rug-weaving and jewelry-making are the most common forms of art among the Navajo. They are also noted for sand paintings, which were traditionally used in healing ceremonies by medicine people and not originally intended for sale.

COMMUNICATIONS

- The Navajo language was not reduced to writing until the 1970s; consequently, many older people speak only their native language, and few are literate in the English language. The few elderly who are bilingual speak limited Spanish or English. The younger populations are usually bilingual, with their native tongue spoken primarily in the home. Be extremely careful when attempting to use the Navajo language, because minor variations in pronunciation may change the entire meaning of a word or phrase. Differences in pronunciation, particularly while speaking with an older Navajo, may cause a misunderstanding. Such misunderstandings make subsequent caring for the individual difficult. It is often safer to use an interpreter.
- Talking loudly among Navajo Indians is considered rude. Voice tones are quiet but not monotone. Their language is full of inflections with different meanings, making the language melodious with a quiet volume.
- Because most individuals generally do not share inner thoughts and feelings with anyone outside their clan, it may take non-tribal health-care providers a long time to build trust.
- Most Indians are comfortable with long periods of silence. Interest in what an individual says is shown through attentive listening skills. One may be considered immature if answers are given quickly or one interrupts another who is forming a response. Failing to allow adequate time for processing information may result in an inaccurate response or no response. Allow time for people to respond to questions.
- Touch among the Navajo is unacceptable unless one knows the person very well. Close observation of body language is very important for determining cues related to the permissibility of touch.
- The acceptable personal space for American Indians is greater than that of most European American cultures.
- Shaking hands is the traditional greeting. The handshake is light, more of a passing of the hands.

- Pointing with the finger is considered rude. Rather than pointing a finger to indicate a direction, individuals shift their lips toward the desired direction. Do not point with your finger.
- Direct eye contact is rude and possibly confrontational. Even close friends do not maintain eye contact, and this rule does not change with socioeconomic status.
- The time sequence is present, past, and future, in that order. Very little planning is done for the future because the Navajo view is that many things are outside of one's control and may affect or change the future. In fact, the Navajo language does not have a future-tense verb. Time is viewed as something that is always with the individual. To plan for the future is sometimes viewed as foolish. Events do not always start on time, but rather time starts when the group gathers. To help prevent frustration in scheduling events, time factors need to be taken into consideration and the speaker made aware of these unique time perceptions. Appointments may not always be kept, especially if someone else in the clan needs help.
- Older people are addressed as grandmother or grandfather or as mother or father by members of their clan. Otherwise, they are called by a nickname. A health-care provider can call an older Navajo client "grandmother" or "grandfather" as a sign of respect.

FAMILY ROLES AND ORGANIZATION

- Most American Indian tribes are matrilineal. The land is not owned, but grazing rights are passed from mothers to daughters. Whereas men are considered important, the grandmothers and mothers are at the center of Navajo society.
- The relationship between brother and sister is often more important than the relationship between husband and wife. When providing family care, it is important to note that no decision is made until the appropriate elderly woman is present. Find the appropriate

gatekeeper; otherwise, time is lost, and the problem must be addressed again later.

- Traditionally, men are expected to care for the livestock, the corral, and the fields. Men move with their sheep grazing over large areas. Women care for and stay close to the hogan, are independent, and often weave.
- Children are looked on with joy and proudly welcomed into the family. Ritual ceremonies and practices occur at various stages for both children and adolescents. Even though children may be named at birth, their names are not revealed until their first laugh, when they are considered to officially have a soul and self-identity. This protects the children and keeps them in tune with the Holy People.
- During the cradleboard phase of child rearing, infants are kept in the cradleboard until they begin walking. However, hip dysplasia may be exacerbated by cradleboards. The use of diapers has decreased the incidence of hip dysplasia because diapers bind the hips in a slightly abducted position. Encourage the use of diapers, and discourage the use of the cradleboard.
- Weaning, toilet training, and disciplining are frequently left to the grandmother. If the grandmother is unavailable, an aunt or a sister assumes this role.
- The use of formula has become popular, resulting in an increased incidence of bottle caries because many babies go to bed with a bottle of juice or soda pop. This practice causes children to lose their teeth by the age of 4 years. Educate parents about dental caries and encourage breast-feeding.
- A primary social premise is that no person has the right to speak for another. Thus, children are allowed to make their own decisions; for example, children may be allowed to decide if they want to take their medicine. Explain the importance of taking medicines as prescribed.
- An important ceremonial ritual for teenage girls is the onset of menarche, which is celebrated with special foods that symbolize passage into adulthood. Men are usually excluded from this celebration, with only aunts and grandmothers participating. There is no similar ritual for men.

Navajo

- Family bonds remain strong even after marriage. The family unit consists of the nuclear family and relatives such as sisters, aunts, and their female descendants.
- Family goals do not center on wealth or the attainment of possessions. In fact, if one person has more wealth than other relatives, the member who has more has a responsibility to assist relatives who have less.
- A sister's children are considered the same as her own children. If a mother dies or for some other reason cannot care for her children, it is assumed that the grandmother or sister will raise the children as her own.
- Older people are looked on with clear deference. Younger adults are faced with the responsibility of caring for relatives.
- There are few nursing homes, and hospitals are forced to keep patients until nursing home placement is found. When nursing home placement is found, it may be at a great distance from the family, making it difficult for family visits.
- Alternative lifestyles are not discussed but are quietly accepted. However, special individuals exist who are not looked on with disfavor but rather are accepted as being different.

BIOCULTURAL ECOLOGY

- Skin color varies from light brown to very dark brown. To assess for oxygenation in darker-skinned people, examine the mucous membranes and nail beds for capillary refill. Anemia is detected by examining the mucous membranes for pallor and the skin for a grayish hue. To assess for jaundice, examine the sclera rather than relying on skin hue. Newborns and infants commonly have Mongolian spots on the sacral area. Do not mistake these spots for bruises, and suspect child abuse.
- The Navajo appear Asian, with epithelial folds over the eyes. They are generally taller and thinner than other American Indian tribes. The Navajo have traditionally been good runners and excel in relay races and long-

distance running. Remember that these characteristics are not seen with everyone; variations in this population do exist.

- The water on the Navajo reservation is often impure and unchlorinated, making those who drink it susceptible to waterborne bacteria such as shigelloses. Salmonella is common because of the lack of refrigeration and hypothermia because of frequent snowstorms and conditions that limit Navajo ability to gather wood.

- Common diseases related to living in close contact with others include upper respiratory illnesses and acute otitis media.

- Conditions that have higher death rates in the American Indian population are shown in Box 25–1.

- The plague, tick fever, and recently the Muerto Canyon Hanta virus have increased due to the area's rodent population, consisting of prairie dogs and deer mice. Teach clients how to protect themselves from rodent-borne diseases.

- Type I diabetes mellitus is almost nonexistent in American Indians; however, type II diabetes mellitus is the third most prevalent disease affecting all American Indian tribes, with the Navajo's rate approaching 30

Navajo

BOX 25–1 • Causes of Increased Incidences of Death Among American Indians

Alcoholism 627 percent higher
Tuberculosis 533 percent higher
Diabetes mellitus 249 percent higher
Unintentional injuries 204 percent higher
Suicide 72 percent higher
Pneumonia and influenza 71 percent higher
Homicide 63 percent higher
Gastrointestinal disease 42 percent higher
Infant mortality 22 percent higher
Heart disease 13 percent higher

percent. Poor control and dietary compliance is associated with major long-term complications such as blindness and kidney failure.

- Unique to the Navajo is severe combined immunodeficiency syndrome (SCIDS), an immunodeficiency syndrome unrelated to AIDS, which results in a failure of the antibody response and cell-mediated immunity. Affected infants who survive initially are sent to tertiary care facilities. Survivors must receive gamma globulin on a regular basis until a bone marrow transplant can be performed.

- Navajo neuropathy is also unique to this population. Characteristics include poor weight gain, short stature, sexual infantilism, serious systemic infections, and liver derangement. Manifestations include weakness, hypotonia, areflexia, loss of sensation in the extremities, corneal ulcerations, acral mutilation, and painless fractures. Individuals who survive have many complications and are generally ventilator-dependent. None have been known to survive past the age of 24 years.

- Albinism, with genetically prone blindness, develops in some individuals during their late teens and early 20s.

- Many of these hereditary and genetic diseases are believed to result from a limited gene pool.

- Lidocaine reactions occur in 29 percent of the population as compared with 11 to 15 percent of European Americans. Carefully observe for lidocaine reactions.

HIGH-RISK HEALTH BEHAVIORS

- Alcohol use is more prevalent than any other form of chemical abuse. Health problems related to alcoholism include motor vehicle accidents, homicide, suicide, and cirrhosis.

- The effects of alcohol abuse are also evidenced in newborns as fetal alcohol syndrome, in teenagers as pregnancies and sexually transmitted diseases, and in adults as liver failure.

- Spousal abuse is common and is frequently related to alcohol use. The wife is the usual recipient of the abuse, but occasionally the husband is abused.
- The use of smokeless tobacco has steadily increased among teenagers and those in their early 20s.
- Suicide is becoming more prevalent among the adolescent population.
- Noncompliance with seat-belt use is high. Teach clients about the importance of using child safety seats, helmets, and seat belts.

NUTRITION

- Food has major significance beyond nourishment. Life events and religious ceremonies are celebrated with food. Food is not generally associated with promoting health or illness. Herbs are used in the treatment of many illnesses to cleanse the body of ill spirits or poisons. Encourage and teach about healthy food choices and preparation practices.
- Sheep are a major source of meat, and sheep brains are a delicacy. Fry bread and mutton are cooked in lard. Access to fresh fruits or vegetables is minimal except during the fall. Squash is common at harvest time. Corn is an important staple. Corn pollen is used in the Blessingway and many other ceremonies.
- Diets may be deficient in vitamin D because many individuals suffer from lactose intolerance or do not drink milk. Recommend nondairy foods that are high in calcium or making stews and purees using animal bones.

PREGNANCY AND CHILDBEARING PRACTICES

- Traditional Navajos do not practice birth control and, thus, do not limit the size of their families. The birth rate among American Indians is 96 percent higher than the birth rate in the overall U.S. population. Large families are considered favorably because, in times past, many children died at an early age. Encourage prenatal

Navajo

care, carefully explaining the detrimental effects on the mother and infant if prenatal care is not sought.

- Twins are not considered favorably and are frequently believed to be the work of a witch, in which case one of the babies must die. Sometimes the mother may have difficulty caring for two infants. Twins may be readmitted to the hospital for neglect and failure to thrive. Culturally sensitive counseling assists adoption. Encourage tribal members to adopt the children.

- It is especially important to adhere to the many prescriptive and restrictive taboo practices related to pregnancy, which involve both husband and wife. See Table 25–1, Navajo Taboos Regarding Expectant Women, and Table 25–2, Taking Care of Yourself During Pregnancy: Navajo Rules for Expectant Couples, which were developed by Ursula Wilson in 1987.

- During labor, the mother wears birthing necklaces made of juniper seeds and beads to assist with a safe birth. Woven belts or sashes are used to help push the baby out. This practice is also used by Navajo midwives in caring for their clients.

- Many Navajo women are reluctant to deliver their babies in hospital settings. They know that people have died in hospitals and thus perceive that pregnant women should not be around the dead or in a place where people have died.

- A taboo practice among the Navajo is purchasing clothes for an infant before birth. Do not interpret not buying clothes for the infant as not wanting the baby.

- Immediately after birth, the placenta is buried as a symbol of the child being tied to the land. Sometimes it is burned in a fire. This is considered a safe place because fire is sacred and protects the baby against evil spirits.

- After birth, the baby is given a mixture with juniper bark to cleanse its insides and rid it of mucus. In addition, a ceremonial food of corn pollen and boiled water is given. Corn symbolizes healthy nutrients and an enduring nature.

TABLE 25–1

Navajo Taboos Regarding Expectant Women

1. Don't wear two hats at once; you'll have twins (or two wives).
2. Don't hit babies in the mouth; they'll be stubborn and slow to talk.
3. Don't have a weaving comb (rug) with more than five points; your baby will have extra fingers.
4. Don't have a baby cross its fingers; its mother will have another one right away.
5. Don't swallow gum while you are pregnant; the baby will have a birthmark.
6. Don't kill animals while your wife is pregnant; the baby will look like a bird.
7. Don't stand in the doorway when a pregnant woman is present.
8. Don't make a slingshot while you are pregnant; the baby will be crippled.
9. Don't go to ceremonies while pregnant; it will have a bad effect on the baby.
10. Don't eat a lot of sweet stuff while you are pregnant; the baby won't be strong.
11. Don't sleep too much when you are about to have a baby; the baby will mark your face with dark spots.
12. Don't look at a dead person or animal while you are pregnant; the baby will be sickly because of bad luck.
13. Don't jump around if you are pregnant or ride a horse; it will induce labor.
14. Don't cut gloves off at the knuckles, the baby will have short round fingers.
15. Don't cut a baby's hair when it is small; it won't think right when it gets older.
16. Don't put on a Yei mask while your wife is pregnant; the baby will have a big head and look strange.
17. Don't let a baby's head stay to one side in the cradle board; it will have a wide head.
18. Don't watch or look at an accident while your wife is present; it will affect the baby.
19. Don't sew on a saddle while your wife is pregnant; it will ruin the baby's mouth.

Ursula Wilson, July 1987. IHS inservice seminar, Tuba City Indian Health Center, Tuba City, AZ, with permission.

Navajo

TABLE 25–2

Taking Care of Yourself during Pregnancy: Navajo Rules for Expectant Couples

DURING PRENATAL PERIOD

Mind/Soul

Do's
- Keep the peace
- Keep thoughts good
- Talk with "corn pollen sprinkled" words
- Say morning (dawn) prayers

- Have shielding prayers done if you have nightmares

Don'ts
- Argue with partner or others
- Scold children
- Allow bad thoughts to occupy mind for long period of time
- Talk negatively or with criticism

Body

Do's
- Eat foods good for baby
- Get up early and walk around
- Have a Blessingway ceremony for a safe delivery

Don'ts
- Drink milk or eat salt or foods taken away by Navajo ceremonies
- Lay around too much
- Tie knots
- Attend funerals or look at body of deceased person
- Be with sick people for long or go to crowded place
- Attend healing ceremonies for sick people like "Yei Bei Chai Dance"
- Look at dead animals or taxidermic trophies
- Look at eclipse of moon or sun
- Make plans for baby or prepare layette sets until after birth
- Lift heavy things
- Kill living things or cut a sheep's throat
- Weave rugs or make pottery

DURING LABOR

Mind/Soul

Do's

- Think about a good delivery
- Have medicine people do "Singing Out Baby" chants
- Have medicine person perform "Unraveling" songs if necessary

Don'ts

- Let too many people observe labor; only people who are helping you in some way

Body

Do's

- Loosen your hair
- Drink corn meal mush
- Wear juniper seed beads
- Burn cedar
- Hold onto sash belt when ready to push
- Have someone apply gentle fundal pressure during pushing effort
- Get in squatting position for pushing
- Drink herbal tea to relax if necessary
- Drink herbal tea to strengthen contractions if necessary

Don'ts

- Braid or tie hair in a knot
- Tie knots

AFTER BIRTH OF BABY (POSTPARTUM PERIOD)

Do's

- Bury the placenta
- Drink juniper/ash tea to cleanse your insides
- Drink blue cornmeal mush
- Smear baby's first stool on your face
- Breast-feed your baby
- Wrap sash belt around waist for 4 days after delivery

Don'ts

- Drink cold liquids or be in cold draft
- Smell afterbirth blood for too long
- Show signs of displeasure if baby soils on you or during diaper change
- Burn placenta or afterbirth blood fluids
- Have sexual intercourse for 3 months after delivery

Navajo

Ursula Wilson, July 1987. IHS inservice seminar, Tuba City Indian Health Center, Tuba City, AZ, with permission.

DEATH RITUALS

- One death taboo involves talking with clients concerning a fatal disease or illness. Effective discussions require that the issue be presented in the third person, as if the illness or disorder occurred with someone else. Never suggest that the client is dying. To do so would imply that the provider wishes the client dead. If the client does die, it would imply that the provider might have evil powers.
- The body must go into the afterlife as whole as possible. The body is not buried for approximately 4 days after death.
- A cleansing ceremony must be performed after an individual dies, or the spirit of the dead person may try to assume control of someone else's spirit. Family members are reluctant to deal with the body because those who work with the dead must have a ceremony to protect themselves from the deceased's spirit.
- If the person dies at home, the hogan must be abandoned, or a ceremony must be held to cleanse it.
- Before burial, a ring is placed on the index finger of each hand, and the shoes are put on the wrong feet. This allows living relatives to recognize individuals if they come back and present themselves at ceremonial dances. Do not wear rings on your index fingers, as older people may not want to be around them.
- Excessive displays of emotion are not considered favorably among some tribes. Support survivors and permit family bereavement and grieving in a culturally congruent and sensitive manner that respects the beliefs of the tribe.

SPIRITUALITY

- The American Indian religion predominates in many tribes. Sometimes hospital admissions are accompanied by traditional ceremonies and consultation with a pastor. Even if people are strong in their adopted beliefs, they honor their parents and families by having a traditional healing ceremony.

- Many Navajo start the day with prayer, meditation, corn pollen, and running in the direction of the sun.
- Spirituality for most is based on harmony with nature. The meaning of life is derived from being in harmony with nature. The individual's source of strength comes from the inner self and also depends on being in harmony with one's surrounding.
- Prayers ask for harmony with nature and for health and invite blessings to help the person exist in harmony with the earth and sky. Along with certain ceremonies, prayer helps the Navajo to attain fulfillment and inner peace with themselves and their environment.
- Spirituality cannot be separated from the healing process in holistic ceremonies. Illness results from not being in harmony with nature, from the spirits of evil people such as witches, or from violation of taboos. Healing ceremonies restore an individual's balance mentally, physically, and spiritually.
- The core concepts of traditional Indian medicine are shown in Box 25–2.

BOX 25–2 • Basic Concepts of Traditional Indian Medicine

- Indians believe in a Supreme Creator.
- Each person is a three-fold being composed of mind, body, and spirit.
- All physical things, living and nonliving, are part of the spiritual world.
- The spirit existed before it came into the body, and it will exist after it leaves the body.
- Illness affects the mind and the spirit as well as the body.
- Wellness is harmony.
- Natural unwellness is caused by violation of a taboo.
- Unnatural wellness is caused by witchcraft.
- Each individual is responsible for his or her own health.

HEALTH-CARE PRACTICES

- Many older people do not understand the theory of germs.
- Asking clients questions in order to make a diagnosis fosters mistrust. This approach is in conflict with the practice of traditional medicine men who tell people what is wrong without their having to say anything.
- The federal government assumes responsibility for the health-care needs of American Indians. Government services respect a blending of both worlds. Few Indians who live on reservations have traditional health insurance.
- When people are ill or out of harmony, the medicine man or, in some cases, a diagnostician tells them what they have done to disrupt their harmony. They are returned to harmony through the use of a healing ceremony. The medicine man is expected to diagnose the illness and prescribe necessary treatments for regaining health. In Western health care, the practitioner asks the client what he or she thinks is wrong and then prescribes a treatment. This practice is sometimes interpreted by American Indians as ignorance on the part of the white healer.
- Often great distances must be traveled to reach hospitals or health-care facilities. Many families do not have adequate transportation and must wait for others to transport them into town. Immunizations may be missed because parents do not have transportation. Pay close attention to the immunization status of clients on their arrival at the emergency department or clinic. If the client is not current with immunizations, scheduling an appointment may be a waste of time because they may not be able to return until a ride is found. Take time to administer the immunization on the spot or make a referral to the public health nursing office.
- Pain control is frequently ineffective because the actual intensity of the Indian's pain is not obvious to the health-care provider and because clients do not request pain medication.

- Pain is viewed as something that is to be endured. Herbal medicines may be used without the knowledge of the health-care provider. Establishing trust will encourage clients to fully disclose herbal treatments used for pain control. Offer pain medicine, and explain that it will promote healing.
- Mental illness is perceived as resulting from witches or witching (placing a curse) on a person. In these instances, a healer who deals with dreams or a crystal-gazer is consulted. Individuals may wear turquoise to ward off evil; however, a person who wears too much turquoise is sometimes thought to be an evil person and, thus, someone to avoid.
- Rehabilitation as a concept is relatively new. Explain concepts of rehabilitation.
- Those with physical or mental handicaps are not considered different; rather, the limitation is accepted, and a role is found for them within the society.
- Cultural perceptions of the sick role for the American Indian are based on the ideal of maintaining harmony with nature and with others. Ill people have obviously done something to place themselves out of harmony or have had a curse placed on them. In either case, support of the sick role is not generally accepted, but rather support is directed at assisting the person with regaining harmony. Older people frequently work even when they are seriously ill and often must be encouraged to rest.
- Autopsy and organ donation are unacceptable practices to traditional American Indians. Explain that autopsy is a legal requirement in some instances.

HEALTH-CARE PRACTITIONERS

- Native healers are divided primarily into three categories: those working with the power of good, the power of evil, or both. Generally, these healers are divinely chosen and promote activities that encourage self-discipline, self-control, and acute body awareness. Some practitioners are endowed with supernatural

Navajo

BOX 25–3 • Traditional American Indian Health-Care Practitioners

1. People who can use their power only for good can transform themselves into other forms of life and can maintain cultural integration in times of stress.
2. People who can use their powers for both evil and good are expected to do evil against someone's enemies. People in this group know witchcraft, poisons, and ceremonies designed to afflict the enemy.
3. The diviner diagnostician, such as a crystal-gazer, can see what caused the problem but cannot implement a treatment. Another example of this type is a hand trembler. These people, instead of using crystals, practice hand trembling over the sick person to determine the cause of an illness.
4. Specialist medicine people treat the disease after it has been diagnosed and specialize in the use of herbs, massage, or midwifery.
5. Those who care for the soul send guardian spirits to restore a lost soul.
6. Singers, who are considered to be the most special, cure through the power of their song. These healers use laying on of hands and usually remove objects or draw disease-causing objects from the body while singing.

powers, whereas others only have knowledge of herbs and specific manipulations.
• Acceptance of Western medicine is variable, with a blending of traditional health-care beliefs.
• Many individuals are suspicious of American Indian physicians. Many health concerns of American Indians can be treated by both traditional and Western healers in a culturally competent manner when these practitioners are willing to work together and respect each other's differences.
• Western practitioners, traditional medicine men, and

herbal healers receive respect on the reservation. However, not all individuals accord equal respect to these groups, and many prefer one group over the other or use all three.

- Navajo tribal practitioners divide their knowledge into preventive measures, treatment regimens, and health maintenance. An example of a preventive measure is carrying an object or a pouch filled with objects prescribed by a medicine man that wards off the evil of a witch. Do not remove medicine pouches from clients.
- The various types of traditional practitioners are shown in Box 25–3.
- Male health-care providers are generally limited in the care they provide to women, especially during menses. Women are generally modest and wear several layers of slips. This practice is very common among elderly women. Provide a same-gender health-care provider for intimate care.

References

Still, O., & Hodgins, D. (2003). Navajo Indians. In L. Purnell and B. Paulanka (Eds.) *Transcultural health care: A culturally competent approach* (2nd ed., pp. 279–284). Philadelphia: F.A. Davis Company.

U.S. Department of Health and Human Services. (1998). *Trends in Indian Health*. Public Health Service: Indian Health Services, Office of Planning and Evaluation. Rockville, MD.

Wilson, U. (1983). Nursing care of the American Indian patient. In M. S. Orque, B. Block, and L. S. A. Monroy, *Ethnic nursing care: A multicultural approach*. St. Louis, MO: Mosby.

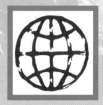

People of Puerto Rican Heritage

Overview and Heritage

Approximately 3 million Puerto Ricans live in the mainland United States as compared with 3.8 million residents in Puerto Rico. More than half live in the northeastern United States. They self-identify as *Puertorriqueños* or *Boricua* (the Taíno Indian word for Puerto Rican) or *Niuyoricans* for those born in New York. Thirty-four percent are age 18 years and younger. More than 25 percent live below the poverty level. Puerto Ricans evolved from interracial marriages among indigenous Indians, Spaniards, and African slaves. During the Spanish-American War, Puerto Rico became a colony of the United States; in 1952, Puerto Rico became a commonwealth. This "status question" is a sensitive topic for most; the perception of many is that the dominant American culture is a potential threat to the Puerto Rican culture, language, and political future.

Most Puerto Ricans come to the United States to seek employment, education, and a better quality of life.

Citizenship status has created a controversial *"va y ven"* (go and come) circular migration in which individuals and families are often caught in a reverse cycle of immigration, alternately living a few months or years in the United States and then returning to Puerto Rico. Education is greatly respected among Puerto Ricans. Although the educational system in Puerto Rico is similar to that in the United States, when children emigrate from Puerto Rico to the United States, many educational organizations place them one grade below their previous academic year as a result of language barriers.

Women are more likely than men to work in managerial and professional positions. Men are more likely to work in technical, sales, administrative support, and services.

COMMUNICATIONS

- The issue of two official languages, English and Spanish, is a sensitive one. Some fear that speaking English will affect their culture, traditions, and practices.
- Most Puerto Ricans speak with a melodic, high-pitched, fast rhythm, which is maintained when speaking English. Avoid making comments about accent, use caution when interpreting voice pitch, and seek clarification when in doubt about the content and nature of a conversation that may seem confrontational.
- Many individuals prefer to read or share sensitive information, options, and decisions with close family members. Some obtain verbal approval from extended family or community members who are knowledgeable in health matters. When consent is needed from a woman, ask if verbal approval or consent from the partner should be obtained first. Seek clarification of the information provided, ask for language preference in verbal and written information, and allow time for the exchange of information with questions and answers when critical decisions need to be made.
- Great value is placed on interpersonal interactions such as *simpatía*, a cultural script according to which an individual is perceived as likeable, attractive, and fun-loving.

- Most individuals enjoy sharing information about their families, heritage, thoughts, and feelings and expect the health-care provider to exchange personal information when beginning a professional relationship.
- If *confianza* (trust) is established, health-care providers can establish open communication channels with individuals and families.
- Most Puerto Ricans readily express their physical ailments and discomforts, with the exception of sexuality, which is taboo. Set boundaries with discretion, emphasizing personal, rather than impersonal and bureaucratic, relationships.
- Personal space may be a significant issue for some older women, particularly those from rural areas who may prefer to maintain a greater distance from men. Those born in the United States may be less self-conscious about personal space.
- Among younger generations and those born in the United States, eye contact is maintained and is often encouraged. With the more traditional, limited eye contact is a sign of respect, especially with older people.
- Hand, leg, head, and body gestures are commonly used to augment messages expressed by words. Feelings and emotions are also expressed through touch.
- Gesturing includes an affirmative nod with an "Aha!" response, which does not necessarily mean agreement or understanding related to the conversation.
- Women greet each other with a strong, familiar hug and if among family or close friends, a kiss is included. Young women may take offense to verbal and nonverbal communications that portray women as nonassertive and passive. Men may greet other men with a strong right handshake and a left hand stroking the greeter's shoulder. Greet Puerto Ricans with a friendly handshake.
- Most individuals are present-oriented, having a relativistic and serene view and way of life. Respect this view, and assist in identifying options, choices, and opportunities to empower individuals to change health-risk behaviors. Carefully explain appointment

times, and explain time limits at the beginning of an interview.

- Respect is reflected in the way children talk, look, and refer to adults and older people. Rather than *Señora* (Mrs.) and *Señor* (Mr.), children and adults are expected to use the term *Doña* (Mrs.) and *Don* (Mr.) for most adults. Aunts and uncles have their name preceded by *tití* or *tío* (auntie/uncle) and *madrina* or *padrino* (godmother or godfather). In health-care settings, individuals expect to be addressed as *Sr., Sra., Don,* and *Doña.* Do not use first names or terms such as "honey" or "sweetheart."

- A single woman may use her name as follows: Sonia López Mendoza, with López being her father's surname and Mendoza her mother's. When she is married, the husband's last name, Pérez, is added with the word *de* to reflect that she is married. This woman's married name would be Sonia López de Pérez; the mother's surname is eliminated. In business and health-care organizations, Señora López de Pérez is the correct formal title to use when promoting conversation or building a relationship. Ask clients their complete name as well as their legal name.

FAMILY ROLES AND ORGANIZATION

- Many traditional values still define women in terms of their reproductive roles, but gender role expectations are strikingly different among more acculturated families. Traditional and newly migrated families may view women as lenient, submissive, and always wanting to please men. Men demand respect and obedience from women and the family. Nevertheless, women play a central role in the family and the community, and the family is moving toward more egalitarian relationships. Accept family decision-making styles without judgment.

- As women become older they gain status for their wisdom.

- Traditional cultural norms discourage an overt sexual-being image for women, but with family assimilation many of these traditional values disappear. When topics such as sex, sexually transmitted diseases, or other infectious diseases are discussed, an environment built on *confianza* and *personalismo* must be established if these sensitive issues are to be addressed effectively.

- Children are the center of Puerto Rican family life. Great significance is given to the concept of *familism*, and any behavior that shifts from this ideal is discouraged and may be perceived as a disgrace.
- Most families expect their children to stay home until they get married or pursue a college education. The mother is expected to assume an active role disciplining, guiding, and advising children. Most fathers expect to be consulted, but they mainly see themselves as financial providers.
- Teen pregnancy, substance abuse, delinquent behaviors, and depression have been associated with the conflict between traditional values and those of mainstream American culture. Address family conflict within the context of the family to resolve adolescents' mental health issues rather than using individual approaches.
- Many families socialize male children to be powerful and strong. This macho behavior encourages dominance over women.
- Female children are socialized with a focus on home economics, family dynamics, and motherhood, which places women in a powerful social status.
- Modesty is highly valued, and issues such as menstruation, birth control, impotence, sexually transmitted diseases, and infertility are rarely discussed.
- Traditional punishments include making the child who has told a lie kneel on rice until the truth is told, washing the mouth vigorously with soap for using profanity, and spanking the buttocks or lower extremities with a belt. Many Puerto Rican mothers use threats of punishment, guilt, and discipline, which can create stress and difficulties for adolescents as they struggle with the more permissive cultural patterns of the United States, such as dating. Assess family disciplining practices, provide counseling, and explain U.S. child abuse laws.

- The family structure may be nuclear or extended. Family members include grandparents, great-grandparents, married children, aunts, uncles, cousins, and even divorced children with their children.
- Two families may live in the same household. Most families want a daughter because traditionally daughters are caretakers when parents reach advanced ages. Grandparents assume an active role in rearing grandchildren, supporting the family, babysitting, teaching traditions, disciplining, and enforcing educational activities. Use and encourage older Puerto Ricans to introduce health promotion and disease prevention education within their families.
- Dependent older people are expected to live with their children and be cared for emotionally and financially. Placements in nursing homes and extended-care facilities may be considered inconsiderate, and family members may feel guilty and experience depression and distress. Explore alternatives for elder care, and provide information to all family members involved in this decision-making process. Address discharge planning and hospice care in a "conference-style" approach to develop strategies for providing emotional support and assistance to family members.
- A family member is expected to be at the bedside of the sick person. Ask the name of the family spokesperson, and document it in the client's chart. Set boundaries about visitation, personal space, and privacy matters with clients' families.
- Some families abide by cultural prescriptions that encourage the initiation of sexual behaviors before marriage, extramarital sexual activity, and control over sexual relationships by men. Less educated families may have great difficulty educating young women about sexuality and reproductive issues. Thus, adolescents depend on educational organizations to learn about menstruation and the reproductive system. Educating the family about sexuality issues gains respect and entrance into the trusted family environment.
- Homosexuality continues to be a taboo topic that carries

Puerto Rican

a great stigma among Puerto Ricans. Homosexual behavior is often undisclosed to avoid family rejection and preserve family links and support. Some men may perceive that sexual intercourse with men is a sign of virility and sexual power rather than a homosexual behavior. When caring for gays and lesbians inquire about their "disclosed" or "undisclosed" status, and act according to client preferences and support resources.

BIOCULTURAL ECOLOGY

- Given the mixed heritage of Native Indian, African, and Spanish, some Puerto Ricans have dark skin, thick kinky hair, and a wide flat nose; others are white-skinned with straight auburn hair and hazel or black eyes. Because of the African heritage of many, drug absorption, metabolism, and excretion differences experienced by African Americans and Native Americans may hold true for black Puerto Ricans.
- Health conditions with increased frequency include heart disease, hypertension, asthma, malignant neoplasm, diabetes mellitus, unintentional injuries, and AIDS (*SIDA* in Spanish). Puerto Ricans have decreased mortality rates for lung, breast, and ovarian cancers and an increased incidence of stomach, prostate, esophageal, pancreatic, and cervical cancers. Educate families about cancer prevention. Discourage smoked, pickled, and spiced foods, and encourage traditional family meals with fruits and vegetables.
- Women have a high incidence of being overweight, increasing the incidence of and mortality from diabetes, the third leading cause of death for Puerto Rican women on the mainland. Develop interventions that are appropriate to gender, age, and socioeconomic status.
- Dengue, a mosquito-transmitted disease, is an endemic disease that migrants may bring to the United States. Advise clients and families traveling to Puerto Rico to avoid exposure to endemic areas and to use mosquito repellent and protective clothing at all times. Become familiar with the signs, symptoms, and current treatment recommendations for dengue fever.

HIGH-RISK HEALTH BEHAVIORS

- Alcoholism is the precursor of increased unintentional injuries, family disruption, spousal abuse, and mental illness among families. Many women smoke tobacco.
- Acculturation, as measured by language use, is significantly associated with marijuana and cocaine use. The longer one lives in the United States, and the more acculturated one becomes, the greater the use of marijuana, smoking, and cocaine. English-speaking Puerto Ricans are five times more likely to use marijuana and two times more likely to use cocaine than Spanish-speaking Puerto Ricans (Amaro et al., 1990). Develop programs that promote early interventions for the use of illicit drugs. Focus on individual psychological differences, gender issues, and other contributing factors.
- Lack of condom use is a significant risk behavior. Issues such as embarrassment, cost, gender or power struggles, and abuse are among some of the barriers. Some men fear that if they use condoms they portray a less macho image, have decreased sexual satisfaction, or portray that they have a sexually transmitted disease or HIV. Some women may refuse a condom, believing that the man thinks she is "dirty." Assess individual perceptions of high-risk behaviors, and intervene with programs designed to meet the particular needs of clients who are at high risk for HIV infection or other sexually transmitted diseases.

NUTRITION

- Most Puerto Ricans celebrate, mourn, and socialize around food. Food is used (a) to honor and recognize visitors, friends, family members, and health-care providers; (b) as an escape from everyday pressures, problems, and challenges; and (c) to prevent and treat illnesses. Clients may bring homemade goods to health-care providers as an expression of appreciation, respect, and gratitude for services rendered. Refusing food offerings may be interpreted as a personal rejection.
- Being overweight is a sign of health and wealth. Some individuals eat to excess believing that if they eat more

Puerto Rican

their health will be better. Efforts directed at weight control may be considered Americans' excessive preoccupation with a thin body image. Negotiate an acceptable weight with clients.

- Many families believe that a healthy child is one who is *gordita* or *llenito* (diminutive for fat or overweight) and has red cheeks. An oversized body image may be perceived as physical and financial wealth. Mothers are often encouraged to add cereal, eggs, and *viandas* (see below) to their infant's milk bottles. Educate mothers about these practices and the health risks for children who are overweight.

- Traditional families emphasize having a complete breakfast that begins with a cup of strong coffee or espresso with lots of sugar. Many families introduce children to coffee as early as 5 or 6 years of age.

- A traditional breakfast includes hot cereal such as oatmeal, corn meal, or rice and wheat cereal cooked with vanilla, cinnamon, sugar, salt, and milk. Although less common, many people also eat corn pancakes or fritters for breakfast. Lunch is served by noon, followed by dinner at around 5 or 6 PM. It is customary to have a cup of espresso-like coffee at 10 AM and 3 PM.

- Rice and stew *habichuelas* (beans) are the main dishes. Rice may be served plain or cooked and served with as many as 12 side dishes. Rice cooked with vegetables or meat is considered a complete meal. *Arroz guisado* (rice stew) is seasoned with *sofrito*, a blend of spices such as cilantro, *recao* (a type of cilantro), onions, green peppers, and other nonspicy ingredients. Rice is cooked with chicken, pork, sausages, codfish, calamari, or shrimp. It is also cooked with corn, several types of beans, and *gandules* (green pigeon peas), a Puerto Rican bean that is rich in iron and protein.

- A great variety of pastas, breads, crackers, vegetables, and fruits are eaten. Fritters are also common foods. Fried green or ripe plantains are a favorite side dish served with almost every meal.

- Families eat a variety of roots called *viandas*, vegetables rich in vitamins and starch. The most common *viandas* are celery roots, sweet potatoes, dasheens, yams, breadfruit, breadnut, green and ripe plantains, green bananas, tanniers, cassava, and chayote squash or christophines. Become familiar with traditional foods and their nutritional content to assist families with dietary practices that integrate their traditional or preferred food selections. Table 26–1 lists a variety of common Puerto Rican foods and their ingredients.

- Many individuals ascribe to the hot-cold classifications of foods for nutritional balance and dietary practices during menstruation, pregnancy, the postpartum period, infant feeding, lactation, and aging. Table 26–2 identifies many of the foods that are considered either "hot" or "cold." Become familiar with these food practices when planning culturally congruent dietary alternatives.

- Understanding that iron is considered a "hot" food that is not usually taken during pregnancy can help

TABLE 26–1

Common Puerto Rican Meals and Fritters

Puerto Rican Meal	English Translation
Alcapurrias	Green plantain fritters filled with meat or crab
Arepas de maíz y queso	Corn meal and cheese fritters
Arroz con pollo	Rice with chicken
Arroz con gandules	Rice with pigeon peas
Arroz blanco (con aceite)	Plain rice (with oil)
Arroz guisado básico	Plain stewed rice
Asopao de pollo	Soupy rice with chicken
Bacalaitos	Codfish fritters
Bocadillo	Grilled sandwich
Mondongo	Tripe stew
Paella de mariscos	Seafood paella
Pastelillos de carne, queso o pasta de guayaba	Turnovers filled with meat, cheese or guava paste
Pollo en fricase con papas	Stewed chicken with potatoes
Relleno de papa	Potato ball filled with meat
Sancocho	Viandas and meats stew
Sofrito	Condiment (1 tbsp)
Surullo de queso	Corn meal fritters filled with cheese

Puerto Rican

TABLE 26 – 2

Puerto Rican Hot-Cold Classification of Health-Illness Status, Medications, Herbs, and Selected Foods

Hot-Cold Classification	Health/ Illnesses Status	Western Medications	Traditional Herbs	Foods
Hot	GI illnesses (constipation, diarrheas, Crohn's colitis, ulcer, bleeding) Gynecologic issues (pregnancy, menopause) Skin disorders (rashes, acne) Neurological disorders (headache) Heart disease Urologic illnesses	Syrups Dark-colored pills Aspirin Anti-inflammatory agents Prednisone Antihypertensives Castor oil Cinnamon Vitamins (iron) Antibiotics	Teas: Cinnamon Dark-leaf teas	Cocoa products Alcoholic beverages Caffeine products Hot cereals (wheat, corn) Salt Spices and condiments Beans Nuts and seeds
Cold	Osteomuscular illnesses (arthritis, rheumatoid arthritis, multiple sclerosis) Menstruation Respiratory illnesses	Diuretics Bicarbonate of soda Antacids Milk of magnesia	Teas: Orange-lemon, chamomile Linden Mint Anise	Rice Rice and barley water Milk Sugar and sugar products Root vegetables Avocado Fruits Vegetables White meat Honey Onions

health-care providers in negotiating approval. Educate women about the importance of maintaining adherence to daily iron recommendations, even during pregnancy and lactation.

- A summary of food habits, reasons for practices, and recommendations for health-care providers during such developmental stages is included in Table 26–3.

TABLE 26–3

Puerto Rican Cultural Nutrition and Health Beliefs and Practices During Health Stages

Behavioral Period	Dietary and Health Practices	Cultural Justification	Recommendation for Health-Care Professionals
Menstru-ation	Food taboos: Avoid spices, cold beverages, acid-citric fruits and substances, chocolate, and coffee.	May induce cramps, hemorrhage, clots, and physical imbalance. May produce acne during menstruation.	Assess individual beliefs and acknowledge them. Incorporate traditional beliefs with treatments as required in the use of non-steroidal anti-inflammatories for dysmenorrhea.
	Foods encouraged: Plenty of hot fluids such as cinnamon tea, milk with cinnamon and sugar. Teas such as chamomile, anise seed, linden tea, mint leaves.	Fluids encourage body cleaning of impurities. Hot beverages encourage circulation and reduce abdominal colic, cramps, and pain. Teas are soothing to all body systems.	Encourage passive exercise. Provide information about the role of exercise in the reduction of menstrual pain. Support other practices.

(Continued)

Puerto Rican

TABLE	2 6 – 3		
Puerto Rican Cultural Nutrition and Health Beliefs and Practices During Health Stages *(Continued)*			
Behavioral Period	Dietary and Health Practices	Cultural Justification	Recommendation for Health-Care Professionals
	Health practices: Avoid exercise, and practice good hygiene. Do not walk bare foot. Avoid wind and rain. Stay as warm as possible.	Exercise may increase pain and bleeding. Good hygiene is important for health. Walking barefoot during menstruation may cause rheumatoid arthritis and other inflammatory diseases. Warm temperatures promote circulation and the health of the reproductive system as well as prevent cramps.	
Pregnancy	Food taboos: Hot foods, sauces, condiments, chocolate products, coffee, beans, pork, fritters, oily foods, and citric products.	May cause excess flatus, acid indigestion, bulging, and constipation. Chocolate and coffee may cause darker skin in fetus. Some believe citric products may be abortive.	Encourage healthy food habits. Provide information about chocolate and coffee myths. Encourage fruits. Discourage the use of raw eggs in beverages because of possibility of salmonella poisoning.

Behavioral Period	Dietary and Health Practices	Cultural Justification	Recommendation for Health-Care Professionals
	Food encouraged: Milk, beef, chicken, vegetables, fruits, ponches.	Considered healthy and nutritious. Increase hemoglobin, strengthen and promote good labor.	Encourage use of food recommended for pregnancy. Provide information about sexual activity.
	Health practices: Rest and get plenty of sleep. Eat plenty of food. Follow diet cautiously. Many avoid sexual intercourse early in pregnancy. Practice good hygiene, and take warm showers.	Enhances health and prevents problems during birth. Sex may cause problems with baby or preterm labor.	Encourage a balanced plan of exercise with emphasis on weight control and the health of the baby.
Lactation	Food taboos: Avoid beans, cabbages, lettuce, seeds, nuts, pork, chocolate, coffee, and hot food items at all times.	These foods cause stomach illnesses for the infant and mother, including baby colic, diarrhea, and flatus.	Include a dietary plan that is balanced with substitute food items. Clarify any myths about infant diarrhea, colic, and flatus.

(Continued)

TABLE 26 – 3

Puerto Rican Cultural Nutrition and Health Beliefs and Practices During Health Stages (Continued)

Behavioral Period	Dietary and Health Practices	Cultural Justification	Recommendation for Health-Care Professionals
	Food encouraged: Milk, water, ponches, chicken soup, chicken, beef, pastas, hot cereals.	Improve health and increase hemoglobin and essential vitamins. Protect mother and infant from illnesses. Fluids and ponches increase milk supply. Red meats reduce cravings.	As above with raw eggs. Provide information about reasons for stroke and facial paralysis. Provide time to ask questions and reduce anxiety during winter season deliveries.
	Health practices: Avoid cold temperatures and wind. A few may avoid showering for several days after birth. Great attention is paid to health of the mother.	Cold temperatures and winds are believed to cause stroke and facial paralysis in a new mother. Showering may cause respiratory diseases. Mother is believed to be at risk and fragile.	
Infant Feeding	Food taboo: Beans, too much rice, and uncooked vegetables.	Believed to cause stomach colic, flatus, and distended abdomen. Too much rice causes constipation.	Provide information about appropriate dietary patterns for infant.

Behavioral Period	Dietary and Health Practices	Cultural Justification	Recommendation for Health-Care Professionals
	Foods encouraged: Hot cereals, ponches, chicken broth or *caldos*. Fresh fruits, cooked vegetables, *viandas* (raw eggs, cereals, baby foods in milk bottle). Fresh fruit juices. Mint, chamomile, and anise tea. Sugar and honey used for hiccups.	Believed to be nutritious, healthy, and to decrease hunger. *Caldos* are fortifying and prevent illness. Cooked vegetables are healthy and prevent constipation. Bottle food fills the baby. Fresh juices and fruits refresh the stomach. Teas help baby sleep and cure flatus. Sugar and honey have curing properties.	Instruct about infant diet and timely introduction of food items to diet. Explain consequences of excessive weight in infants. Discourage food in bottle to prevent choking. Discourage raw eggs because of the risk of salmonella and egg allergies and the use of honey because of the risk of botulism. Teas are harmless and provide additional fluid when used in moderation without sugar.
	Health practices: Keep baby warm while feeding.	Warm babies eat, chew, and digest food better, and choking is decreased.	Provide information about choking and babies.

- Many clients use relaxation, massage, acupuncture, guided imagery, chelation, biofeedback, and therapeutic touch in addition to or as an alternative to allopathic medicine.
- Black cohosh, evening primrose, St. John's wort, gingko,

ginseng, valerian root, sarsaparilla, chamomile, red clover, and passionflower are the most common herbs and botanical alternatives used by Puerto Rican women. Discuss the safety and efficacy of the most frequently used alternatives. Include use of complementary and alternative therapies in routine health assessments.

- For older clients, a good diet includes meats, traditional meals, and vitamin supplements. Beverages such as fresh-squeezed orange juice, grape juice, and ponches are used as additional nutritional support, particularly for those who are immunosuppressed or chronically or terminally ill.

- If the individual is believed to have low blood pressure and is weak or tired, a small daily portion of brandy may be added to black coffee to enhance the work of "an old heart." Do not criticize folk practices; it deters clients from seeking follow-up care and decreases trust and confidence. Inquire about nutritional practices, and incorporate harmless or nonconflicting practices into the diet.

- During illness, chicken soups and *caldos* (broth) are used as a hot meal to provide essential nutrients.

- A mixture of equal amounts of honey, lemon, and rum are used as an expectorant and antitussive. A malt drink, *malta* (grape juice), or milk is often added to an egg yolk mixed with plenty of sugar to increase the hemoglobin level and provide strength. Ulcers, acid indigestion, and stomach illnesses are treated with warm milk, with or without sugar.

- Herbal teas are used to treat illnesses and to promote health. Most herbal teas do not interfere with medical prescriptions. Incorporating herbal tea with traditional Western medicine may enhance compliance.

- From the onset of menstruation, young girls are encouraged to avoid foods believed to produce flatus, abdominal cramps, and colic. Hot drinks are encouraged to increase circulation and promote the elimination of metabolic waste.

PREGNANCY AND CHILDBEARING PRACTICES

- Because the Catholic Church condones only the rhythm method and sexual abstinence, women do not commonly use birth control methods such as foams, creams, and diaphragms, which are perceived as immoral. Traditionally, abortion has never been accepted except in cases in which the life of the mother was in danger. Nevertheless, this view is changing, and many women now ascribe to this practice. Women have fertility rates, teenage and unmarried pregnancy rates, and live birth rates that are greater than any other Hispanic group in the United States.

- Pregnancy is a time of indulgence for women when favors and wishes are for their well-being and that of their babies. Many women do not begin prenatal care until later in their pregnancies.

- Men are socialized to be tolerant, understanding, and patient regarding pregnant women and their preferences. Women are encouraged to rest, consume large quantities of food, and carefully watch what they eat. Some individuals expect women to "get fat" and place little emphasis on weight control.

- Strenuous physical activity and exercise are discouraged, and lifting heavy objects is prohibited.

- Women are strongly discouraged from consuming aspirin, Alka-Seltzer, and malt beverages because these substances are believed to cause abortion.

- Many women refrain from *tener relaciones* (having sexual intercourse) after the first trimester to avoid hurting the fetus or causing preterm labor.

- Women prefer the bed position for labor, wish to have their bodies covered, and prefer a limited number of internal examinations. They welcome the support of their husbands, mothers, or sisters to assist during labor.

- Loud and verbally expressive behaviors are a culturally accepted and an encouraged method of coping with pain and discomfort. Pain medications are welcomed. Most women oppose having a cesarean section because it portrays a "weak woman." Discuss the possibility of

Puerto Rican

a cesarean section early in the pregnancy. Explain reasons for the necessity of invasive interventions during labor.

- The first postpartum meal should be homemade chicken soup to provide energy and strength.
- Women are encouraged to avoid exposure to wind and cold temperatures, not to lift heavy objects, and not to do housework for 40 days after delivery. Some traditional women do not wash their hair during this time.
- Mothers who breast-feed are encouraged to drink lots of fluids such as milk and chicken soup; if feeling weak or tired, they drink *ponches*, beverages consisting of milk or fresh juices mixed with a raw egg yolk and sugar. Hot foods such as chocolate, beans, lentils, and coffee are discouraged because they are believed to cause stomach irritability, flatus, and colic for the mother and infant.
- Because some women believe that breast-feeding increases their weight, disfigures the breast, and makes them less sexually attractive, they undervalue the benefits of breast-feeding. Provide information about breast-feeding, and educate women about myths and misconceptions. Because maternal grandmothers have a great influence on practices related to breast-feeding, maternal grandmothers should be included along with significant others in educational programs that encourage breast-feeding.

DEATH RITUALS

- Death is perceived as a time of crisis. The body is considered sacred and is guarded with great respect.
- Give news about the deceased to the head of the family first, usually the oldest daughter or son. Use a private room to communicate such news, and have clergy or a minister present when the news is disclosed. Allow time for the family to view, touch, and stay with the body before it is removed.
- Some families keep the body in their home before

burial. Funeral homes are considered impersonal, financially unnecessary, and detrimental to the mourning process because they detract from family intimacy. Burial rituals may be delayed until all close family members can be present.

- Cremation is rarely practiced.
- Among Catholics, religious ceremonies such as praying of the rosary, *velorio* (wake), novenas, and 9 days of saying the rosary following the death are included.
- Families freely express themselves through loud crying and verbal expressions of grief. Some may talk in a thunderous way to God. Others may express their grief through a sensitive but continuous crying or sobbing. Some believe that not expressing their feelings could mean a lack of love and respect for the deceased. Some develop psychosomatic symptoms, and others may experience nausea, vomiting, or fainting spells as a result of an *ataque de nervios* (nervous attack). Be nonjudgmental with clients' psychosomatic or other expressions of grief by providing a private environment and helping to minimize interruptions.

SPIRITUALITY

- Most Puerto Ricans on the mainland are Catholic; however, many have joined Evangelical churches because they offer a more personal spiritual approach.
- A few individuals practice *espiritismo*, a blend of Native Indian, African, and Catholic beliefs that deal with rituals related to spiritual communications with spirits and evil forces. *Espiritistas* (individuals who communicate with spirits) may be consulted to promote spiritual wellness and treat mental illnesses. *Espiritistas* treat clients with mental health conditions and are often consulted to determine folk remedies compatible with Western medical treatments. Older people, those who have limited access to health care, and those who are dissatisfied with or distrust the Western medical system commonly use spiritual healers.
- Because the elderly may consider illness a result of sins,

Puerto Rican

a cure should be sought through prayer or by the "laying on of hands."

- Among Catholics, candles, rosary beads, or a special patron or figurine might accompany the client to the health-care facility and be used during prayer rituals. Inquire about the family's wishes regarding the Sacrament of the Sick.

- Many see the quality of life as a harmonious balance among the mind, body, and spirit. Most are very religious and, when confronted with situations related to health, illness, work, death, or the prognosis of a terminal illness, maintain their trust in spiritual forces.

- Rather than a fatalistic approach to life during illness, death, or health promotion, most use coping mechanisms such as religious practices that are instrumental in providing control in their lives. God, who is their highest source of strength, guides life. For some, scripture readings, praise, and prayer bring inner spiritual power to the soul.

- Clergy and ministers are a resource for spiritual wisdom and help with a host of spiritual needs.

- Although amulets have lost their popularity, some still use them. An *azabache* (small black fist) or a rabbit's foot might be used for good luck, to drive away bad spirits, and to protect a child's health. Rosary beads and patron saint figures may be placed at the head or side of the bed or on the client to protect him or her from outside evil sources. Ask permission before removing, cleaning, or moving amulets; a benediction may be requested before removing amulets or religious objects, giving the Sacrament of the Sick, or providing spiritual support. Assess individual and family religious preferences, and support spiritual resources according to the client or family's request.

HEALTH-CARE PRACTICES

- Most Puerto Ricans have a curative view of health. They tend to underuse health promotion and preventive services such as regular dental or physical examinations and Pap smears. Many use emergency services for acute problems rather than preventive health. The primary and secondary characteristics of culture (see Chapter 1) influence health-seeking beliefs and behaviors. Develop mechanisms to integrate individual, family, and community resources to encourage a focus on health promotion and enhance early health screening and disease prevention. Offering weekend, evening, and late-night health-care services in community-based settings increases the use of preventive services.

- After surgery, some individuals prefer to bathe using a basin of water instead of taking a shower or tub bath. Most prefer to shower and wash their hair daily; however, some women may avoid these activities during menstruation.

- During hospitalization, some refrain from having a bowel movement if they have to use a bedside commode or bedpan. Provide a private, nonintrusive environment when providing personal care.

- Most Puerto Ricans believe in "family care" rather than self-care. Women are considered the main caregivers and promoters of family health and are the source of spiritual and physical strength. Incorporate the participation of the family in the care of the ill.

- Natural herbs, teas, and over-the-counter medications are often used as initial interventions for symptoms of illness. Many consult family and friends before consulting a health-care provider.

- Pharmacists play a vital role in symptom management. Although Puerto Rico is subject to U.S. drug administration regulations and practices, many are able to obtain controlled prescriptions from their pharmacists in Puerto Rico. When they are in the United States, they try to obtain the same kind of services from local pharmacists, creating distress and frustration for both the client and the pharmacist.

- Over-the-counter medications and folk remedies are often used to treat mental health symptoms, acute illnesses, and chronic diseases. Inquire about folk

Puerto Rican

remedies and over-the-counter medicines, and encourage clients to bring their medications to every visit.

- Clients who use folk practices visit *botánicas* (folk religious stores), and use natural herbs, aromatic incenses, special bathing herbs, prayer books, prayers, and figurines for treating illness and promoting good health. Refrain from making prejudicial comments that may inhibit collaboration with folk healers.
- Most families prefer to keep chronically or terminally ill family members at home.
- Asphyxia (shortness of breath) is believed to be caused by lack of air in the body. Fanning the face or blowing into the client is believed to provide oxygen and relieve dyspnea.
- Some individuals may use tea from an alligator's tail, snails, or *savila* (plant leaves) for illnesses such as asthma and congestive heart failure.
- Nausea and vomiting may be embarrassing and cause alarm.
- Many believe that smelling or rubbing isopropyl alcohol (*alcolado*) may help alleviate these symptoms. Some place a damp cloth on the forehead to refresh the "hot" inside the body and relieve nausea. Some put the head between the legs to stop vomiting. Mint, orange, or lemon-tree leaves are boiled and used as tea to relieve nausea and vomiting.
- Rectal suppositories are believed to induce diarrhea. Provide clear information about suppositories and the etiology of symptoms.
- Barriers to using health-care services include poor English-language skills, low acculturation, poor socioeconomic status, lack of insurance, and lack of transportation and child care. Provide interpreters as needed, and offer transportation services, if available.
- Most Puerto Ricans tend to be loud and outspoken in expressing pain. Some prefer oral or intravenous medications for pain relief rather than intramuscular injections or rectal medications. Herbal teas, heat, and prayer are often used to manage pain. Do not censure expression of pain, or judge it as an exaggeration. This

expressive behavior is a socially learned mechanism to cope with pain. *¡Ay!* is a common verbal moaning expression for *dolor* (pain). Because rural elderly individuals might have difficulty interpreting and quantifying pain, the use of numerical pain-identifying scales may be inappropriate.

- Because mental illness carries a stigma, obtaining information or talking about mental illness may be difficult. Some families might not disclose the presence or history of mental illnesses, even in a trusting environment. Mental illness may result from a terrible experience, a crisis, or the action of evil forces or spirits.

- Symptoms of mental illness are often perceived as the result of *nervios* (nerves), having done something wrong, or failing God's commandments. When someone is anxious or overcome with emotions or problems, he or she is just *nervioso*. Similarly, someone who is experiencing despair, anorexia, bulimia, melancholy, anxiety, or lack of sleep may be *nervioso(a)* or suffering from an *ataque de nervios* (attack of nerves) rather than being clinically depressed, manic-depressive, or mentally ill. These conditions may be used to camouflage mental illness. Acknowledge the confidentiality of information when obtaining a history. If trust is developed, practitioners may get a more accurate response to their questions. Community-based settings such as churches, schools, and child-care centers are excellent environments for promoting physical and mental health.

- Genetic or physical defects among Puerto Ricans may be considered a result of heredity, suffering, or lack of care during pregnancy. Less educated individuals may place guilt and blame on the mother or father. Provide information about the causes of genetic defects to reduce stress and guilt for parents. Supply information about community resources, support groups, and culturally appropriate mental health services.

- Organ donation is considered an act of goodwill and a gift of life. Autopsy may be considered a violation of the body. When discussions regarding autopsies and organ donations are necessary, proceed with patience, and

Puerto Rican

provide precise and simple information. A priest or minister is often helpful and may be expected to be present at the time of death. Many individuals are reluctant to receive or donate blood for fear of contracting HIV. Carefully explore beliefs about blood donation and transfusions to dispel myths.

HEALTH-CARE PRACTITIONERS

- Most hold health-care providers in high regard; that is, they are considered wise figures of authority. Distrust may develop if the health-care provider (a) lacks respect for issues related to traditional health practices, (b) ignores personalism in the relationship, (c) does not use advanced technological assessment tools, and (d) has a physical or personal image that differs from the traditional "well-groomed white attire" image.
- Many Puerto Ricans use traditional and folk healers such as *espiritistas* and *santeros* in conjunction with Western health-care providers. Some *espiritismo* practices are used to deal with the power of good and evil spirits in the physical and emotional development of the individual. *Santeros*, individuals prepared to practice *Santería*, are consulted in matters related to the belief of object intrusion, diseases caused by evil spirits, the loss of the soul, the insertion of a spirit, or the anger of God. See Chapter 10, People of Cuban Heritage, for a more complete explanation of Santería.
- Some individuals may have a gender or age bias against health-care providers. Men prefer male physicians for care and may feel embarrassed and uncomfortable with a female physician.
- A few individuals discount the academic and intellectual competencies of female physicians and may distrust their judgment and treatment.
- Some women feel uncomfortable with a male physician; a few prefer a male doctor.
- Older people may prefer older health-care providers because they are considered wise and mature in matters related to health, life experiences, and the use of folk

practices and remedies. To build the client's confidence, younger and female health-care providers must demonstrate an overall concern for the client and develop respect and understanding by acknowledging and incorporating traditional healing practices into treatment regimens.

References

Amaro, H., Whitaker, R., Coffman, G., & Heeren, T. (1990). Acculturation and marijuana and cocaine use: Findings from the HHANES 1982–1984. *American Journal of Public Health, 80,* (Suppl), 54–60.

Juarbe, T. (2003). People of Puerto Rican heritage. In L. Purnell and B. Paulanka (Eds.), *Transcultural health care: A culturally competent approach* (2nd ed., pp. 307–326). Philadelphia: F.A. Davis Company.

Therrien, M., & Ramirez, R. (2001). *The Hispanic population in the United States: Population characteristics.* U.S. Department of Commerce. Economics and Statistics Administration. U.S. Census Bureau. Washington, DC: U.S. Government Printing Office.

U.S. Bureau of the Census. (2000). *U.S. Hispanic Population: 2000.* Current Population Survey, March 2000, PG-4. U.S. Department of Commerce. Economics and Statistics Administration. U.S. Census Bureau. Washington, DC: U.S. Government Printing Office.

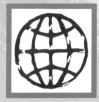

People of Russian Heritage

Overview and Heritage

The Russian Federation, the largest country in the world, with a population of more than 146 million people, is composed of 21 republics and covers parts of two continents, Asia and Europe. The capital and largest city, Moscow, has more than 13 million people. The Russian Federation has a landmass of 6,592,800 square miles, almost twice that of the United States. The diversity of Russia's people reflects the primary and secondary characteristics of its culture and ethnicity as described in Chapter 1. This chapter focuses on Russians who are immigrants to the United States, most of whom are well educated. The name Russia is used to refer to the former communist Union of Soviet Socialists Republics (USSR) established in 1917, which later became a Federation in 1924. From 1917 to 1991, when communism collapsed, travel, the ability to emigrate, and receiving news and information from outside the USSR were severely restricted. Communism controlled all media, disseminating only information that they wanted people to know. Russian Jewish immigrants, like other Russian ethnoreligious groups, may not adhere to their dominant religious practices because much was lost when they were not able to openly practice their faith. There were more than 3 million Russian Americans before 1971; approximately 181,000 more came as refugee and asylum seekers between 1971 and 1991. Immigration to the United States continues with 21,000 to 36,000 immigrants per year. Most are in California, Massachusetts, Illinois, Pennsylvania, and New York.

Although Russia is rich in natural resources, the lack of an infrastructure deters access to, and the refining of, these resources. Under Communism, everyone could attend higher education institutions, resulting in a well-educated population. Many scientists, physicians, and other professionals who have immigrated to the United States have difficulty in practicing their profession, necessitating employment in blue-collar jobs that lower their self-esteem.

COMMUNICATIONS

- The official language of Russia is Russian. However, most educated Russians in the United States speak English to some extent because professional literature in Russia was printed in English. Many do not understand medical jargon and have difficulty communicating abstract concepts. Speak slowly and clearly with exaggerated mouthing or using a loud voice volume, which changes the tone of words. Even though the client may appear to understand the fundamentals of the English language, provide an interpreter if in doubt.

- Many older Russian Jewish immigrants speak Yiddish. Younger Jewish immigrants usually do not speak Yiddish because it was strongly discouraged in Russia.

- Punctuality is the norm, and many arrive early. Temporality is toward present and future orientation because in Russia the concern for many was to have food and other necessities not just for that day but also for the following days and weeks ahead. Thus, some may take medicine until the symptoms disappear and then save the remainder for future use. Explain the necessity of taking all medicine as prescribed. Also explain that some prescriptions can be refilled and that it is not necessary to hoard medicine in the United States.

- Direct eye-to-eye contact is the norm among family, friends, and others, without distinction between genders. Some, however, may avoid eye contact when speaking with government officials, a practice common in Russia where making eye contact with government officials could lead to questioning.
- Most individuals accept touch regardless of age and gender.
- Tone of voice may be loud, extending to those nearby who are not part of the conversation. Do not interpret direct eye contact as aggression or a loud voice volume as anger.
- Until trust is established, many Russians stand at a distance and are aloof when speaking with health-care providers. Greet clients with a handshake, and call them by their surname and title such as Mr., Mrs., Miss, Ms., or Dr.
- Many educated women keep their maiden names when they marry.

FAMILY ROLES AND ORGANIZATION

- Family, children, and older adults are highly valued. Russians, accustomed to extended family living in their home country, continue the practice in the United States. Even though both parents usually work, women maintain the home and care for children. Men do heavier labor and care for the outside of the home.
- Decision-making among current immigrants is usually egalitarian, with decisions being made by the parents or by the oldest child. Ask clients whom they want included in making medical decisions.
- While parents work, grandparents care for grandchildren. Include grandparents and older family members in health education.
- Older people live with their children when self-care is a

concern. Nursing homes are rare and are of poor quality in Russia; thus, children may fear placing parents in long-term care facilities. Help families find long-term care facilities if needed, and encourage visiting the facility before a decision is made to place a family member there.

- Children of all ages are expected to do well in school, go on for higher education, help care for older family members, and tend to household chores according to traditional gender roles.
- Teens are not expected to engage in sexuality activity. Sex and contraceptive education are not traditionally provided.
- Singleness and divorce are accepted without stigma. Gay and lesbian relationships are not recognized or discussed. Do not disclose same-sex relationships to family members.

BIOCULTURAL ECOLOGY

- Russians who immigrate to the United States are predominately white and have a physical structure similar to other white Americans, making them prone to skin cancer. Encourage the use of sun block, which is unknown in Russia, and instruct all family members about the dangers of skin cancer.
- There are no known enzymatic deficiencies for this group.

HIGH-RISK HEALTH BEHAVIORS

- Both men and women have high smoking rates. Encourage ceasing smoking or decreasing the number of cigarettes smoked each day. Assist with finding smoking cessation programs.
- Domestic violence is common and is related mostly to high rates of alcohol consumption. Domestic violence support services are not available in Russia; thus, patients are reluctant to report or seek help for domestic violence in the United States. Explain support services in

the United States for domestic abuse, and help clients access them.

- Male life expectancy is 58 years, 10 years lower than it was a decade ago; female life expectancy is 72 years, with the discrepancy between the two among the widest in the world.
- The number of disabled children in Russia has doubled in the last 10 years.
- Prevalent diseases among this group include alcoholism, depression, diabetes, hypertension, respiratory conditions and tuberculosis, gastrointestinal disorders, dental disease, and obesity. Screen all newer immigrants for conditions common in their home country. Provide scientific, factual information, and assist in finding appropriate services and resources.
- Many who come from Eastern Europe were exposed to the radiation effects of the Chernobyl disaster, resulting in a high incidence of cancer among this immigrant group.

NUTRITION

- Common foods include cucumbers in sour cream, pickles, hard-boiled eggs as well as eggs served in a variety of other ways, marinated or pickled vegetables, soup made from beets (borscht), cabbage, buckwheat, potatoes, yogurt, soups, stews, and hot milk with honey. Cold drinks are not favored.
- Meat choices include pickled herring, smoked fish, anchovies, sardines, cold tongue, chicken, ham, sausage, and salami. Bread is a staple with every meal. The diet overall is high in fat and salt. Determine preferred foods and preparation practices before providing dietary counseling. Incorporate traditional foods into prescriptions.

PREGNANCY AND THE CHILDBEARING FAMILY

- Many new immigrants may not be aware of different methods of fertility control. Abortion is very common in

Russia, and some may choose this option in the United States. Russian condoms are made of thick rubber, discouraging their use by men. Inform clients of the variety of birth control methods common in the United States, understanding that cost may be a factor for some.

- Pregnant women have regular prenatal check-ups, which are mandatory in Russia. During pregnancy, women are discouraged from heavy lifting and from engaging in strenuous physical activities; they are also protected from bad news that can be harmful to the fetus. They are encouraged to eat foods that are high in iron, calcium, and vitamins. Strawberries, citrus fruits, peanuts, and chocolate are avoided to prevent allergies in the newborn.
- As labor approaches, women take laxatives and enemas to facilitate delivery. Traditionally in Russia, husbands and relatives could not participate in the delivery or visit the hospital postpartum. There are no cultural restrictions for fathers or female relatives not to participate in delivery. Ask clients who they wish to be involved in the delivery.
- The delivery room should not have bright lights because many individuals believe that bright lights will harm the newborn's eyes.
- Many women breast-feed until the infant reaches the toddler stage. Many women believe the breasts must be kept warm during feeding lest the mother get breast cancer later in life.
- Peri-care with warm water is important, and a binder is worn to help the mother's figure return to normal.
- In Russia, women were accustomed to 8 weeks of maternity leave before delivery and up to 3 years leave following delivery. Explain family leave practices in the United States.

DEATH RITUALS

- Families want to be notified about impending death first, before the patient is told.

Russian

- Most families prefer to have the dying family member cared for at home. Facilitate transferring the dying person to the home if the family wishes and has the means to provide terminal care. Assist with obtaining hospice home care.
- Do-not-resuscitate orders are appropriate; many families want their loved one to die in comfort.
- Ask permission from the family before contacting clergy.
- Few families believe in cremation; most prefer interment.
- Both men and women may wear black as a sign of mourning. Black wreaths are hung on the door of the deceased's home. Expression of grief varies greatly. Recognize a wide variety of grieving and bereavement behaviors.

SPIRITUALITY

- Most who practice a religion are Eastern Orthodox or Jewish, with smaller numbers of Molokans, Tartar Muslims, Seventh Day Adventists, Pentecostals, and Baptists. Sixty percent of Russian people are nonreligious.
- The state-controlled Russian Orthodox Church was the only accepted religion in Russia (other religions were prohibited) until *perestroika* and *glasnost*. Russian Americans pray in their own way, which may be different from that of the dominant religion with which they identify. Discuss individual religious practices with clients and family on admission.

HEALTH-CARE PRACTICES

- Because health care is free at the point of entry in Russia, newer immigrants might not be aware of the need for insurance in the United States. Explain health reimbursement procedures in the United States, and elicit assistance from social workers as needed.
- Hospital stays in Russia average 3 weeks. Some clients may expect this in the United States. Explain shorter

hospital stays in the United States. Elicit the help of home health nurses, and teach extended family how to care for members at home.

- Unmarried women are not accustomed to Pap tests because in Russia only married women get them. Mammography is uncommon in Russia. Encourage and explain the importance of Pap tests and mammography, regardless of the woman's marital status.

- Many individuals are preoccupied with remaining warm to prevent colds and other illnesses. Most do not want breezes from fans or drafts from an open window to blow directly on them. They may also be reluctant to apply ice at the recommendation of a health-care provider. Explain the necessity of treatments with ice in factual terms. Do not assume that the client wants ice in drinks.

- Some individuals may be reluctant to wash their hair for fear of catching a cold if the room is not warm or has a draft.

- Most Russians are stoical with pain and may not ask for pain medicine. Offer and encourage pain medicine, indicating that it will help the healing process.

- Because of high radiation in Russia, many fear having an x-ray. Explain the necessity of x-rays and the lower radiation x-rays used in the United States.

- Clients are not accustomed to being told about cancer, terminal illnesses, or grave diagnoses because it is believed to make the condition worse. Inform clients about grave diagnoses gradually, on their terms, and preferably in several meetings. Consult with family members, and listen for verbal and nonverbal cues for readiness to receive news about a grave diagnosis.

- A primary treatment for a variety of respiratory illnesses is cupping. Physicians, nurses, and family members use cupping in Russia and the United States. Do not mistake round ecchymotic areas on children or adults as abuse. Ask if they have been practicing cupping. A small glass cup, a *bonzuk* or *bonki*, has alcohol-saturated cotton or other materials in it. The material is lighted, and then the lighted cup turned upside down on the patient's back. The skin is drawn into the cup. The cup is then pulled off the skin, leaving round ecchymotic areas 1 to $1\frac{1}{2}$ inches wide.

- Common cultural practices include taking vodka with sugar for a cough; soaking one's feet in warm water for a sore throat; aromatherapy for a variety of respiratory illnesses; mud and mineral baths to promote healing; and herbs and teas for fever, colds, and minor ailments. Incorporate nonharmful folk practices into allopathic prescriptions.

- Most Russians are accustomed to seeing more than one health-care provider without the other's knowledge. Each provider may give prescriptions. Clients rarely inform the provider about seeing other providers. Specifically ask clients if they are seeing other health-care providers and taking any prescription medicine, over-the-counter medicines, or traditional herbs and teas.

- People are accustomed to not telling health-care providers about depression or any other emotional or mental health concerns because mental illness carries a significant stigma and mental health facilities are very poor in Russia. Be alert for post-refugee stress and anxieties. Establish trust before eliciting information about mental health concerns.

- Based on inadequate screening in Russia, many have great fear of contracting HIV from blood transfusions. Most Russians do not believe in organ donation. Explain U.S. safety procedures with blood donations and transfusion.

HEALTH-CARE PRACTITIONERS

- Health-care providers are respected. Because nurses function in higher roles in the United States than in Russia, they may be mistaken for physicians. Explain the roles and education of nurses in the United States.

- Men and women are accustomed to living together in very small physical quarters; thus, most do not have a problem with privacy. Gender is not generally a concern in delivering care. Always ask about gender concerns before providing intimate care to clients.

References

Andrews, M., & Boyle, J. (1999). *Transcultural concepts in nursing care,* 3rd ed., Philadelphia: Lippincott.

Aorian, F. (2003). Russians (former Soviets). In P. St. Hill, J. Lipson, and A. Meleis, *Caring for women cross-culturally* (pp. 249–263). Philadelphia: F.A. Davis Company.

Culture Clues: Communicating with Your Russian Patient. Retrieved September 3, 2003, from http://healthlinks.washington.edu/clinical/ethnomed/

Evanikoff, L. (1996). Russians. In J. Lipson, S. Dibble, and A. Meleis, *Culture & nursing care* (pp. 239–250). San Francisco: UCSF Nursing Press.

Information please: Almanac. (2003). Retrieved September 3, 2003, from www.infoplease.com

Kittler, P., & Sucher, K. (1998). *Food and culture in America.* Albany, NY: West/Wentworth Publishing.

Smith, L. (1999). Russian Americans. In Giger, J., and Davidhizar, R. *Transcultural nursing assessment and intervention* (4th ed., pp. 379–407). St. Louis: Mosby.

Twenty percent of Russians healthy; 60% of children sick. (2003). *Russia Weekly, 4*(21).

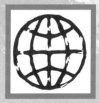

People of Turkish Heritage

Overview and Heritage

Türkiye, as it is written in Turkish, means "land of Turks." Referred to as a geographic, religious, and cultural crossroads, the Republic of Turkey is situated at the geographic intersection of Europe, Asia, the Middle East, and Africa. The land borders of Turkey include Armenia, Georgia, Iran, Iraq, Syria, Greece, and Bulgaria. However, three-quarters of this land mass is bordered by water: the Black Sea, the Aegean Sea, and the Mediterranean Sea. In its northwest corner, one-thirtieth of Turkey lies in Europe and is referred to as Thrace. The remainder of the country's landmass, located in Asia, is commonly called Asia Minor or Anatolia and is separated from Thrace by a waterway including the Dardanelles Straits, the Sea of Marmara, and the Bosphorus Strait. This waterway also separates Istanbul, the country's most populous city with 10.2 million inhabitants, into "Asian" and "European" sides.

At 300,000 square miles, Turkey is slightly larger than Texas, but it has a diverse terrain where mountainous and coastal areas create significant variations in climate. Among its estimated 65.6 million inhabitants, more than half live in urban areas. A large "Turkic belt" stretches from the Balkans across Turkey, Iran, and Central Asia and the former republics of the USSR and deep into the borders of Mongolia. This belt includes many ethnic Turks who may share cultural, linguistic, religious, and historical links with the people of Turkey.

An armistice at the end of World War I left the Empire stripped of all but present-day Turkey occupied by Greek, French, British, and Italian armies and established independence for Armenia and autonomy for Kurds in eastern Anatolia. However, the Treaty of Lausanne in 1923 officially ended Allied occupation, partitioned Armenia between Russia and Turkey, reinstated the Kurds, and proclaimed an independent Republic of Turkey, with Ankara as its new capital. Because of its geopolitical location and its cultural and religious ties, Turkey remains strategically important to the West and is a strong ally of the United States.

More than 202,000 people of Turkish descent live in the United States. They live in 42 states, with over half living in New York, California, New Jersey, and Florida. Just over half the individuals in this group were born outside the United States, arriving before 1980. Many come from the elite and upper-middle classes, interspersed with smaller groups of middle-class students and skilled laborers who are supported privately or by the government. Education is highly valued in Turkey, and significant numbers of Turks in the United States hold advanced degrees. Most are employed in professional, managerial, and technical occupations.

COMMUNICATIONS

- Turkish, a Uralic-Altaic language, is spoken by 90 percent of the Turkish population. Through the centuries, the Turks borrowed from the Arabic and Persian languages, and bits of "turkified" French and English can also be found. Until 1928, Turkish was written in Arabic script.
- The Turkish language does not distinguish gender pronouns, such as "he" from "she" or "her" from "his." However, Turkish does distinguish a formal from

an informal "you," signifying the importance of status in Turkish society.

- Speaking in loud voices is common, signifying excitement or involvement in a discussion. It may also be common for more than one person to speak at the same time or to interrupt another person; this is not necessarily considered rude. However, someone of lower status should not interrupt someone of higher status. Do not confuse speaking in a loud voice as anger.

- Group affiliation is valued over individualism in Turkish society. Identity may be determined by family membership or group, school, and work associations. An individual's behavior is expected to conform to the norms or traditions of the group. In this group-oriented culture, Turks generally do not desire much privacy and tend to rely on cooperation between family and friends, although competition between groups can be fierce.

- Turks value harmony over confrontation, with the outward show of feelings being less restrained. For women, expressions of anger are usually acceptable only within same-sex friendships and kinship networks or toward those of lower social status. Generally, women are not free to vent their anger toward their husbands or other powerful men.

- Touching, holding hands, and patting one another on the back are acceptable behaviors between same-sex friends and opposite-sex partners. Likewise, personal space is closer between same-sex friends than opposite-sex partners; physical proximity is valued as a sign of emotional closeness. Touch, when necessary, is allowed and expected from health-care professionals. However, strict Muslims may not shake hands or touch members of the opposite sex, especially if they are not related.

- Eye contact may be used as a way of demonstrating respect. When interacting with someone of higher status, one is expected to maintain occasional eye contact to show attention; however, prolonged eye contact may be considered rude or may be interpreted as flirting. Maintain eye contact with clients, demonstrating respect and truthfulness.

- Turkish people tend to dress formally; men wear suits

rather than sports jackets and slacks on social occasions. Women tend to dress modestly, wearing skirts and
dresses rather than slacks. More traditional Muslim
women may wear very modest clothing and cover their
heads with either a black or a colorful print scarf.
However, styles continue to change, and denim jeans
and casual dress are becoming common among young
people for less formal occasions. Expect a wide variety
of dress among Turks, depending on religiosity,
acculturation, and age.

- Turks tend to display emotions openly, such as
  happiness, disgust, approval, disapproval, and sadness,
  through facial expressions and gestures. "No" is
  indicated by raising the eyebrows or lifting the chin
  slightly while making a snapping or "tsk" sound with
  the mouth. Appreciation may be expressed by holding
  the tips of the fingers and thumb together and kissing
  them. This signal is commonly used to express
  appreciation for food.

- Turkish people take pride in keeping their homes
  immaculately clean; one is expected to remove one's
  shoes inside the home. Most Turkish hosts in Turkey
  and many in the United States offer slippers to their
  guests. Whether wearing shoes or not, showing the sole
  of one's foot is considered to be offensive in Turkish
  culture. Women are expected to sit modestly with knees
  together and not crossed. Home health-care providers
  should look for cues and ask if they should remove their
  shoes when entering the home of a Turkish family.

- Most Turks tend to have a relaxed attitude about time;
  social visits can begin late and continue well into the
  night. However, in business relationships, punctuality
  among Turkish Americans is gaining in importance.
  Explain the necessity of being punctual for health-care
  appointments.

- A variety of titles are used to show respect and
  acknowledge status. Strangers are always greeted with
  their title, such as *Bey* (Mr.), *Hanim* (Mrs., Miss, or
  Ms.), *Doktor*, or *Profesör*. Members of the family are
  also addressed using specific titles that recognize
  relationships, such as *agbi* (older brother or older close

male friend), *amca* (uncle or elderly male relative or stranger), *abla* (older sister or older close female friend), *teyze* (maternal aunt or older female relative or older female stranger), and *yenge* (wife of a brother or paternal uncle). Greet clients formally with a title or Mr., Mrs., or Ms.

- When friends or family members greet, it is customary for each to shake hands and to kiss one another on each cheek. Traditionally, when greeting someone of very high status or an elderly person, one might grasp his or her hand and kiss it and then bring it to touch one's forehead in a gesture of respect.

FAMILY ROLES AND ORGANIZATION

- In a very traditional Turkish home, the father is considered the absolute ruler. The concept of *izin* (permission or leave to do something specific) captures this significance. In traditional families, women may require *izin* from the head of household for shopping, traveling, and seeing a nurse midwife, physician, or dentist. The rationale is that the one who earns the money may spend the money. *Izin* exhibits a structure of authority that is both hierarchical and patriarchal; therefore, women typically require *izin* more often than men. Less traditional families show more equality between spouses, especially in nuclear families in which the wife is well educated and works outside the home. Yet remnants of traditional family structure prevail, with the husband taking on the role of ultimate decision-maker, especially in matters of finance. Women may work full-time outside the home in addition to assuming full responsibility for running the daily activities inside the home. Modern Turkish women tend to be more Westernized than some of their Middle Eastern or Muslim counterparts. Ascertain the family spokesperson before eliciting health-care decisions. Accept family decision-making patterns without judgment.
- A woman's age, as well as the number, ages, and gender of her living children, influence her status in the family

and the community. Women gain respect but not power as they age, although this varies according to education, religious practice, socioeconomic level, urbanization, and professional achievement.

- Children are held very dear in the Turkish family, and they are expected to act as young children, not small adults. They are accustomed to receiving attention from family, friends, and visitors. Once children enter school, they are expected to study hard, show respect, and obey their elders, including older siblings. Traditionally, children are not allowed to act out or talk back to their superiors. Light corporal punishment is generally acceptable. Explain legalities of child abuse in the United States.

- As children age, they are socialized into more traditional gender roles. Girls are expected to help care for younger siblings, to help at mealtimes, and to learn to cook.

- Circumcision is a major rite of passage for a male child. This is a time of celebration within the extended family, and newly circumcised boys are honored with gifts. Traditionally, boys can be circumcised up to the age of about 12 years, although the modern trend is to perform the circumcision in the hospital shortly after birth.

- Although not common among rural Turks, urban adolescents begin to date in pairs in addition to the more traditionally accepted practice of group outings. However, sexual interaction is strongly discouraged among youth and the unmarried, especially for young women, for whom virginity is a strong cultural value.

- Although financial independence is valued in Turkish culture, independence from the family is not encouraged. Adult children, especially men, remain an integral part of their parents' lives, and parents expect their children to care for them in their old age.

- Because respect is highly valued in Turkish society, maintaining or improving status in the community is of key importance. Family members' accomplishments raise the entire family's status, and failures have an equally broad effect. Parents or other family members

Turkish

are often consulted before major decisions are made. Arranging for a family conference with the family spokesperson is a useful tactic in order to obtain compliance with health prescription and health teaching.

- Marriage is perhaps the most important developmental task for adulthood. Young people generally live in their parents' home until they are married, unless school or work necessitates other arrangements. This practice may be quite different among assimilated Turks in America. Although one study showed that more than half of marriages in Turkey were arranged by families, with a greater prevalence of this practice in rural areas, it is unknown how extensive this practice is among Turks in other parts of the world.

- Elders in Turkish culture are attributed authority and respect until they become weak or they retire, at which time their authoritative roles diminish. Individuals are socialized to take care of elderly parents, regarding it as normal, not as an added burden, and grandparents play a significant role in raising their grandchildren, especially if they live in the same home.

- The extended family is very important in Turkish culture. In many Turkish families, aunts, uncles, cousins, and in-laws form the extended family. Extended family members have a social relationship that may also play an authoritative role within the network. A cooperative relationship is essential between women in an extended family or neighborhood, which includes sharing child care, labor, and food when necessary and providing companionship. Use the extended family arrangement for health teaching.

- Marriages into a "good family," maintaining a high-status occupation, and achieving wealth are means of attaining higher social status for the individual and the entire family. Teachers, health-care personnel, and similar professionals have always held prestige and commanded a relatively high income in Turkey.

- Divorce is becoming more common among Turks but remains socially undesirable, especially for women, for whom remarriage opportunities may be limited to divorced or widowed men. Widows, however, are generally taken care of by their late husband's families; depending on their age and socioeconomic background, they may have the option to remarry.

- Homosexuality is only beginning to be received "at a distance." Most Turks would be hesitant to associate themselves with the gay community. Do not disclose same-sex relationships to family members or others.

BIOCULTURAL ECOLOGY

- Because of historical migration and inhabitance patterns, the Turkish population is a mosaic in terms of appearance, complexion, and coloration. Appearances range from light-skinned with blue or green eyes to olive or darker skin tones with brown eyes. Mongolian spots, usually found at or near the sacrum, are common among Turkish babies and should not be confused with bruising.
- Because of the diversity in climate, topography, and culture in Turkey, it is essential to ascertain the specific geographic origin of a Turkish immigrant. The Black Sea region tends to have a relatively high incidence of helminthiasis (intestinal worm) and goiter.
- Endemic goiter associated with iodine deficiency is a major health problem in Turkey despite iodine prophylaxis. Screen newer immigrants for helminthiasis and goiter.
- Behçet's disease, a syndrome of unknown etiology, is prevalent in Mediterranean countries and the Middle East and affects primarily males between the ages of 20 and 40 years. This chronic inflammatory disorder involving the small blood vessels is characterized by recurrent aphthous ulceration of the oral and pharyngeal mucous membranes and the genitalia. Also seen are skin lesions, severe uveitis, retinal vasculitis, and optic atrophy, with frequent involvement of the joints and the gastrointestinal and central nervous systems. Assess for Behçet's disease with Turkish clients.
- Lactose intolerance is common among Turks. Assess for

lactose intolerance as part of the intake interviews, and help clients identify alternative sources of calcium.

- Thalassemia, a cause of growth and endocrine problems, is a major health concern in Turkey. The overall incidence of β-thalassemia in Turkey is estimated at 2 percent, with 0.6 percent in eastern Turkey and 10.8 percent in northwestern Turkey (Aksoy, 1991). Assess Turkish clients for β-thalassemia before prescribing medications.

- A high rate of cardiovascular heart disease (CHD) among Turkish women may be related to a high prevalence of obesity, hypertension, and diabetes. CHD risk factors, such as high total cholesterol, low high-density lipoprotein (HDL) levels, high triglycerides, hypertension, and smoking, vary across regions and socioeconomic levels and suggest that low HDL levels may in part be caused by genetic factors.

- Turks in Turkey have high rates of occupational injuries because of a lack of educational programs. Provide education regarding safety issues in occupational health.

HIGH-RISK HEALTH BEHAVIORS

- Cigarette smoking is widespread in Turkey and tends to start at an early age. Turkey, a major producer of tobacco in the world, has instituted very limited antitobacco activities. Encourage clients to cease smoking, and help them access smoking cessation programs.

- Turks tend to consume less alcohol than Americans or Europeans, perhaps as a result of the Muslim culture, which discourages more than moderate alcohol use. Despite stereotypes promoted in the American film *Midnight Express*, drug use is not common among mainstream Turks. In fact, some Turkish people try to avoid drug addiction even to the extent of refraining from taking medically prescribed drugs.

NUTRITION

- Turks take great pride in the fact that French, Chinese, and Turkish cooking are reportedly the three foremost cuisines in the world. Turkish cuisine is influenced by the many civilizations encountered by nomadic Turks over the centuries as well as by a mixture of delicacies from different regions of the vast Ottoman Empire. Therefore, food choices are varied and tend to provide a healthy, balanced diet. Turkish cooking is quite delicious, not terribly spicy, and is prepared artfully and fastidiously.

- Food is a highly valued symbol of hospitality and communicates love and respect to those for whom it is prepared. While a typical family dinner may be simple, guests are generally served a bountiful array of dishes. More food is always better, and dinner guests may have difficulty finishing everything on their plates because Turkish hostesses may relentlessly offer to replace what has been eaten. Polite guests refuse the first offer.

- Breakfast is typically a simple meal of *beyaz peynir* (white feta cheese), olives, tomatoes, eggs, cucumbers, toast, jam, honey, and Turkish tea. Turks typically eat their evening meal at about 8 PM. Take mealtimes into consideration when teaching Turkish American clients about medication therapies. Hot midday or evening meals may include any of the foods described below.

- Soups range from light to substantial. Hors d'oeuvres include a great variety of small dishes, either hot or cold, such as stuffed grape leaves in olive oil, olives, circassian or chicken with walnut sauce, dried mackerel, roasted chick peas, or a savory cheese pastry fried until crispy. Hors d'oeuvres may be accompanied by *rakí*, a traditional anisette liquor distilled from grapes served with water over ice and drunk slowly.

- Salads include lettuce, tomatoes, cucumbers, onions, and other raw vegetables, with a dressing of olive oil and lemon juice or vinegar. Turks generally prepare meat in small pieces in combination with other vegetables, potatoes, or rice. Famous Turkish cuisine includes *köfte*, small spicy meatballs, and *kebab*, skewered beef or lamb and vegetables.

- Turkey is the birthplace of yogurt, which is an essential

part of the Turkish diet and is generally served with hot meals rather than as cold breakfast food.

- Rice and *börek* are important parts of Turkish culinary tradition. *Börek* is made by wrapping *yufka* (thin sheets of flour-based dough) around meat, cheese, or spinach and then frying or baking until the dough is flaky.

- Turkish desserts fall into four categories: rich and sweet pastry, such as *baklava*; puddings; cooked fruits; and fresh fruits. Most meals are concluded with fresh fruit and coffee or tea.

- Turkish *kahve*, from which the English word coffee is derived, is famous for its dark, thick, sweet taste. *Ayran*, a mixture of yogurt and milk, is the national cold drink and is drunk by children and adults alike. The Muslim religion requires abstinence from eating pork and drinking alcohol, but not all Muslims abstain, depending on their degree of religious practice. Given the diversity among food options for Turks in America, health-care providers need to provide dietary counseling according to the individual's unique food choices and practices.

- The Islamic tradition of Ramazan (Ramadan in Arabic countries) is a month of fasting observed by practicing Muslims throughout the world. During Ramazan, one is not allowed to eat or drink anything from sunrise to sunset as a test of will power and as a reminder of the preciousness of the food provided by a gracious Allah (God). Many Muslims also stop smoking during this month. Unleavened bread called *pide* is sold only during Ramazan in Turkey. Observance of this tradition varies, from some not observing to others who observe the ritual strictly.

- Sunni Muslims, most Muslims in Turkey, start practicing Ramazan at age 10 or 11 years, and some believe that women have the duty to fast even during pregnancy and the postnatal period. Alevi Muslims do not require fasting for men or women. Generally, pregnant and postpartum women, travelers, and those who are ill are excused from fasting but may be required to make up lost time at a later date. Health teaching strategies for Turks in America should include the recognition and prevention of dehydration, bloating, constipation, and fatigue during periods of Ramazan fasting.

- Ramazan is determined by the lunar calendar and, therefore, can take place at various times in the year. Typically, Turks who are fasting eat breakfast before dawn and before the call to prayer. The evening meal is something to which all look forward with great anticipation, and Turkish women, who almost invariably do all the cooking, create veritable feasts each night. Ramazan is a spiritual and physical cleansing that brings the community together.

- Fasting also can cause a variety of digestive problems and may endanger the health of a pregnant or postnatal woman and her baby. Provide factual information regarding fasting and the potential effect on some health conditions.

- Molasses and *baklava*, *lokom* (Turkish delight), tahini, and honey and nuts and raisins are believed to increase strength and sexual vigor.

- Fruits, especially bananas, oranges, tangerines, and apples, are brought to convalescing people, helping them to regain their strength and aid in the healing process.

- Milk, which is not commonly drunk by adults, is considered more medicinal than yogurt. Chicken soup is a common remedy for cold and flu symptoms. An *ebe* (a traditional midwife or healer in Turkey) relies on various herbs and home remedies to heal clients. *Ebegömeci* (a spinach-like leaf or herb) may be prepared for topical or oral use to treat inflammation, infection, and sometimes infertility.

- Tea, cinnamon, hot sugar water, ginger, mint, and various roots are used separately or in various combinations to treat rheumatism, low blood pressure, intestinal gas, or colds and flu. Nettles may be used topically for rheumatism, arthritis, and varicose veins.

- A folk remedy for diabetes is boiling olive leaves and, after refrigeration, drinking the juice.

Turkish

- *Lapa,* a watery rice mixture with a gruel-like texture, or a boiled potato may be used to treat diarrhea and is followed by yogurt to replace the natural flora of the intestines. Ask Turkish clients if they are using folk dietary practices, and incorporate them into prescription therapies. Because malnutrition may be a significant problem among economically disadvantaged Turks immigrating to the United States, consider extensive nutritional assessments for more recent immigrants.

PREGNANCY AND CHILDBEARING PRACTICES

- Before the 1960s, the sale of contraceptives and birth control education were prohibited in Turkey. Abortion and sterilization, except for medical reasons, were illegal until 1983. Currently, common methods of contraception used by Turkish women include withdrawal, intrauterine devices, and birth control pills. Only recently has Turkish society become more open about sexuality, which has increased men's willingness to seek assistance for fertility problems. Given the history of family planning in Turkey, be open in culturally congruent ways to discussions of family planning with Turks in America.

- Motherhood, and therefore pregnancy, is accorded great respect, and pregnant women are usually made comfortable in any way possible, including satisfying their cravings. Pregnant women may continue their daily activities or work as long as they are comfortable.

- Many pregnant women take prenatal vitamins, drink a lot of milk, and apply salves such as Vaseline to avoid stretch marks. Light exercise, such as walking, is encouraged, but weather conditions often hamper such efforts because Turks generally tend to avoid wet or cold weather, fearing its ill effects on one's health.

- Most Turks prefer hospitals for physician-assisted child delivery. In Turkey it is acceptable, although not common, for the husband and the birth mother's father to be present during the birthing process. However, in immigrant populations, especially in countries such as the United States, where partner support is encouraged, this situation is changing. Expressions of discomfort and pain are quite acceptable.

- The postpartum period can last up to 40 days. Light exercise is encouraged during this period, and bathing, an important part of the Muslim tradition, is strongly encouraged.

- A special food called *loğusalik* is served to the postpartum woman. *Loğusalik* is a sweet sherbety foodstuff, which is prepared by dissolving *loğusalik* beads in hot water. This high-carbohydrate mixture is said to increase the woman's strength. Postpartum women drink hot soups and other fluids such as milk, especially when breast-feeding. Most Turks value breast-feeding, which is commonly but modestly practiced. Encourage incorporation of non-harmful postpartum practices with Western interventions.

- Newborns are treated as cherished gifts. A small blue bead called a *nazar boncuk*, believed to protect the child from the "evil eye," is usually placed on the child's left shoulder to protect the child from the evil angel whispering in the left ear. Other traditional practices include placing iron under the baby's mattress to protect against anemia, tying a yellow ribbon to the crib to ward against jaundice, and placing a red bow on the crib to distract any envy or negativity. Do not remove protective beads or ribbons from the infant's bedside.

- Swaddling, a common practice, has been linked to congenital hip dislocation, pneumonia, and upper respiratory infections among young infants. Explain the harmful effect of swaddling.

DEATH RITUALS

- Turkish Muslims do not generally practice cremation because of their belief that the body must remain whole. After death, the body is washed in a ritual manner and wrapped in a white sheet.

- The traditional mourning period is 40 days, during

Turkish

which time traditional women may wear black clothes or a black scarf.

- Although Muslim Turks believe in the afterlife, death is always an occasion of great sorrow and mourning. An expression of sympathy to one who has just lost someone to death is *Basiniz sağ olsun* (May your head be healthy), hoping that one is not overwhelmed with grief.

SPIRITUALITY

- Most Turks are Sunni Muslim, with a minority from the Alevi Muslim group. Other religious minority groups include Jews (mostly Sephardic), Christians, Armenians, Greeks, and Assyrians. Most Turks who emigrate to the West tend to be very moderate Muslims.
- Traditional prayer is practiced five times each day and can take place anywhere, as long as one is facing the holy city of Mecca. A special small rug called *seccade* is used for praying in places other than the *cami*. When entering the *cami*, shoes are always removed, and women must cover their heads. Men and women go to separate parts of the *cami* for prayer. One prepares for prayer by ritual cleansing, which, at minimum, includes washing the face, ears, nostrils, neck, hands to the elbow, and feet and legs to the knee, three times each. Caregivers may need to make special arrangements so that Muslims can practice their religious obligations when they are in a health-care facility.
- Turks rely on their religious beliefs and practices and their family and friends for strength and meaning in life. One's degree of religiosity influences the importance of prayer in giving meaning to life.
- Religious beliefs intertwined with folk beliefs continue to influence Turkish lifestyle. Spiritual leaders or healers are sought most often for assistance with relationships or emotional problems and, less frequently, for physical problems. A *muska*, a paper inscribed by a *hoca* (spiritual teacher) with a prayer in Arabic, is wrapped in fabric and hidden in the home or worn by the person

seeking help. *Turbe* and *yatir* are the practice of going to the saints' graves to pray about wishes, mental or emotional problems, or fertility problems. *Tesbih* (small beads traditionally used for praying) now take a more secular meaning and are often referred to as "worry beads." Religious or folk items should not be removed from the health-care facility because they provide comfort for the client, and removal may increase anxiety.

HEALTH-CARE PRACTICES

- Most Turks rely on Western medicine and highly trained professionals for health and curative care. However, remnants of traditional beliefs continue to have an impact on health-care practices. A common explanation for the cause of illness is an imbalance of hot and cold. For example, diarrhea is thought to come from too much cold or heat; pneumonia results from extreme cold. When asked how to best treat a child's fever or cough, the most common response is to seek care from a physician; in reality, however, distance, poor economic conditions, and limited education present barriers to this care.
- Many Turks have a traditional fatalistic worldview, which is more common among those living in extended households that believe "You cannot change what God has written." Incorporate factual information for the entire family regarding disease causation and treatment in patient education.
- Terminally ill clients are generally not told the severity of their condition. Informing a client of a terminal illness may take away hope, motivation, and energy that should be directed toward healing, or it may cause the client additional anxiety related to the fear of dying and concern for those being left behind. Furthermore, it may be believed that no one can second-guess Allah. Take cues from the patient, and discuss the patient's condition with the family before disclosing the severity of the condition to the patient.

Turkish

- In general, women are responsible for the actual care-taking of the ill in the home. However, in traditional households, the mother-in-law or father-in-law, depending on who controls the finances in the family, makes decisions about going to the physician. In many situations, the person who is respected as the most educated has primary input into decisions about health care. Determine the family spokesperson for decision-making on health issues, and incorporate group interventions whenever possible.

- Turkey has high rates of consumption of over-the-counter antibiotics and painkillers; aspirin is commonly used as a panacea for a variety of ailments, including gastric upset. Turks, especially those who have difficulty affording the services of a physician, commonly consult a pharmacist before visiting a physician. Fever and pain reducing medicines and cough syrups are frequently purchased without professional medical consultation. Assess Turkish American clients for their use of over-the-counter medications to prevent conflicting or potentiating effects with prescription medications.

- The concept of the "evil eye" is prevalent. Specific to health, it is a cultural inclination not to speak too well of one's health for fear that one may incur misfortune through others' *nazar* (envy). So pervasive is this concept that taxi drivers and medical doctors alike respect the *nazar boncuk;* a blue bead that is used as protection from the evil eye. Some Turks may believe that excessive complaining may bring the benefit of closer medical attention. However, when describing an illness, one avoids using oneself or another person as an example for fear that it may invite the illness or condition upon that person.

- *Kolonya* (cologne) is part of a traditional practice that crosses religious and secular lines. Originally derived from the religious value of cleanliness, cologne is sprinkled on the hands of guests before and after eating to provide cleanliness and a fresh lemon scent. Inhaling from a cloth or handkerchief doused with cologne may be used for relief from motion sickness. In the hospital,

clients may offer cologne to a physician or nurse prior
to examination. Respect this custom as appropriate.
Other home remedies that may be used to treat illness
or symptoms include using rubbing alcohol or a wet
cloth to bring down a fever and warming the back to
treat coughing.

- Although the amount of pain expression varies, Turkish
culture allows freedom to express pain, through either
emotional outbursts or verbal complaints. Accept a
wide range of pain expression among Turkish patients.
- Although stigma is attached to mental illness, many
families seek treatment or care for the client at home.
The most common reasons given for mental illness
include discord among family members, marital and
love problems, gossip, and other familial problems.
Social causes include financial inadequacies, societal
disorders, and a "struggle with life." Men more
frequently blame social causes for mental illness, and
women often give psychological causes. Including the
family in therapy may add to therapeutic effectiveness.
- Epidemiological evidence deems depression to be a
major public health problem in Turkey, with high-risk
groups including women, individuals in middle
adulthood, and those in nuclear families rather than
extended families. Such groups may well describe a
large portion of Turkish immigrants in the United
States. Holding in anger, somatic expression of anger,
and not discussing anger are linked to elevated blood
pressure, rheumatoid arthritis, breast cancer, poorer
health status, and depression. Address somatization
among Turkish American clients with mental health
concerns, and encourage expression of their feelings.
Incorporate group interventions whenever possible.
- Seriously ill people are expected to conserve their energy
to allow their minds and bodies to fight their illnesses;
thus, reducing their workload and unnecessary energy
expenditure is acceptable.
- During hospitalization, *refakatçí* refers to the person
who stays overnight with the client, providing
emotional and physical support and comfort. A show of

concern and compassion for the client eases his or her fears and reduces loneliness. Family members may also attend to physical needs such as bathing. A balanced healthy diet is considered essential to regaining one's health; Turks frequently bring food from home for the patient. Encourage family-assisted care as well as having families bring food from home.

- While blood transfusions are gaining acceptance, Turkish people usually prefer to receive blood from family members. Muslims traditionally prefer that the body remain intact after death, a belief that may conflict with organ donation.

HEALTH-CARE PRACTITIONERS

- Although Turkish people are inclined toward Western health-seeking behaviors, medical care tends to be holistic. Great value is placed on emotional well-being, especially as it affects physical well-being. Physicians may be "adopted" as members of their clients' families, and it is common to give gifts (usually food) to the physician as an expression of gratitude.
- Generally, treating someone of the opposite sex is not an issue among Turks. Ask each client for preference on gender issues in health care.
- Physicians, and to a lesser extent nurses and midwifes, have historically been held in very high esteem. Clients rarely question the authority of physicians, but the notion of obtaining a second opinion is gaining popularity.

References

Aksoy, M. (1991). The history of beta-thalassemia in Turkey. *Turkish Journal of Pediatrics, 33,* 195–197.

Arkar, H., & Eker, D. (1992). Influence of having a hospitalized mentally ill member in the family on attitudes toward mental patients in Turkey. *Social Psychiatry and Psychiatric Epidemiology, 27,* 151–155.

Bedük, T. (1991). Pain management in oncological patients: A Turkish perspective. *Cancer Nursing, 14*(2), 112–114.

Eker, D. (1989). Attitudes toward mental illness: Recognition, desired social distance, expected burden and negative influence on mental health among Turkish freshmen. *Social Psychiatry and Psychiatric Epidemiology, 24*, 146–150.

Ibis, E., Erbay, G., Aras, G., & Akin, A. (1991). Postoperative goitre recurrence rate in Turkey. *Acta Endocrinologica, 125*, 33–37.

İçli, F., Içli, T., Gunel, N., & Arikan, R. (1992). Cigarette smoking among young physicians and their approach to the smoking problem of the patients. *Journal of Cancer Education, 7*(3), 237–240.

Kandela, P. (1993). Sexuality goes public in Turkey. *The Lancet, 342*, 42.

Karanci, N. (1993). Causal attributions for illness among Turkish psychiatric out-patients and differences between diagnostic groups. *Social Psychiatry and Psychiatric Epidemiology, 28*, 292–295.

Kutlu, A., Memik, R., Mutlu, M., Kutlu, R., & Arslan, A. (1992). Congenital dislocation of the hip and its relation to swaddling used in Turkey. *Journal of Pediatric Orthopedics, 12*(5), 598–602.

Mahley, R. W., Palaogh, K. E., Atak, Z., Dawson-Pepin, J., Langlois, A. M, Chung, V., et al. (1995). Turkish heart study: Lipids, lipoproteins, and apolipoproteins. *Journal of Lipid Research, 36*(4), 839–859.

Purnell, L. (2003). People of Turkish heritage. In L. Purnell and B. Paulanka (Eds.), *Transcultural health care: A culturally competent approach* (2nd ed., chapter on CD). Philadelphia: F.A. Davis Company.

Şaatçí, I., Özmen, M., Balkanci, F., Akhan, O., & Şenaati, S. (1993). Behçet's disease in the etiology of Budd-Chiari disease. *Angiology, 44*(5), 392–398.

Thomas, S., & Atakan, S. (1993). Trait anger, anger expression, stress, and health status of American and Turkish mid-life women. *Health Care for Women International, 14*, 129–143.

Time Almanac. (2002). Boston: Time Inc.

U.S. Census Bureau. (2000). Retrieved December 26, 2003, from *www.census.gov*

Turkish

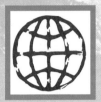

People of Vietnamese Heritage

Overview and Heritage

Vietnam, located at the extreme southeastern corner of the Asian mainland along the South China Sea, is bordered by China on the north and Laos and Cambodia on the west. With a population of more than 78 million people and a landmass of 127,330 square miles, it is the 14th most populous country in the world. The Vietnamese, a Mongolian racial group, make up approximately 85 percent of the population of Vietnam. The Vietnamese in America differ substantially, depending on the primary and secondary characteristics of culture as described in Chapter 1.

Approximately 1.2 million Vietnamese people live in the United States, the majority having arrived since 1975. Their departures were often precipitous and tragic. Escape attempts were long, harrowing and, for many, fatal. Survivors were often placed in squalid refugee camps for years. More than 100,000 left their homeland in 1978, and more than 150,000 left in 1979. For more than a decade, many others, known as the "boat people," departed Vietnam in small, often unseaworthy and overcrowded vessels in hopes of reaching a non-

Communist port. Half died during their journey. Many were forcibly repatriated to Vietnam or eventually returned voluntarily; others continue to languish in camps. The 1979 Orderly Departure Program provided safe and legal exit for the Vietnamese to reunite with family members already in America. In 1987, The Amerasian Homecoming Act provided for the entry of former South Vietnamese military officers, other political detainees, children of American servicemen, and Vietnamese women and their close relatives.

Vietnamese people place a high value on education and accord scholars an honored place in society. The teacher is highly respected as a symbol of learning and culture.

COMMUNICATIONS

- Vietnamese is a single distinctive language with northern, central, and southern dialects, all of which can be understood by individuals speaking any one of these dialects. Vietnamese is the only language of the Asian mainland that is regularly written in the Roman alphabet.
- All words in Vietnamese consist of a single syllable, although two words are commonly joined with a hyphen to form a new word. Each vowel can be spoken in five or six tones that may completely change the meaning of the word. One perennial stumbling point with potential medical connotations is that the word for "blue" and "green" is the same. Do not give directions such as take one "blue" pill at a specified time. Instead, provide the name and dosage of the medication.
- Many individuals cannot easily give a blunt "no" as an answer because they feel that such an answer may create disharmony. A "yes" response, rather than expressing a positive answer or agreement, may simply reflect an avoidance of confrontation or a desire to please the other person. Ask open-ended questions, and have clients demonstrate rather than verbalize their understanding of treatments.
- The terms "hot" and "cold", rather than expressing physical feelings associated with fever and chills, may

Vietnamese

actually relate to other conditions associated with perceived bodily imbalances. See the sections on Nutrition and Health-Care Practices in this chapter for a more thorough understanding of the hot and cold theory.

- English skills may not be sufficient to communicate in psychiatric interviews, which are usually carried out at a highly abstract level. Open discussions with small talk, and direct the initial conversation to the oldest member of the group to facilitate communication. Watch clients for behavioral cues, use simple sentences, paraphrase words with multiple meanings, and avoid metaphors and idiomatic expressions. Explain all points carefully. Approach clients in a quiet, unhurried manner.

- Self-control, another traditional value, encourages keeping to oneself. Expressions of disagreement that may irritate or offend another person are avoided. Individuals may be in pain, distraught, or unhappy yet rarely complain except perhaps to friends or relatives.

- Expressions of emotion are considered a weakness that may interfere with self-control. Negative emotions and expressions may be conveyed by silence or a reluctant smile. A smile may express joy or convey stoicism in the face of difficulty or may indicate an apology for a minor social offense. A smile may also be a response to a scolding to show sincere acknowledgment for the wrongdoing or merely convey the absence of ill feelings. Clarify the meaning of a client's smile.

- The head is a sacred part of the body that should not be touched. To place one's feet on a desk is considered offensive. If it is medically necessary to touch the head, provide an explanation, and ask permission. Do not place feet on a table or desk.

- Looking another person directly in the eyes may be deemed disrespectful.

- To signal for someone to come by using an upturned finger is considered a provocation, usually used to call a dog; waving the hand is considered more proper. Do not point when beckoning clients; call them by name.

- Hugging and kissing are not seen outside the privacy of the home. Men greet each other with a handshake, but they do not shake hands with a woman unless she offers her hand first. Women do not usually shake hands. Greet men with a handshake. Men should wait for the woman to extend her hand for a greeting.

- Two men or two women can walk hand in hand without implying sexual connotations. However, for a man to touch a woman in the presence of others is insulting.

- Women may be reluctant to discuss sex, childbearing, or contraception when men are present. They may demonstrate this unwillingness by giggling, shrugging their shoulders, or averting their eyes.

- Traditional Vietnamese people prefer more distance during personal and social relationships than other cultures, but extended families of many individuals live comfortably together in close quarters.

- Noncompliance in keeping appointments may relate to not understanding oral or written instructions or not knowing how to use the telephone. The more acculturated understand the significance of punctuality.

- Little attention is given to one's precise age. Birth dates may pass unnoticed, with everyone celebrating birthdays together during the Lunar New Year (*Tet*) in January or February. A person's age is calculated from the time of conception; children are considered to be already a year old at birth and gain a year each *Tet*. A child born just before *Tet* could be regarded as 2 years old when only a few days old. Because of the difficulty in determining age, many immigrants may use January 1 as a date of birth for official records.

- Most names consist of a family name, a middle name, and a given name of one or two words, always written in that order. There are relatively few family names, with Nguyen (pronounced "nwin") and Tran accounting for more than half of all Vietnamese names. Other common family names are Cao, Dinh, Hoang, Le, Ly, Ngo, Phan, and Pho. There are relatively few middle names, with Van being used regularly for men and Thi (pronounced "tee") for women. A typical woman's name is Tran Thi Thu. That is how she would write or give her name if requested. She would expect to be called simply Thu or sometimes *Chi* (sister) Thu by friends and family. In other situations, she would expect to be addressed as *Cô* (Miss) or *Ba* (Mrs.) Thu. If married to a man named Nguyen Van Kha, the proper way to address her would be as Mrs. Kha, but she would retain her full three-part maiden name for formal purposes. The man would always be known as *Kha* or *Ong* (Mr.) Kha. Some Vietnamese American women have adopted their husband's family name. Children always take the father's family name. Ask women their preferred name as well as their legal name.

FAMILY ROLES AND ORGANIZATION

- The family is the main reference point for the individual throughout life, superseding obligations to country, religion, and self. The family, as the fundamental social unit and the primary source of cohesion and continuity, is responsible for all decisions and individual actions.
- The traditional family is patriarchal, with an extended family structure. Men deal with matters outside the home. Women are responsible for the actual care of the home. A wife is expected to be dutiful and respectful toward her husband and his parents. Women often make family health-care decisions.
- Children are expected to be obedient and devoted to their parents and to worship their memory after death. The eldest son is usually responsible for rituals honoring the memory and invoking the blessings of departed ancestors.
- For the first 2 years of life, mothers primarily care for their children; thereafter, grandmothers and others take on much of this responsibility.
- A son's obligations and duties to his parents may assume a higher value than those to his wife, children, or siblings. Sibling relationships are considered permanent.
- Exposure of the younger generation to American culture can become a source of conflict with considerable family strain when adolescents are influenced by the perceived

American values of individuality, independence, self-assertion, and egalitarian relationships.

- Traditional Vietnamese are class-conscious and rarely associate with individuals at different levels of society. Respect is accorded to people in authoritative positions who are well educated or otherwise successful or who have professional titles.

BIOCULTURAL ECOLOGY

- Skin color ranges from pale ivory to dark brown. Mongolian spots, bluish discolorations on the lower back of a newborn child, are normal hyperpigmented areas in many Asians. To assess for oxygenation and cyanosis in dark-skinned Vietnamese, examine the sclera, conjunctiva, buccal mucosa, tongue, lips, nail beds, palms of the hands, and soles of the feet. Assess for patches of melanin in the buccal mucosa and the conjunctiva for petechiae and rashes. Assess for jaundice by observing for yellow discoloration of the conjunctiva.
- Most Vietnamese are small in physical stature and light in build relative to European Americans. Adult women average 5 feet tall and weigh 80 to 100 lbs. Men average a few inches taller and weigh 110 to 130 lbs.
- Typical physical features include inner eye folds that make the eyes look almond shaped, sparse body hair, and coarse head hair. They also have dry earwax, which is gray and brittle. People with dry earwax have few apocrine glands, especially in the underarm area, and thus produce less sweat and associated body odor. Asians generally have larger teeth than European Americans, creating a normal tendency towards a prognathic profile, the mouth area coming out farther than the upper part of the face.
- Vietnamese children are small by American standards. American growth charts do not provide adequate assessments for evaluating the physical development of Vietnamese children. Standing, walking, and language skills begin at a slightly later age in Vietnamese children,

but they rapidly catch up with European American norms by the age of $1\frac{1}{2}$ to 2 years.

- Betel-nut pigmentation may be found in some adults, resulting from the practice of chewing *chau* (betel leaves), which is common among older women for its narcotic effect on diseased gums. Some elderly women lacquer their teeth, believing that it strengthens the teeth and symbolizes beauty and wealth.

- Women have high rates of cervical cancer resulting from a lack of education, reluctance to seek early treatment, fear that nothing can be done, low utilization of annual Pap smears, and failure to follow up on abnormal Pap smears.

- Cancer and other problems common to this group may be associated with the widespread application of chemical agents during the Vietnam War. Explain the importance of cancer screening.

- Refugees have high rates of depression, generalized anxiety disorders, and post-traumatic stress associated with military combat, political imprisonment, harrowing events during escapes by sea, and brutal pirate attacks.

- Many refugees have a high incidence of tuberculosis, intestinal parasitism, anemia, malaria, and hepatitis B, which is hyperendemic in Indochina. Assess clients for tuberculosis, parasitism, anemia, malaria, and hepatitis B. HBV vaccination is recommended for all newborn refugee children.

- Melioidosis and paragonimiasis may mimic tuberculosis. Microcytosis may be misdiagnosed as iron deficiency, and inappropriate treatment with iron may be initiated. Erythrocytic microcytosis is a reflection of the presence of thalassemia or of hemoglobin E trait. Screen for these disorders in people with findings consistent with tuberculosis but with a negative purified protein derivative response.

- Most Vietnamese people are slow metabolizers of alcohol, making them more sensitive to the adverse effects of alcohol as expressed by facial flushing, palpitation, and tachycardia. Asians are twice as sensitive to the effects of propranolol on blood pressure and heart rate, experience a greater increase in heart rate from atropine and require lower doses of benzodiazepines, diazepam, and alprazolam. Because of their increased sensitivity to the sedative effects of these drugs, many may require lower doses of imipramine, desipramine, amitriptyline, and clomipramine. They are less sensitive to cardiovascular and respiratory side effects of analgesics (for example, morphine) but are more sensitive to their gastrointestinal side effects. Asians require lower doses of neuroleptics. Because Vietnamese people are considerably smaller than most white Americans, medication dosages may need to be reduced. Vietnamese people generally consider American medicines more concentrated than Asian medicines; thus, they may take only half the dosage prescribed.

HIGH-RISK HEALTH BEHAVIORS

- Some newer immigrants have never heard of cancer; among those who have heard of it, some believe it is contagious. Many women have never heard of or had a Pap test. Many have never performed a breast self-examination or had a mammogram. Explain the necessity of Pap tests, mammograms, and self-breast exams.
- Liver cancer is 12 times higher among Southeast Asian men and women than among the general population and is associated with the prevalence of hepatitis B. High rates of gastrointestinal cancer may be due to asbestos that, in some parts of the world, is used in the process of "polishing" rice. Remind clients that polished, imported rice should always be washed.
- Many individuals do not know that cigarette smoking can cause cancer. Explain the adverse effects of cigarette smoking, and encourage cessation.
- Trichinosis risk is 25 times greater in Southeast Asian refugees than in the general population. This increased risk is related to undercooking pork and purchasing pigs directly from farms. Screen newer immigrants for the possibility of trichinosis.

Vietnamese

NUTRITION

- Meals are a time for the entire family to come together and share a common activity. Preparation is precise and may occupy much of the day. Celebrations and holidays involve elaborately prepared meals.
- The normal daily caloric intake of the Vietnamese is approximately two-thirds that of average Americans. White or polished rice is the main staple in the diet, providing up to 80 percent of daily calories. Other common foods are fish (including shellfish), pork, chicken, soybean curd (tofu), noodles, various soups, and green vegetables. Preferred fruits are bananas, mangoes, papayas, oranges, coconuts, pineapples, and grapefruit. Soy sauce, garlic, onions, ginger root, lemon, and chili peppers are used as seasoning. Rice and other foods are commonly served with *nuoc mam* (a salty, marinated fish sauce). A meal typically consists of rice, *nuoc mam*, and a variety of other seasonings, green vegetables, and sometimes meat cut into slivers. Chicken and duck eggs may be used.
- The Vietnamese prefer white bread, particularly French loaves and rolls, and pastry. A regular dish is *pho*, a soup containing rice noodles, thinly sliced beef or chicken, and scallions.
- Food preparation similar to Chinese cooking includes *com chien* (fried rice) and *thit bo xau ca chua* (beef fried with tomatoes). *Cha gio* (pronounced "cha-yuh") is a combination of finely chopped vegetables, mushrooms, meat, or bean curd that is rolled in delicate rice paper and deep-fried.
- Stir-frying, steaming, roasting, and boiling are the preferred methods of cooking. Hot tea is the usual beverage.
- A predominant aspect of the traditional Asian system of health maintenance is the principle of balance between two opposing natural forces, known as *am* (cold) and *duong* (hot) in Vietnamese. The terms have nothing to do with temperature and are only partly associated with seasoning. Rice, flour, potatoes, most fruits and vegeta-

bles, fish, duck, and other things that grow in water are considered cold. Most other meats, fish sauce, eggs, spices, peppers, onions, candies, and sweets are hot. Tea is cold, coffee is hot, water is cold, and ice is hot.

- Illness or trauma may require therapeutic adjustment of hot-cold balance to restore equilibrium. Hot foods and beverages, used to replace and strengthen the blood, are preferred after surgery or childbirth. During illness, certain foods, such as *chao* (light rice gruel) mixed with sugar or sweetened condensed milk and a few pieces of salty pork cooked with fish sauce, are consumed in greater quantity. Fresh fruits and vegetables are usually avoided, being considered too cold. Water, juices, and other cold drinks are restricted. Nutritional counseling should take into consideration these factors and other aspects of the usual Vietnamese diet, because advice to simply eat certain kinds of American foods may be ignored.

- Anemia in children is associated with an iron deficiency. The diet, which may be exceedingly high in sodium, may also be deficient in calcium and zinc. These conditions have implications relevant to hypertension.

- Most adults and many children suffer from lactose intolerance, which may cause problems in schools, other institutional settings, and adoptive families. Encourage the use of substitute milk products that use soybeans for those who are lactose-intolerant.

PREGNANCY AND CHILDBEARING PRACTICES

- Women have high fertility rates (average of 6 pregnancies, with 4 live births) and commonly have children until their early to middle 40s. Many know little about contraception. Abortions are commonly performed in their homeland because pregnancy outside of marriage is considered a disgrace to the family. More acculturated individuals practice some form of birth control. Avoid family planning issues on the first encounter; but such information is usually well received on subsequent visits.

- Prescriptive food practices for a healthy pregnancy

include noodles, sweets, sour foods, and fruit and exclude fish, salty foods, and rice. After birth, to restore equilibrium and provide adequate warmth to the breast milk, women consume soups with chili peppers, salty fish and meat dishes, and wine steeped with herbs.

- Foods are also classified as *tonic* and *wind*. Tonic foods include animal protein, fat, sugar, and carbohydrates; they are usually also hot and sweet. Sour and sometimes raw and cold foods are classified as *antitonic*. Wind foods, often classified as cold, include leafy vegetables, fruit, beef, mutton, fowl, fish, and glutinous rice. It is considered critical to increase or decrease foods in various categories to restore bodily balances upset by unusual or stressful conditions such as pregnancy. While the balance of foods may be followed, the terminology is not used consistently.

- During the first trimester, the expectant mother is considered to be in a weak, cold, and antitonic state. Therefore, she should correct the imbalance by eating and drinking hot foods, such as ripe mangoes, grapes, ginger, peppers, alcohol, and coffee. To provide energy and food for the fetus, she is prescribed tonic foods, including a basic diet of steamed rice and pork.

- Cold foods, including mung beans, green coconut, spinach, and melon, and antitonic foods, such as vinegar, pineapple, and lemon, are avoided during the first trimester. In the second trimester, the pregnant woman is considered to be in a neutral state. Cold foods are introduced, and the tonic diet is continued.

- During the third trimester, when the woman may feel hot and suffer from indigestion and constipation, cold foods are prescribed, and hot foods are avoided or strictly limited. Tonic foods, which are believed to increase birth weight, are restricted to reduce the chances of a large baby. Wind foods are generally avoided throughout pregnancy, as they are associated with convulsions, allergic reactions, asthma, and other problems. This regimen may appear more complex and restrictive than it actually is in practice. Most women use it only as a general guide, commonly restricting, rather than totally abstaining from, the restricted foods. A great variety of food, including rice, many kinds of vegetables and fruits, various seasonings, and certain meats and fish are generally permissible throughout pregnancy. Ask women at each stage of their pregnancy about preferred foods before initiating dietary counseling and recommendations. Dispel any myths, and recommend foods that are congruent with beliefs.

- Many women do not seek medical attention until the third trimester because of cost, fear, or lack of perceived need. Women who are generally better educated seek early prenatal care. For obstetric and gynecologic matters, they tend to feel more comfortable with a female physician or midwife.
- Women maintain physical activity to keep the fetus moving and to prevent edema, miscarriage, or premature delivery. Prolonged labor may result from idleness. An undesirably large baby may result from afternoon napping.
- Restrictive beliefs include avoiding heavy lifting and strenuous work and raising the arms above the head, which pulls on the placenta, causing it to break. Sexual relations late in pregnancy may cause respiratory stress in the infant.
- Many consider it taboo for pregnant women to attend weddings or funerals.
- Some pregnant women look at pictures of happy families and healthy children, believing that it helps give birth to healthy babies.
- Women generally dislike invasive procedures, such as episiotomies, cesarean sections, circumcisions, nasal oxygen, and intravenous fluids. However, anesthesia during labor and delivery is usually accepted. Once in labor, the woman tries to maintain self-control and may even smile continuously. Her period of labor is usually short, and there may be no warning of impending delivery. Because the head is considered sacred, neither that of the mother nor of the infant should be touched or stroked. Removal of vernix from the infant's head can cause distress. If necessary to touch the head for

Vietnamese

medical treatment, an explanation is essential. Stress the importance and necessity of invasive procedures, and select other venous routes if possible.

- Because body heat is lost during delivery, women avoid cold foods and beverages and increase consumption of hot foods to replace and strengthen their blood. Ice water and other cold drinks are usually not welcome, and most raw vegetables, fruits, and sour items are consumed in lesser amounts. Prescriptive foods include steamed rice, fish sauce, pork, chicken, eggs, soups with chili or black peppers, other highly seasoned and salty items, wine, and sweets.

- Because water is *am* (cold), women traditionally do not fully bathe, shower, or wash their hair for a month after delivery. Some women have complained that they were adversely affected by showering shortly after delivery in American hospitals; others, however, welcomed the opportunity to shower and seemed willing to give up some traditional practices.

- Postpartum women avoid drafts and strenuous activity; wear warm clothing; stay in bed, indoors, or both for about a month; some avoid sexual intercourse for months. Many use hot water bottles or electric blankets to combat the cold forces of childbirth.

- Other women in the family assume responsibility for the baby's care. Do not interpret the mother's inactivity and dependence on others as apathy or depression. A newborn is often dressed in old clothes. Do not praise the baby lest jealous spirits steal the infant. Do not cut the child's hair or nails for fear that this might cause illness.

- The infant is generally maintained on a diet of milk for the first year, with the introduction of rice gruel at around 6 months.

- Some women discard colostrum and feed the baby rice paste or boiled sugar water for several days. This does not indicate a decision against breast-feeding.

- After the milk comes in, the mother and baby benefit from the hot foods consumed by the mother for the first month. Then, however, a conflict arises: the mother believes that hot foods benefit her health but that cold foods ensure healthy breast milk. Having the mother change from breast-feeding to formula can easily solve this dilemma. However, if the mother cannot afford formula, she may use fresh milk or rice boiled with water, which may result in anemia and growth retardation. Reinforce the benefits of colostrum.

- There is little formal toilet training; the child usually learns by imitating an older child.

DEATH RITUALS

- Most Vietnamese people accept death as a normal part of life. Ancestors are commonly honored and worshipped and are believed to bestow protection on the living.
- Most individuals have an aversion to hospitals and prefer to die at home. Some believe that a person who dies outside the home becomes a wandering soul with no place to rest.
- Many do not want to artificially prolong life and suffering, but it may still be difficult for relatives to consent to terminating active intervention, which might be considered contributing to the death of an ancestor who shapes the fate of the living. Having a family conference and providing factual information is appreciated.
- Clergy visitation is usually associated with last rites; rites influenced by Catholicism can actually be upsetting to hospitalized clients. Sending flowers may be startling, as flowers are usually reserved for the rites of the dead. Do not place flowers in the patient's room until getting permission from the patient or family. Contact religious leaders only with the permission or request of the client or family.
- Families gather around the body of a deceased relative and express great emotion. Traditional mourning practices include the wearing of white clothes for 14 days, the subsequent wearing of black armbands by men and white headbands by women, and the yearly celebration of the anniversary of a person's death.
- Few families consent to autopsy unless they know and agree with the reasons for it. Cremation is an acceptable practice to some families.

Vietnamese

SPIRITUALITY

- The major religions practiced are Buddhism, Confucianism, and Taoism; a few are Christians, of whom most are Catholic. Many are Buddhists, but some almost never visit temples or perform rituals. Others, both Buddhist and Christian, may maintain a religious altar in the home and conduct regular religious observances. Animism is found mainly among people from the highland tribes. Many believe that deities and spirits control the universe and that the spirits of dead relatives continue to dwell in the home.

HEALTH-CARE PRACTICES

- Good health is achieved by having harmony and balance with the two basic opposing forces, *am* (cold, dark, female) and *duong* (hot, light, male). An excess of either force may lead to discomfort or illness. The forces of *am* (cold) and *duong* (hot) are pervasive forces in the practice of traditional Vietnamese medicine. *Am* represents factors that are considered negative, feminine, dark, and empty, whereas *duong* represents those that are positive, masculine, light, and full. *Am* stores strength, and care must be taken not to use it up too quickly. *Duong* protects the body from outside forces and, if the body is not cared for, the organs are thrown into disorder. Proper balance of these two life forces ensures the correct circulation of blood and good health. If the balance is not proper, life is short.
- Diseases and other debilitating conditions result from either cold or hot influences. For example, diarrhea and some febrile diseases are due to an excess of cold, whereas pimples and other skin problems result from an excess of hot. Countermeasures involve using foods, medications, and treatments that have properties opposite those of the problem and avoiding foods that would intensify the problem. Asian herbs are cold, and Western medicines are hot. Common Vietnamese medical practices are discussed in Box 29–1.

BOX 29–1 • Traditional Vietnamese Medicine

- *Cao gio* (literally, "rubbing out the wind") is used for treating colds, sore throats, flu, sinusitis, and similar ailments. An ointment or hot balm oil is spread across the back, chest, or shoulders and rubbed with the edge of a coin (preferably silver) in short, firm strokes. This technique brings blood under the skin, resulting in dark ecchymotic stripes, so the offending wind can escape. Dermabrasion may provide a portal for infection. **Do not interpret these ecchymotic areas as evidence of abuse.**

- *Be bao* or *bar gio* (skin pinching) is a treatment for headache or sore throat. The skin of the affected area is repeatedly squeezed between the thumb and forefinger of both hands, as the hands converge towards the center of the face. The objective is to produce ecchymoses or petechiae. **Do not interpret these ecchymotic areas as evidence of abuse.**

- *Giac* (cup suctioning), another dermabrasive procedure, is used to relieve stress, headaches, and joint and muscle pain. A small cup is heated and placed on the skin with the open side down. As the cup cools, it contracts the skin and draws unwanted hot energy into the cup. This treatment leaves marks that may appear as large bruises. **Do not interpret these ecchymotic areas as evidence of abuse.**

- *Xong* (an herbal preparation) relieves motion sickness or cold-related problems. Herbs or an agent such as Vicks Vaporub is put into boiling water, and the vapor is inhaled. Small containers of aromatic oils or liniments are sometimes carried and inhaled directly.

- Moxibustion is used to counter conditions associated with excess cold, including labor and delivery. Pulverized wormwood or incense is heated and placed directly on the skin at certain meridians.

Vietnamese

(Continued)

> ### BOX 29–1 • Traditional Vietnamese Medicine (Continued)
>
> - Acupuncture, acupressure, and acumassage relieve symptomatic stress and pain (see Chapter 9, People of Chinese Heritage, for a description of these healing practices).
> - Balms and oils, such as Red Tiger balm, available in Asian shops, are applied to affected areas for relief of bone and muscle ailments.
> - Herbal teas, soups, and other concoctions are taken for various problems, generally in the sense of using cold measures to overcome hot illnesses. Eating organ meats such as liver, kidneys, testes, brains, and bones of an animal is said to increase the strength of the corresponding human part. Two additional practices are consuming gelatinized tiger bones to gain strength and taking powdered rhinoceros horn to reduce fever.

- Many Vietnamese people try home remedies, allowing the condition to become serious before seeking professional assistance. Once a physician or nurse has been consulted, the Vietnamese are usually quite cooperative and respect the wisdom and experience of health-care professionals.
- The belief that life is predetermined is a deterrent to seeking health care. Diagnostic tests may be baffling, and invasive procedures are frightening. The prospect of surgery can be terrifying. Explain procedures in simple, realistic terms, and reinforce information as necessary. Hospitalization is considered a last resort and is acceptable only in case of emergency when everything else has failed.
- Naturalistic explanations for poor health include eating spoiled food and exposure to inclement weather. Natural elements are associated with bad weather and cold drafts and cause problems such as the common cold, mild fever, and headache. Countermeasures

involve dietary, herbal, hygienic, and simple medical practices. Collectively, these measures are categorized as *thuoc nam*, the traditional southern medicine of Vietnam, and *thuoc bac*, the more formal northern or Chinese medicine.

- Supernaturalistic causes, such as gods, spirits, or demons, may cause illness. Illness may be considered a punishment for offending such an entity or violating some religious or moral code.

- A "weak heart" may refer to palpitations or dizziness, a "weak kidney" to sexual dysfunction, a "weak nervous system" to headaches, and a "weak stomach or liver" to indigestion.

- Loss of blood from any route is feared, and some may refuse to have blood drawn for laboratory tests. The client may complain, although not to the health-care worker, of feeling weak for months. A client may fear that any body tissue or fluid removed cannot be replaced and that the body suffers the loss in this life as well as into the next life. Explain that blood is naturally replenished.

- Most individuals deal with illness by means of self-care, self-medication, and use of herbal medicines. Many believe that Western medicine is very powerful and cures quickly, but few understand the risks of over- or underdosages. The concept of long-term medication for chronic illnesses and acceptance of unpleasant side effects and increased autonomic symptoms are not congruent with traditional notions of safe and effective treatment of illnesses. Some people politely accept a prescription but may not fill it. Even if they have filled it, they may not take the medicine, or they may adjust the dosage without telling the health-care provider. Extensive education, repetition of instructions, and home visitations are necessary to ensure compliance.

- Persistent reminding, as part of an overall effort to improve communication and information dissemination, has been suggested as the best way to encourage Vietnamese women to undergo regular cancer screening and follow-up treatment. Include family members in all major treatment decisions regarding physical and mental health.

- Common problems that pose barriers to health care are discussed in Box 29–2.
- Fatalistic attitudes and the belief that problems are punishment may reduce the amount of complaining and expression of pain among those who view endurance as an indicator of strong character. Many Vietnamese people accept pain as part of life and attempt to maintain self-control as a means of relief. A deep cultural restraint against showing weakness limits the use of pain medication. However, the sick person is allowed to depend on family and receives a great deal of attention

BOX 29–2 • Barriers to Health Care for Vietnamese People

- Subjective beliefs and the cost of health care
- Lack of a primary provider
- Differences between Western and Asian health-care practices
- Caregivers' judgment of Vietnamese as deviant and unmotivated because of noncompliance with medication schedules, diagnostic tests, follow-up care, and failure to keep appointments
- Inability to communicate effectively in the English language with recent immigrants, who lack confidence in their ability to communicate their needs; failure of providers to communicate
- Avoidance of Western practitioners out of fear that traditional methods will be criticized
- Fear of conflicts and ridicule, resulting in loss of face
- Lack of knowledge of the available resources
- Fear of stigmatization, difficulty in locating agencies that can provide assistance without distorted professional and cultural communication, and unwillingness to express inner feelings

and care. Explain that accepting pain medication will hasten the healing process.

- Most individuals are unaccustomed to discussing their personal feelings openly with others. In times of distress or loss, they often complain of physical discomforts, such as headaches, backaches, or insomnia.
- Mental illness is believed to result from offending a deity. It brings disgrace to the family and, therefore, must be concealed. A shaman may be enlisted to help, and additional therapy is sought only with the greatest discretion and often after a dangerous delay.
- Emotional disturbance is usually attributed to possession by malicious spirits, bad luck of familial inheritance or, for Buddhists, bad karma accumulated by misdeeds in past lives.
- The term *psychiatrist* has no direct translation in Vietnamese and may be interpreted to mean nerve physician or specialist who treats crazy people. The nervous system is sometimes considered the source of mental problems, neurosis being thought of as "weakness of the nerves" and psychosis as "turmoil of the nerves." A mentally disabled person may be stigmatized by the family and society, which can jeopardize the ability of relatives to find marriage partners. The mentally disabled are usually harbored within their families unless they become destructive; then they may be admitted to a hospital. Health-care providers should use the depression scale developed by Kinzie and Associates and Buchwald when working with Vietnamese clients.
- Physically disabled people are commonly accepted and are treated well and cared for by their families.
- Because many believe that the body must be kept intact even after death, they are averse to blood transfusions and organ donation. Those who prefer cremation will donate body parts under certain circumstances.

HEALTH-CARE PRACTITIONERS

- Four kinds of traditional and folk practitioners exist in Vietnam, as shown in Box 29–3. Many consult one or more of these healers in an attempt to find a cure.

BOX 29–3 • Folk Practitioners

- Asian physicians who are learned individuals who use herbal medication and acupuncture.
- Informal folk healers who use special herbs and diets as cures based on natural or pragmatic approaches. The secrets of folk medicine are passed down through the generations.
- Spiritual healers, some of whom have a specific religious outlook, and others who have powers to drive away malevolent spirits.
- Magicians or sorcerers have magical, curative powers but no communication with the spirits.

- Acknowledgment and support of traditional belief systems are important in building a trusting relationship. Traditional healers often provide the Vietnamese with necessary social support.
- Traditional Asian male practitioners usually do not touch the bodies of female clients and sometimes use a doll to point out the nature of a problem. Although most Vietnamese might no longer insist on the use of this practice, adults, particularly young and unmarried women, are more comfortable with health-care providers of the same gender, especially for obstetrical and gynecological conditions.
- Some Vietnamese people are not accustomed to female authority figures and may have difficulty relating to women as professional health-care providers.
- While many individuals have great respect for professional, well-educated people, they may be distrustful of outside authority figures. Most have come to America to escape oppressive authority. Refugees generally expect health-care professionals to be experts. A common suspicion is that divulging personal information for a medical history may jeopardize their legal rights. Respect and mistrust are not mutually exclusive concepts.

- Women may not want to discuss sexual problems,
  reproductive matters, and birth control techniques until
  after an initial visit and confidence has been established
  in the practitioner. Pelvic examinations on unmarried
  women should not be made on the first visit or without
  careful advance explanation and preparation. When
  such an examination is necessary, the woman may want
  her husband present. If possible, the practitioner and an
  interpreter should both be female.

References

Buchwald, D., Manson, S. M., Dinges, N. G., Keane, E. M., &
Kinzie, J. D. (1993). Prevalence of depressive symptoms among
established Vietnamese refugees in the United States. *Journal of
General Internal Medicine, 8*(2), 76–81.

Kinzie, J. D., Manson, S. M., Vinh, D. T., Tolan, N. T., Anh, B., &
Pho, T. N. (1982). Development and validation of a Vietnamese-
language depression rating scale. *American Journal of Psychiatry,
139*(10), 1276–1281.

Nowak, T. (2003). People of Vietnamese heritage. In L. Purnell and
B. Paulanka (Eds.), *Transcultural health care: A culturally com-
petent approach* (2nd ed., pp. 327–343). Philadelphia: F.A. Davis
Company.

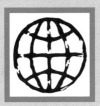

Index

Page numbers followed by "b," "i," *and* "t," *indicate boxed material, illustrations, and tables, respectively.*